MULTIPLE MYELOMA - A QUICK REFLECTION ON THE FAST PROGRESS

Edited by **Roman Hajek**

Multiple Myeloma - A Quick Reflection on the Fast Progress
http://dx.doi.org/10.5772/56515
Edited by Roman Hajek

Contributors

Meral Beksac, Artur Jurczyszyn, Ana Muñoz, Cristina Riber, Katy Satue, Pablo Trigo, Manuel Gómez-Díez, Francisco Castejon, Lucie Rihova, Emine Ozyuvaci, Tolga Sitilci, Onat Akyol, Taner Demirer, Pervin Topcuoglu, Sinem Civriz Bozdag, Saad Usmani, Stephen Harding, Marie-Christine Kyrtsonis, Magdalena Cortes, Raul Vinet, Svachova, Plesner, Thomas Lund, Maja Hinge, Jean-Marie Delaisse, Klara Gadó, Elisabetta Ferrero, Nathalie Steimberg, Giovanna Mazzoleni, Marina Ferrarini, Daniela Belloni, Je-Jung Lee, Roman Hajek

Published by InTech

Janeza Trdine 9, 51000 Rijeka, Croatia

Publishing Process Manager Ana Pantar
Technical Editor InTech DTP team
Cover InTech Design team

Additional hard copies can be obtained from orders@intechopen.com

Multiple Myeloma - A Quick Reflection on the Fast Progress, Edited by Roman Hajek
p. cm.
ISBN 978-953-51-1083-5

For EU product safety concerns:
IN TECH d.o.o., Prolaz Marije Krucifikse Kozulić 3, 51000 Rijeka, Croatia,
info@intechopen.com or visit our website at intechopen.com.

Meet the editor

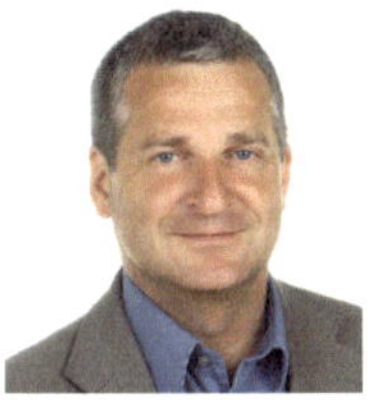

Roman Hajek is the Professor of Oncology, Head of Department of Haemato-Oncology at the University Hospital Ostrava and School of Medicine University Ostrava and Head of Babak Myeloma Research Group of MU Brno in Czech Republic. After qualifying in medicine in 1988 from J.E. Purkyne University Brno, Dr. Hajek completed degrees in Internal Medicine, Medical Oncology and Hematology & Transfusiology and received a PhD in 1995. Dr Hajek was a founder member of the Czech Myeloma Group and an active chairman of the Czech Myeloma Group. He is also the founder of Amyloidosis Diagnostic and Treatment Center in Ostrava. He is a member of the Scientific Advisory Board of International Myeloma Foundation. Dr. Hajek has published over 200 scientific articles and book chapters.

Contents

Preface

Multiple myeloma is the second most common haematological malignancy. This book does not provide a comprehensive overview of the disease but offers a collection of chapters with in-depth information on distinct hot topics in the diagnostic, research and therapeutic fields. On the biological side, the authors show plasticity of myeloma cells and describe the innovative models to assess multiple myeloma biology. On the clinical side, the authors analyse current therapeutic development. Pharmacotherapy of multiple myeloma is an example of the fast introduction of scientific discoveries into clinics. The dynamics of testing new drugs for multiple myeloma treatment in clinical trials is breathtaking. Scientific discoveries have uncovered complicated pathogenesis of multiple myeloma; complicated reactions to treatment lead to creation of super cocktails. This strategy is most beneficial for the patient, but it is not yet personalized medicine. The curability of multiple myeloma is a question that is being discussed by the entire professional myeloma world. Regardless of your position in this debate, some professionals are missing the vital point in this debate - the incredible improvement in treatment options. Consequently, improvement of prognosis is a fact which is most important from a patient's perspective.

This book will be of interest to medical professionals specializing in hematooncology, researchers, as well as many others.

Prof. Roman Hajek
Department of Pathological Physiology,
Faculty of Medicine, Masaryk University,
Czech Republic

Chapter 1

Strategies for the Treatment of Multiple Myeloma in 2013: Moving Toward the Cure

Roman Hajek

Additional information is available at the end of the chapter

http://dx.doi.org/10.5772/55366

1. Introduction

Multiple myeloma (MM) is a hematooncological disease, and in recent years, overall survival of patients has been significantly increased. Improvement of treatment results is connected not only to the introduction of autologous transplantation of hematopoietic cells into the treatment strategy for younger patients in the 90s but also to the introduction of new beneficial drugs into clinics; in the first decade of this century, bortezomib, thalidomide and lenalidomide were introduced in [1]. These new drugs have repeatedly proven their high treatment efficacy in clinics in all age groups of patients, in primotherapy as well as refractory disease. There are also newer drugs currently under investigation, such as new proteasome inhibitors (carfilzomib, MLN9708 and other peroral proteasome inhibitors) and other immunomodulatory drugs (pomalidomide) with the aim to improve or maintain treatment effects and decrease unfavorable effects in [2]. Using drugs from both these groups together with glucocorticoids and alkylating cytostatics had a major impact on prolonging survival of our patients as previously published. On the other hand, it is clear that use of only one of the new efficient drugs in combination with glucocorticoids and alkylating cytostatics does not lead to a cure in [3-7]. Optimization of dosage in combination with other drugs and the length of treatment have been clarified for thalidomide and bortezomib. Current dosage levels are different from recorded dosages in registration studies which in certain cases led to common or higher level of side effects than is acceptable; these side effects are reduced after optimization. Side effects, especially the long-term ones, may fundamentally influence the quality of life of patients after successful treatment. Nowadays, optimization of thalidomide and bortezomib treatments is almost completed and lenalidomide optimization is currently being processed in [5]. It is logical to think that optimization of efficient drugs is a never ending process that waits for each new efficient drug, for example carfilzomib and pomalidomide in the near future. A variety of new drugs are being tested in clinical studies at phases I/II. In MM treatment, modern target therapies are being tested, such as monoclonal antibodies, kinase inhibitors or inhibitors of other target molecules connected to one of the signaling pathways important for malignant cells. Although treatment results of this group of drugs failed to reach expectations, we feel that they will produce very promising results in the future. Current treatment strategies will lead to a cure – a topic which is being discussed very seriously. In this chapter, the current state of affairs as well as the potentials of pharmacotherapy in MM will be discussed.

2. Basic scientific data influencing current treatment strategies

Our current treatment strategies originate from a variety of research data that may be shortly described as follows:

a. Every MM is preceded by a precancerosis called monoclonal gammopathy of undetermined significance (MGUS) in [8]. Individual stages starting from the occurrence of first clonal plasmocyte to MGUS, MM, refractory MM up to plasmocellular leukemia are concurrent; in one individual, they may be described as disease progression changing in time. Many internal and external factors influence the phase when the initial plasmocyte will develop into hematological malignancy requiring therapy (Fig.1).

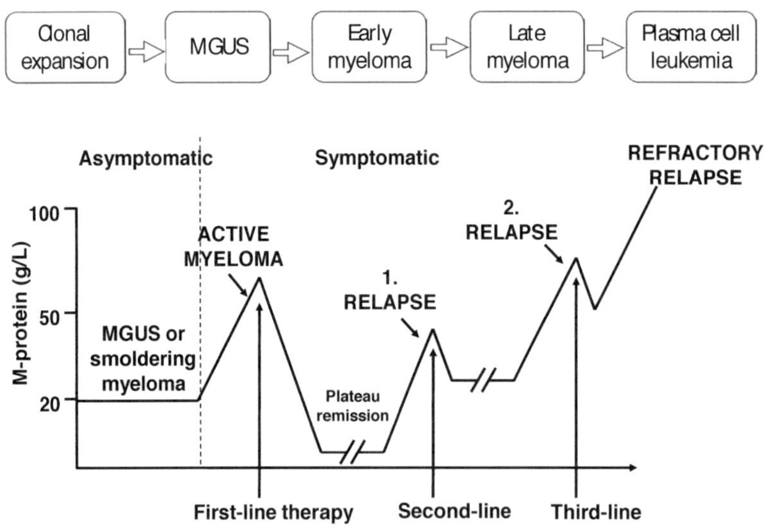

MGUS, monoclonal gammopathy of undetermined significance

Figure 1. Natural history of multiple myeloma

b. There is a variety of subtypes of multiple myeloma as this disease is very heterogenous. Thus, MM patients have various prognoses. All currently available classifications (based on ISS, cytogenetics, gene expression profiling, etc.) allow for classification of patients into groups with high, low or sometimes also intermediate risk for long-term survival. Unfortunately, no classification is specific enough to allow for prediction of treatment success and prognosis for each individual patient in [9-11].

c. Based on the subclonal theory as well as new proofs, it seems probable that there are more clones of plasmocytes present at the time of diagnosis in one patient. Various subclones exist in a dynamic equilibrium, competing for limited resources with alternating dominance of various subclones at different time points. These clones have various characteristics including treatment sensitivity, and their ratio is significantly influenced by the treatment given to patients. It seems that new subclones may originate even during treatment and/or course of the disease in [12,13]. This finding has completely changed our view of efficacy of simple combination treatments with one novel agent. On the other hand, it is in complete harmony with important successes in the treatment including the cure in patients treated with intensive sequences of treatment protocols consisting of most efficient drugs. Drug combinations are essential to overcome resistance and the impact of intra-clonal heterogeneity in [14].

d. Treatment resistance to a specific drug does not have to be absolute. From the above mentioned subclonal theory, it is obvious that disease resistance to a certain drug in first progression does not have to be resistant to the same drug in the fourth progression. Then, the subclone sensitive to the drug may or may not be prevalent over resistant subclones. In case there are no other treatment options available, it is suitable to test sensitivity to previously used drugs.

3. Treatment strategy and treatment line

When deciding on a treatment, it is necessary to plan a complex treatment – not only anticancer treatment but also supportive treatment; it is important to think about relapse at the time of initial treatment, which drugs to use so that initial treatment does not block further steps in the future. Autologous transplantation is a basic part of treatment wherever possible. Today, treatment strategies use optimal choices of treatment lines, in an individual that should cover 5-7 disease activities within 10 years of treatment if necessary.

4. Newly diagnosed multiple myeloma

Current treatment strategies for newly diagnosed patients are always aiming to reach deepest complete remission - molecular or immunophenotypic in [15,16]. In the first decade of this century, therapeutic regimens with one novel agent as backbone together with glucocorticoids and alkylating cytostatics were used as high standard based on randomized trials (Tab. 1).

Modern protocols of second decade use intensive treatment strategies in the clinical trials called "Multi Agent Sequential Therapy Targeting Different Clones" with at least two novel agens based on the strong evidence of curative potential of such approaches such as Total Therapy trials pioneered by Bart Barlogie in the Little Rock in [14].

MPT	>	MP	Randomized trial 6
MPV	>	MP	Randomized trial 1
MPR - R	>	MP	Randomized trial 1
VMPT - VT	>	MP	Randomized trial 1

M – melfalan, P – prednison, T – thalidomide, V – Velcade (bortezomib); R – Revlimid (lenalidomide)

Table 1. Better PFS on randomized trials with one novel agent based regimen vs. melphalan prednisolon (MP)

1. Induction therapy (2-6 lines of combined therapy) in [17]
2. Myeloablative treatment (1-2 autologous transplantation)
3. Consolidation therapy (3-4 cycles of combined treatment, if possible different from entry induction therapy) in [18,19]
4. Maintenance therapy by lenalidomide and possible combination of drugs should ensure maintenance of remission due to probable immunomodulatory effect in [20,21].

A similar course without myeloablative regimen but with extension of the induction phase of therapy should be evaluated for seniors not indicated for a myeloablative regimen. Unfortunately, in this group of patients, proof of curability is still anecdotal; treatment is less intensive and more modified based on status of the patient. It is important to treat the patient and not the disease. Adequate intensity of therapies in fragile patients is one of the more important aspects for a final positive outcome (Tab. 2) in [22]. Novel combinative fully peroral regimens with two novel agens will further improve prognosis in patients not indicated for myeloablative treatment.

5. Relapse of multiple myeloma

Aims of treatment for patients with relapsed/progressed disease are more limited. Key targets of intensive therapeutic strategies regarding the first and second relapse should be to make the disease chronic again for several years. Balance between efficacy and toxicity as well as long-term toxicity (peripheral polyneuropathy) are main issues in this setting in [23]. Re-

Agent	Dose level 0	Dose level -1	Dose level -2
Dexamethasone	40 mg/d d 1,8,15,22 / 4 wk	20 mg/d d 1,8,15,22 / 4 wk	10 mg/d d 1,8,15,22 / 4 wk
Melphalan	0.25 mg/kg d 1-4 / 4-6 wks	0.18 mg/kg d 1-4 / 4-6 wks	0.13 mg/kg d 1-4 / 4-6 wks
Prednisone	50 mg qod	25 mg qod	12.5 mg qod
Cyclophosphamide	100 mg/d d 1-21 / 4 wks	50 mg/d d 1-21 / 4 wks	50 mg qod d 1-21 / 4 wks
Bortezomib	1.3 mg/m^2 twice/wk d 1,4,8,11 / 3 wks	1.3 mg/m^2 once/wk d 1,8,15,22 / 5 wks	1.0 mg/m^2 once/wk d 1,8,15,22 / 5 wks
Thalidomide	100 mg/d	50 mg/d	50 mg qod
Lenalidomide	25 mg/d d 1-21 / 4 wks	15 mg/d d 1-21 / 4 wks	10 mg/d d 1-21 / 4 wks

Wk, week; d, day; qod, every other day

Adopted from Palumbo & Anderson, New Engl J Med 2011

Table 2. Dose reductions algorithm for frail patients

transplantation is always one of the most effective treatment options during the relapse setting and can be very safely used based on the individual history of the patient in [24]. There is a reduced chance to achieve complete remission if compared to first line therapy. However, combinative regimens using two novel agents (carfilzomib or bortezomib with lenalidomide or thalidomide) are able to induce even higher proportions of remission including complete remission than older types of therapy without the use of imunomodulatory drugs and proteasome inhibitors in newly diagnosed patients (personal experience with lenalidomide and carfilzomib). Generalized benefits for patients in further relapses from a similar number of treatment cycles using one novel agent (IMiD or proteasome inhibitor) is in median at least 1 year in [25]. Thus, the main benefit is not due to overcoming the natural course of the disease but rather to the possibility of using other novel agents in the next relapse. In the advanced disease stage, the treatment is very individualized and reaches a state of stability for a longer period of time (> 6 months) is considered to be acceptable treatment outcome. Long term survival of more than 10 years is currently reached for more than one third of multiple myeloma patients; this has been achieved due to new efficient drugs that can be offered to patients in relapse. It is important to create long-term treatment strategies so that the patient is offered efficient treatment even in third, fourth and further relapses of the disease. The patients who have relapsed after at least two new drugs have a very poor outcome if no other new drug is available, and they should receive the best palliative care in [26].

6. Drugs available for intensive treatments

It is necessary to note that novel agents, imunomodulatory drugs (thalidomide, lenalidomide, pomalidomide) and proteasome inhibitors (bortezomib, carfilzomib), are key players currently used in therapeutical protocols and/or in the clinical trials. The 'old' drugs, such as alkylating cytostatics and glucocorticoids, still belong to the most effective group of drugs in multiple myeloma. These old drugs are used in most treatment protocols. The therapeutic strategy in newly diagnosed patients is described in details in another chapter (Induction Therapy in Multiple Myeloma). The same drugs could be used in a relapse setting depending on the components of initial therapy, efficacy and toxicity of the initial therapy, patient status and circumstances of relapse (age, performance status, glucose metabolism, aggressive vs non-aggressive relapse, bone marrow reserve, renal function impairment, pre-existing peripheral neuropathy and quality of life considerations).

7. Drugs available for the maintenance part of treatment regimen

Decade after decade, there is a change in opinion about benefits of maintenance therapy. While conventional cytostatics and glucocorticoids were used because of lack of any other option, the era of interferon alpha ended with the introduction of immunomodulatory drugs. It is also true that worldwide, interferon alpha had never been accepted as routine maintenance therapy because of its comparatively high toxicity as well as minimal benefit for the unclassified subgroup of patients in [28].

8. Immunomodulatory drugs (IMiDs)

Meta-analysis of randomized clinical studies of phase III with thalidomide as maintenance therapy confirms the benefits of use after autologous transplantation. Statistically significant increase of PFS in six studies and overall survival prolongation in three studies were noted. On the other hand, only one third of patients tolerated thalidomide maintenance therapy for more than a year. At this point, when there are less toxic drugs available for maintenance therapy, thalidomide is recommended as a part of short-term intensive consolidation therapies in [29,28,30].

Lenalidomide was tested in two independent randomized clinical trials of phase III as maintenance treatment after autologous transplantation. Both these trials, CALGB 100104 and IFM 2005-02, demonstrated benefit from lenalidomide compared to placebo, which showed a major decrease in risk of progression by 60% in [21] and an improvement of three-year PFS in the group with lenalidomide (61% vs. 34%) in [20]. Based on new analyses (follow-up of 28 months), there was a statistically significant improvement in overall survival in Len/Dex treated groups of patients in comparison to the placebo treated group of patients, regardless of short follow-ups in [21]. Its role in maintenance therapy is highlighted by improved results when RMP-R treatment is used with maintenance therapy compared to RMP without maintenance therapy in a study of seniors MM-015 in [31]. RMP-R treatment ensured one of the longest median of PFS (31 months). Maintenance therapy of lenalidomide was generally well tolerated with no signs of cumulative toxicity as in the case of thalidomide. Although the occurrence of secondary malignancies after lenalidomide treatment was increased, the risk of disease progression or death by MM overcame this risk in [5]. Despite superb results of maintenance therapy by lenalidomide, it is not yet approved for maintenance therapy till the end of the year 2012 mainly due to safety reasons, although long-term results are also limited.

9. Inhibitors of proteasomes

In the study GEM/Pethema, patients were induced by VMP (bortezomib, melphalan, prednisolon) or VTP (bortezomib, thalidomid, prednisolon) and randomized for maintenance treatment (VT or VP) for 3 years. Maintenance treatment with bortezomib increased IF-CR from 24% to 42% in [32]. Maintenance treatment with bortezomib was better after autologous transplantation in comparison to thalidomide (PFS 28 vs. 35 months; $p=0.002$), and overall survival benefit was seen not only for the whole group ($p = 0.049$) but also for high risk patients in [33]. So far, there is not enough information about maintenance therapy with bortezomib although the data are promising. The change in the route of bortezomib administration from intravenous to subcutaneous significantly reduced toxicity, mainly peripheral polyneuropathy in [34]. Thus, long-term use of bortezomib will be more suitable for patients starting at the end of the year 2012. Moreover, novel proteasome inhibitors that undergo clinical trials have limited toxicity and per oral route of administration that further increased their potential for maintenance therapy in [35].

10. Curability of available treatment options

Multiple myeloma is curable if an intensive combination regime is used upfront. Long-term complete remission becomes a more important factor than reaching complete remission. Complete remission that lasts more than three years is the first milestone on the road towards curability in [36]. It is necessary to accentuate that in the light of current knowledge and long-term experience with intensive regimens, the possibility of curing MM patients is being discussed from the end of 2011 in [37]. The first report, at the time very provocative, was presented at ASH in 2009 suggesting the possibility of a cure in 2009 in [29]. This was a major breakthrough in the observation of this malignant disease.

Which MM patients have a chance of a cure and what is that chance? Curability depends on reaching a deep and constant complete remission which is most probable and possible in MM patients with a favorable prognosis suitable for autologous transplantation. Of which are treated by an intensive combination treatment composed of the most effectively available drugs. These drugs are set into a complex block of entry induction therapy followed by maintenance therapy. Curability is possible only in patients with a low-risk based on gene expression profiles and cytogenetics based on experience from Total Therapy 3 treatment protocols in [30]. It is important to realize how many patients really have this chance. Of all MM patients, about 40% are involved in intensive treatments. Out of these patients, about 80% are low risk which means about 32% of entry number. To simplify the calculation, about 75% of these patients reach complete remission (24% of entry numbers), and up to 85-90% of these patients reach long-term complete remission (21% of entry numbers) with a chance of curability at about 50-60% (10-12% of entry numbers) in [29,36,30]. Thus, based on available data, a qualified estimate would suggest that a chance for cure is possible for 10% of MM patients and 25% of patients who are able to undergo intensive treatments including myeloablation. These results changed natural course of the disease (Fig.2); moreover, they were impossible 20 years ago.

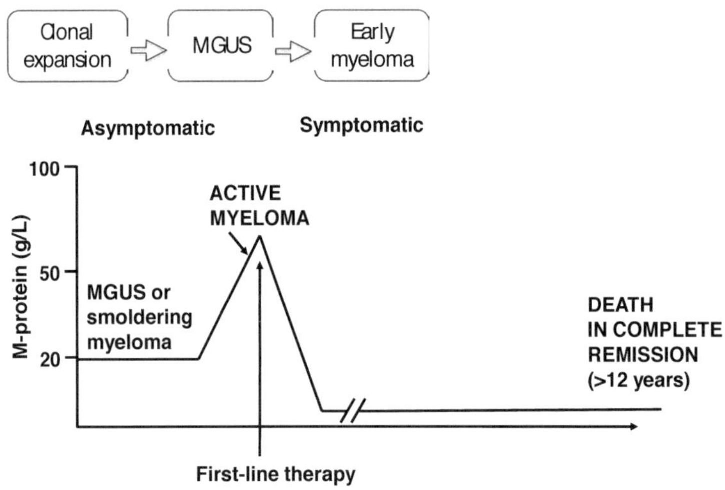

Figure 2. Natural history of multiple myeloma can be changed

11. Summary

In 2012, we can announce MM to be a curable disease under favorable prognostic conditions at the time of diagnosis and using intensive therapy in about 10% of MM patients. Relapsed MM or disease progression is not curable using current treatment options with the exception of allogeneic transplants in some cases. Due to highly efficient drugs, especially proteasome inhibitors and immunomodulatory drugs, our current treatment options are such that we can modulate another 5-6 active parts of the disease and offer long-term survival of more than 10 years to more than 1/3 of the patients.

Author details

Roman Hajek

Faculty of Medicine University Ostrava and Faculty Hospital Ostrava, Czech Republic

References

[1] Kumar, S. K, Rajkumar, S. V, Dispenzieri, A, et al. Improved Survival in Multiple Myeloma and the Impact of Novel Therapies. Blood (2008). , 111(5), 2516-20.

[2] Offidani, M, Corvatta, L, Morabito, F, et al. How to Treat Patients with Relapsed/ Refractory Multiple Myeloma: Evidence-Based Information and Opinions. Expert Opin Investig Drugs (2011). , 20(6), 779-93.

[3] San Miguel JF., Schlag R., Khuageva N.K. et al. VISTA Trial Investigators. Bortezomib Plus Melphalan and Prednisone for Initial Treatment of Multiple Myeloma. N Engl J Med (2008). , 359(9), 906-17.

[4] Palumbo, A, Bringhen, S, Liberati, A. M, et al. Oral Melphalan, Prednisone, and Thalidomide in Elderly Patients with Multiple Myeloma: Updated Results of a Randomized Controlled Trial. Blood (2008). , 112(8), 3107-14.

[5] Palumbo, A, Adam, Z, Kropff, M, et al. A Phase 3 Study Evaluating the Eficacy and Safety of Lenalidomide(Len) Combined with Melphalan and Prednisone Folowed by Continoues Lenalidomide Maintenance (MPR-R) in Patients ? 65 Years(Yrs) with Newly Diagnosed Multiple Myeloma(NDMM): Updated Results from Pts Aged Yrs Enrolled in MM-015. Blood (2011). Abstract 475., 65-75.

[6] Morgan, G. J, Davies, F. E, Gregory, W. M, et al. Cyclophosphamide, Thalidomide, and Dexamethasone (CTD) as Initial Therapy for Patients with Multiple Myeloma Unsuitable for Autologous Transplantation. Blood (2011). , 118(5), 1231-1238.

[7] Morgan, G. J, Davies, F. E, Gregory, W. M, et al. Cyclophosphamide, Thalidomide, and Dexamethasone as Induction Therapy for Newly Diagnosed Multiple Myeloma Patients Destined for Autologous Stem-cell Transplantation: MRC Myeloma IX Randomized Trial Results. Haematologica (2012). , 97(3), 442-50.

[8] Landgren, O, Kyle, R. A, Pfeiffer, R. M, et al. Monoclonal Gammopathy of Undetermined Significance (MGUS) Consistently Precedes Multiple Myeloma: a Prospective Study. Blood (2009). , 113, 5412-5417.

[9] Fonseca, R, Bergsagel, P. L, Drach, J, et al. International Myeloma Working Group Molecular Classification of Multiple Myeloma: Spotlight Review. Leukemia (2009). , 23(12), 2210-21.

[10] Munshi, N. C, Anderson, K. C, Bergsagel, P. L, et al. Consensus Recommendations for Risk Stratification in Multiple Myeloma: Report of the International Myeloma Workshop Consensus Panel 2. Blood (2011). , 117(18), 4696-700.

[11] Shaughnessy, J. D. Jr, Haessler J., van Rhee F. et al. Testing Standard and Genetic Parameters in 220 Patients with Multiple Myeloma with Complete Data Sets: Superiority of Molecular Genetics. Br J Haematol (2007). , 137(6), 530-6.

[12] Keats, J. J, Chesi, M, Egan, J. B, et al. Clonal Competition with Alternating Dominance in Multiple Myeloma. Blood (2012).

[13] Walker, B. A, Wardell, C. P, Melchor, L, et al. Intraclonal Heterogeneity and Distinct Molecular Mechanisms Characterize the Development of t(4;14) and t(11;14) Myeloma. Blood (2012). , 120(5), 1077-86.

[14] Usmani, S. Z, Crowley, J, Hoering, A, et al. Improvement in Long-term Outcomes with Successive Total Therapy Trials for Multiple Myeloma: are Patients Now Being Cured? Leukemia (2012).

[15] Ladetto, M, Pagliano, G, Fererro, S, et al. Correlation Between Clinical Outcome and Disease Kinetics by Quantitative PCR in Myeloma Patiens Following Post-transplant Consolidation with Bortezomib, Thalidomide and Dexamethasone. Blood (2011).

[16] Paiva, B, Martinez-lopez, J, Vidriales, M. B, et al. Comparison of Immunofixation, Serum Free Light Chain, and Immunophenotyping for Response Evaluation and Prognostication in Multiple Myeloma. J Clin Oncol. (2011). , 29(12), 1627-33.

[17] Richardson, P, Keller, E, Lonial, S, et al. Lenalidomide, Bortezomib, and Dexamethasone Combination Therapy in Patiens with Newly Diagnose Multiple Myeloma. Blood (2010). , 116, 679-686.

[18] Mellqvist, U. H, Gimsing, P, Hjertner, O, et al. Improved Progression Free Surfoval with Bortezomib Consolidation after High Dose Melphalan; Results of a Randomized Phase III Trial. Haematologica (2011). , 96(1), 31-11.

[19] Cavo, M, Pantani, L, Patriarca, F, et al. Superior Complete Response Rate (CR) and Progression-Free surfoval (PFS) with Bortezomib-Thalidomide-Dexamethasone (VTD) versus Thalidomide-Dexamethasone (TD) as Consolidation Therapy after Autologus Stem-cell Transplantation (ASCT in Multiple Myeloma (MM). Blood (2011).

[20] Attal, M, Olivier, P, Cances-lauwers, V, et al. Maintenance Treatment with Lenalidomide after Transplantation for Myeloma: Analysis for Secondary Malignancies within the IFM trial. Haematologica (2011). , 2005-02.

[21] Mccarthy, P, Lazar, K, Anderson, K, et al. Phase III Intergroup Study of Lenalidomide versus Placebo Maintanance Therapy following Single Autologous Stem Cell

Transplant (ASCT) for Multiple Myeloma (MM): CALB ECOG BMT-CTN 100104. Haematologica (2011). SS24., 23.

[22] Palumbo, A, & Anderson, K. Multiple myeloma. N Engl J Med. (2011). , 364(11), 1046-60.

[23] Garderet, L, Iacobelli, S, Moreau, P, et al. Superiority of the Triple Combination of Bortezomib-Thalidomide-Dexamethasone over the Dual Combination of Thalidomide-Dexamethasone in Patients with Multiple Myeloma Progressing or Relapsing after Autologous Transplantation: the MMVAR/IFM 2005-04 Randomized Phase III Trial from the Chronic Leukemia Working Party of the European Group for Blood and Marrow Transplantation. J Clin Oncol (2012). , 30(20), 2475-82.

[24] Gonsalves, W. I, Gertz, M. A, Lacy, M. Q, et al. Second Auto-SCT for Treatment of Relapsed Multiple Myeloma. Bone Marrow Transplant (2012).

[25] Krejci, M, Gregora, E, Straub, J, et al. Similar Efficacy of Thalidomide- and Bortezomib-Based Regimens for First Relapse of Multiple Myeloma. Ann Hematol (2011). , 90(12), 1441-7.

[26] Kumar, S. K, Lee, J. H, Lahuerta, J. J, et al. International Myeloma Working Group: Risk of Progression and Survival in Multiple Myeloma Relapsing after Therapy with IMiDs and Bortezomib: a Multicenter International Myeloma Working Group Study. Leukemia (2012). , 26(1), 149-57.

[27] Cavo, M, Tacchetti, P, Patriarca, F, et al. Bortezomib with Thalidomide Plus Dexamethasone Compared with Thalidomide Plus Dexamethasone as Induction Therapy before, and Consolidation Therapy after, Double Autologous Stem-cell Transplantation in Newly Diagnosed Multiple Myeloma: a Randomised Phase 3 Study. Lancet (2010). , 376(9758), 2075-85.

[28] Ludwig, H, Durie, B. G, Mccarthy, P, et al. IMWG Consensus on Maintenance Therapy in Multiple Myeloma. Blood (2012). , 119(13), 3003-3015.

[29] Barlogie, B, & Shaughnessy, J. D. Jr, Anaissie E. et al. Modeling for Cure with Total Therapy (TT) Trials for Newly Diagnosed Multiple Myeloma (MM): Let the Math Speak. Blood (2009). Abstract 744.

[30] Van Rhee, F, Szymonifka, J, Anaissie, E, et al. Total Therapy 3 for Multiple Myeloma: Prognostic Implications of Cumulative Dosing and Premature Discontinuation of VTD Maintenance Components, Bortezomib, Thalidomide, and Dexamethasone, Relevant to all Phases of Therapy. Blood (2010). , 116(8), 1220-7.

[31] Palumbo, A, Hajek, R, Delforge, M, et al. Continuous Lenalidomide Treatment for Newly Diagnosed Multiple Myeloma. N Engl J Med. (2012). , 366(19), 1759-69.

[32] Mateos, M. V, Oriol, A, Teruel, A. I, et al. Maintenance Therapy with Bortezomib plus Thalidomide (VT) or Bortezomib Plus Prednisone (VP) in Elderly Myeloma Patiens Included in the GEM2005MAS65 Spanish Randomized Trial. Blood (2011).

[33] Sonneveld, P, Schmidt-wolf, I. G, Van Der Holt, B, et al. Bortezomib Induction and Maintenance Treatment in Patients with Newly Diagnosed Multiple Myeloma: Results of the Randomized Phase III HOVON-65/ GMMG-HD4 trial. J Clin Oncol. (2012). , 30(24), 2946-55.

[34] Moreau, P, Pylypenko, H, Grosicki, S, et al. Subcutaneous Versus Intravenous Administration of Bortezomib in Patients with Relapsed Multiple Myeloma: a Randomised, Phase 3, Non-inferiority Study. Lancet Oncol. (2011). , 12, 431-40.

[35] Moreau, P, Richardson, P. G, Cavo, M, et al. Proteasome Inhibitors in Multiple Myeloma: 10 Years Later. Blood (2012). , 120(5), 947-59.

[36] Hoering, A, Crowley, J, Shaughnessy, J. D, et al. Complete Remission in Multiple Myeloma Examined as Time-dependent Variable in Terms of Both Onset and Duration in Total Therapy Protocols. Blood (2009). , 114(7), 1299-1305.

[37] San-miguel, J. F, & Mateos, M. V. Can Multiple Myeloma Become a Curable Disease? Haematologica (2011). , 96(9), 1246-8.

Chapter 2

Monoclonal Immunoglobulin

Marie-Christine Kyrtsonis, Efstathios Koulieris,
Vassiliki Bartzis, Ilias Pessah, Eftychia Nikolaou,
Vassiliki Karalis, Dimitrios Maltezas,
Panayiotis Panayiotidis and Stephen J. Harding

Additional information is available at the end of the chapter

http://dx.doi.org/10.5772/55855

1. Introduction

Secretion of monoclonal immunoglobulins (M-Ig) may be associated with several malignant conditions, also called M-protein, paraprotein, or M-component they are produced by an abnormally expanded single (''mono-'') clone of plasma cells in an amount that can be detected in serum, urine, or rarely in other body fluids [1]. The M-Ig can be an intact immunoglobulin (Ig) (containing both heavy and light chains), or light chains in the absence of heavy chain (encountered in light chain myeloma, light chain deposition disease, AL amyloidosis), or rarely heavy chains in the absence of light chains only (heavy chain disease).

All intact Igs have the same structure, made up of mirror imaged identical light and heavy chains. There are five classes of heavy chain, γ, α, μ, δ and ε with two classes of light chain κ and λ. Igs are secreted by terminally differentiated B-lymphocytes and their normal function is to act as antibodies recognizing a specific antigen.

During B-cell maturation, the rearrangement of Ig heavy and light chain genes takes place early in pre-B-cell development and ends in memory B-cells or Ig producing plasma cells that have a unique heavy and light chain gene rearrangement, thus being selected to recognize a given antigen. During, oncogenic events which occur randomly during this process, the B cell may acquire a survival advantage, and proliferate into identical (clonal) daughter B-cells able to differentiate into Ig producing cells secreting a monoclonal component. With additional oncogenic events a mature B-cell neoplasm may develop, carrying the inherent ability to produce a monoclonal Ig. Multiple myeloma and Waldenstrom's macroglobulinaemia are architypical of Ig-secreting B-cell disorders.

The purpose of this present chapter is to describe the properties of M-Igs and discuss the biologic, clinical and other implications of their presence in the course of B-cell disease entities.

2. Ontogeny of normal and monoclonal Ig-producing B-cells

2.1. B-cell development

B-cell maturation is a complex process that comprises both cell differentiation into Ig secreting plasma cells and, in parallel, the rearrangement of the genes responsible for Ig synthesis. Furthermore it includes inherent risks of genetic derailment because it is associated with DNA remodelling with intrinsic instability, thus presenting the possibility of malignant development.

B cell development begins in the bone marrow (BM) from gestation week 18 and throughout life. The generation of pro-B cells from a common lymphoid progenitor cell depends on two main transcription factors, E12 and E47 and on the contribution of the transcriptional regulators EBF and Pax-5 [5]. During B-cell evolution the rearrangement of Ig heavy and light chain genes takes place [2]. The Ig heavy gene (IgH) is located on chromosome 14 while Ig light chain (IgL) genes are on chromosomes 2 and 22 for κ (1-40 vκ, 1-5 jκ and 1cκ) and λ (1-30 vλ, 1-4 jλ and 1-4cλ) light chain respectively. Rearrangement of IgH and IgL genes allows variable (V), diversity (D) and joining (J) gene segments rearrangement. V(D)J recombination starts in precursor B cells (pre B-I); recombinase activating genes 1 and 2 (RAG-1 and RAG-2), are essential for this step. The resulting IgVH is frequently not functional therefore the pre-B cell initiates V(D)J recombination at the other allele. If this is successful, the complete IgVH will be expressed as an Igμ H chain in the cytoplasm (Cy-Igμ) and on the membrane, together with a surrogate light chain, the pre B cell receptor complex (pre-BCR). Accordingly the pre-B-II cell proliferates, then looses its pre-BCR and re-express RAG proteins [7]. At that point, the B-cell is transformed into a small pre B-II cell that will subsequently rearrange the IgL variable gene segments and expresses a mature membrane BCR. If the BCR is not strongly self-reactive, the immature B cell leaves the BM as transitional B cell that evolves into naive B cell in the spleen; alternatively, it may mature in the periphery. However, if the immature B cell is still self-reactive, it will remain in the BM for additional IgVL recombination, replacing the self-reactive IgVL by another IgVL and so on. B cells producing self-reactive BCRs are removed from the repertoire during maturation by BM silencing mechanisms [3;4]. Splenic transitional B cells (CD27- CD5+ CD10+ CD24^{hi} CD38^{hi} and L-selectin^{lo}) undergo differentiation into mature naive B2, also called follicular (FO) B cells, or marginal zone (MZ) B cells [5]. The aforementioned B-cell population is characterized by limited proliferative capacity and survival upon BCR stimulation; it comprises less than 2% of the peripheral B cells [6]. While maturating in the spleen, transitional B cells loose CD10 and CD5 and start expressing higher levels of L selectin and CD44. Following which the B cell transforms into conventional naive B2 cells that recirculate via the blood to the secondary lymphoid tissues or organs [7]. MZ cells could represent the normal counterpart of marginal zone lymphoma cells and CD5+ B-cells the one of mantle cell lymphoma (MCL) and chronic lymphocytic leukemia (CLL). Blood also contains a small normal population of naive CD5+ CD27- cells that frequently produce poly-/self-reactive antibodies (Abs) [8]. The CD5 molecule negatively regulates BCR signals [9] and CD5 B cells represent 50% of poly-/self-reactive cells [10].

Lymph node (LN) colonization depends on the expression of L-selectin and integrin $\alpha L\beta 2$ (LFA-1), while recruitment to mucosa-associated lymphoid tissues (MALT) depends on expression of L-selectin and integrin $\alpha 4\beta 7$. Without antigenic stimulation, the naive B cells recirculate again.

Activation of mature naive B cells into Ig secreting plasma cells can be T-helper independent (TI) and antigen free, via invariant receptors (TI-1), or derives from crosslinking of the BCR by polyvalent Ags (TI-2). More frequently, it is performed in close collaboration with CD4-expressing T cells (T-helper dependant: TD), and results from a monovalent Ag aggression. MZ B cells of the spleen and other mucosal sites, mostly respond to TI-2 Ags, such as polysaccharides of bacterial cell walls and other bacterial components, able to crosslink BCRs [11]. IgM+ MZ B cells that are CD27+ are memory cells while CD27- are naïve; their BCRs display poly- and self- reactivity.

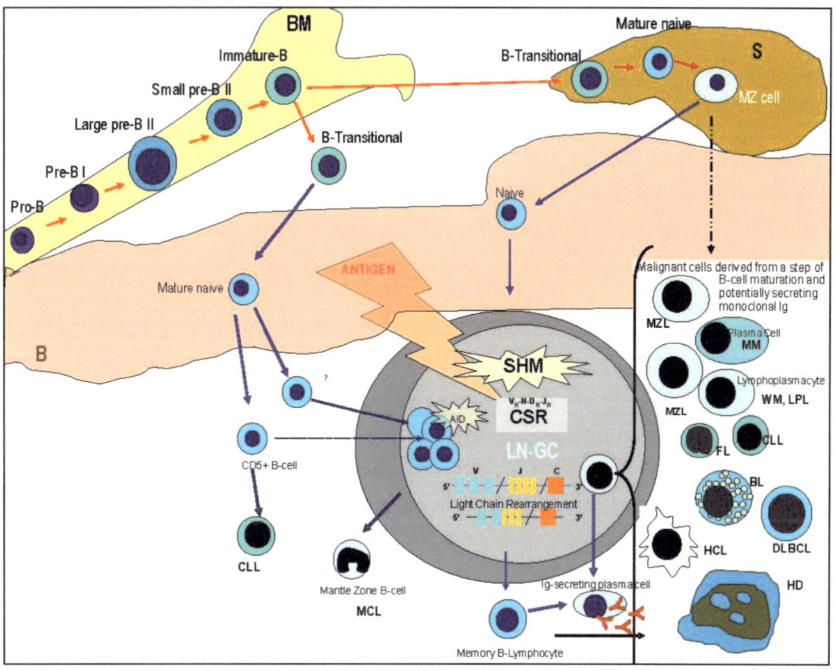

BM: Bone Marrow, S: Spleen, B: Blood, LN-GC: Lymph Node-Germinal Center, MZL: Mantle Cell Lymphoma, MM: Multiple Myeloma, LPL: Lymphoplasmacytic Lymphoma, WM: Waldenstroms Macroglobulinaemia, FL: Follicular Lymphoma, CLL: Chronic Lymphocytic Leukemia, BL: Burkitt Lymphoma, HCL: Hairy Cell Leukemia, DLBCL: Diffuse Large B Cell Lymphoma, HD: Hodgkin Lymphoma, SHM: Somatic Hypermutations, CSR: Class Switch Recombination.

Figure 1. Schematic of B-cell Maturation and B-Lymphoproliferative Disorders Origin

T-helper-cell dependent (TD) B-cell activation takes place in germinal centers (GC) in response to the presence of free Ags, as part of immune complexes or at the surface of Ag presenting cells (APC). B-cells then differentiate into short-lived, Ab-forming plasma cells or proliferate as centroblasts expressing CD10+, CD38+ and BCL-6. These centroblasts express low amounts of the BCR at their surface and undergo somatic hypermutations (SHM), by accumulating nucleotide substitutions in their Ig variable (*IgV*) genes [12;13]. GC activated B-cells are meant to be short-lived, except for the few with a high affinity IgV region (BCR) for the Ag. These high-affinity B cells are selected in the GC light zone, and may undergo class switch recombination (CSR), switching the IgM/IgD sequence with any of the other downstream region sequences [14]. Igs formed early in the context of normal response to an Ag aggression are of IgM and IgD isotypes; these are located on the B-cell surface as recognition receptors. Then activated B cells divide, and class switching from the IgD and IgM heavy chains to IgG, IgE or IgA classes takes place [15;16]. The process is regulated by various cytokines [16] while both SHM and CSR depend on the B-cell-specific enzyme activation-induced cytidine deaminase (AID) which is highly expressed by GC B cells [17]. Cytokines and costimulatory soluble factors stimulate the transcriptional activation of individual I promoters and determine the S region and Ig isotype involved in the CSR event. SHM depends on transcription of the variable (IgVH and IgVL) regions and leads to point mutations and, to a lower extent, insertions and deletions. The rate of SHM is about 1 mutation on 1000 nucleotides per cell division. CSR consists on transcription of the S regions that started upstream of an I exon that is located 5′ of each S region, giving rise to non-coding germline transcripts that span the I exon, the S region and downstream CH exons [7].

Terminally differentiated B cells become either Ab-producing mature plasma cells that home to the bone marrow or memory cells [18]. Memory B cells (CD27+) are Ag-selected B cells, derived from TD GC responses and usually express either IgM- IgD- or IgM+ IgD+, comprising about 20% of all peripheral B cells. A small percentage of IgM only (IgM+ IgD-) and IgD only (IgM- IgD+) also exists. IgD-only B cells have undergone a Cμ deletion due to a non-canonical CSR event, express Igλ, contain extremely high levels of somatic IgV mutations [19] and show a strongly biased V3-30 IgVH gene usage [20], that can be seen in some malignant B-cell disorders [2]. Memory B-cells are long-lived, prone to Ig class switch (to IgG, IgA or IgE) and contain hypermutated IgV genes. Following stimulation, they present a competitive advantage over naive B cells in rapidly transforming themselves into plasma cells producing high affinity, class switched, IgG/IgA Abs [21]. They may hide in BM niches and recirculate numerous times. It is believed that in most indolent B-cell lymphoproliferative disorders, a proneoplastic condition precedes where the precursor neoplastic B-cell circulates and recirculates as a memory cell.

2.2. Malignant transformation

Where one or more oncogenic events occur during B-cell maturation, the resulting daughter cell will be identical and, if it has the ability to differentiate into an Ig producing cell, it will secrete a monoclonal component. Consequently, all B-cell mature neoplasms [22] have a common origin as well as the inherent ability to produce a monoclonal Ig.

Malignant B-cell Non-Hodgkin's lymphoma (NHL) possibly develops because risks for genetic derailment are increased during SHM and CSR that are associated with DNA remodelling. Thus, the initiating steps of the malignant B-cell transformation concern erroneous V(D)J rearrangement. Recurrent translocations involving the IgH or IgL locus and observed in B-cell lymphoproliferative disorders are shown in table 1, in relation to their biologic repercussions in disease entities concerned.

Disease Entity	IgH Translocation	Gene Involved	Biologic Consequences
MCL/MM	t(11;14)	Cyclin D1 encoded by CCND1	Regulator of CDKs CDK4/CDK6 required for cell cycle transition G1→S
FL	t(14;18)	Bcl2	Antiapoptotic
MM	t(4;14)	FGFR3	Signal transduction, pathways activation, cell proliferation regulation & differentiation
MM	t(6;14)	Cyclin D3	Cell cycle: G1→S transition
MM	t(14;20)	MAFB	Transcription factor, lineage specific hematopoiesis regulation
MM	t(14;16)	c-MAF	Cell cycle Stimulation. Promote interactions of tumor & stromal cells
BL/MM	t(8;14)	myc	Transcription factor, cell proliferation, differentiation, apoptosis, stem cell self renewal

Table 1. Main Recurrent Translocations Involving The IgH Locus

Monoclonal gammopathy of undetermined significance (MGUS) is a pro-neoplastic condition that may evolve into multiple myeloma (MM) or other B-cell lymphoproliferative disorders. MGUS represent a first step in the development of monoclonal diseases while the progression of MGUS to MM or other entities may be secondary to a random second genetic event. Several studies indicate that the majority of IgH locus aberrations reported in MM are already present in MGUS, favoring the hypothesis that these are early genetic events in the progression leading to MM [23].

In MM, the most frequent partners in reciprocal translocations involving the IgH locus on chromosome 14q32, are 11q13 (15%), 4p16 (5%), 16q23 (5%), 21q12 (2%) and 6p21 (2%); two additional partners are also found rarely 12p13 (<1%) and 8q24 (<1%). Thus, the aforementioned translocations may deregulate seven oncogenes involved, CCND1, CCND2, CCND3, MAF, MAFB, MAFA and FGFR3/MMSET [24]. The overall rate of 14q32 translocations increases with disease progression and reaches 90% in advanced tumors. Light chain translocations are rather rare in MM, particularly Igκ, which seem to be very infrequent [25]. Changes in the expression of gene subsets could be partly responsible for disease heterogeneity, as well as for further disease transformation. Moreover, with the 11q13 partner, constitutive upregulation of cyclin D1 results, deregulating the cell cycle [26]; t(11;14) is accompanied with a higher frequency of CD20 expression, hyposecretory disease and λ light chain usage. This subtype is increasingly encountered in AL amyloidosis, with or without MM, and in the rare IgM MM and is associated with favorable outcome. Translocation t(4;14)(p16;q32), is cryptic because of its telomeric location [27] and has been associated with IgA isotype, λ chain usage, deletion or monosomy of chromosome 13, immature plasma morphology, more aggressive disease and shortened survival. It leads to deregulation of fibroblast growth factor receptor 3 (FGFR3) gene on der(14) and of Multiple Myeloma SET (MMSET) domain gene on der(4); the latter may be a critical transforming event. t(4;14) was found characterized by deregulation of chromatin organization, actin filament and microfilament movement [28].

The t(14;16)(q32;q23) leads to the dysregulation of the c-maf oncogene; it is more frequently encountered in IgA isotope and is associated with chromosome 13 deletion whereas t(14;20)(q32;q11) results in maf-B deregulation that like c-maf is a basic zipper transcription factor. The clinical significance of these rare IgH translocations is unknown and under investigation. However, the oncogenic process is continually going on during disease course and secondary IgH translocations can be observed such as those involving the myc oncogene (8q24), that are associated with advanced and aggressive disease. Especially in patients with cytogenetically high-risk disease, more changes are observed, including heterogeneous clonal mixtures with shifting predominant competitive clones [29].

It is interesting to observe that the abnormalities observed are not disease specific and can occur in different B-cell disorders in which they may confer different phenotypes, suggesting a role for additional factors [24].

A hallmark of Burkitt lymphoma (BL) is the expression of the myc oncogene, which has an essential role in cell proliferation, cell growth, protein synthesis, metabolism and apoptosis [30]. myc deregulated expression arises from t(8;14)(q24;q32), juxtaposing myc to the IgH locus, in 80% of cases, whereas in the remaining, myc is translocated to the κ- (2p12), or λ- (22q11) light chain respectively. In endemic BL, most myc/IgH breakpoints originate from aberrant somatic hypermutation, in contrast to sporadic cases where the translocation mostly involves the Ig switch regions of the IgH locus at 14q32. The discrepancies are perhaps due to differences in Epstein Bar Virus positivity between endemic and sporadic forms [31]. myc translocations are not completely specific for BL and have been reported in other B-cell entities.

Almost 70% of mantle cell lymphoma (MCL) patients are genetically characterized by the chromosomal translocation t(11;14). In several cases, patients also have point mutations and / or deletion of the ATM (ataxia telangiectasia mutated) gene. In addition, blastic forms or subtypes with more aggressive clinical behavior, may have additional mutations in genes that act as negative regulators of the cell cycle such as p16, p18 and p53 [32]. Rarer MCL cases are negative for cyclin D1, lack t(11; 14) and stand out of the usual clinical picture of MCL [33]; in such cases, cyclin D2 or cyclin D3 are overexpressed, a different permutation t(2; 12) (p12; p13) which connects cyclin D2 to the IgL-k locus may be present; it does not cause loss or quantitative disorder of genetic material, but at a molecular level, reconnecting two chromosomal regions can disrupt important genetic sequences, causing inactivation or gene mutation. Moreover, in this permutation, the protooncogene PRAD1 (Parathyroid Adenomatosis 1, or bcl1) which is normally found on chromosome 11, is swapped in the heavy chain Ig gene on chromosome 14 [34]. The resulting oncogene bcl1/IGH encodes cyclin D1 that is an important cell cycle regulator, particularly during the transition from the G1 to the S phase (the same applies for cyclins D2 and D3). Under normal conditions, cyclin D1 acts through its interaction with cyclin dependent kinases (CDKs). CDKs are enzymes that add phosphate groups to protein-targets in order to make them inactive. The resulting complexes CDK4-D1 and CDK6-D3, promote the progress to cell cycle phase S, resulting in an uncontrolled proliferation.

Follicular lymphoma (FL) is characterized by the presence of chromosomal translocation t(14;18), which promotes protein bcl2 overexpression that in turn, leads to the suspension of apoptosis and survival increment of B cells that harbor the translocation. Less commonly, bcl2 is deregulated by translocation to the Igκ t(2;8) and Igλ t(8;22) loci [35]. The t(14;18) is apparently mediated by the RAG recombinase proteins, which cleave at J segments in the IgH locus and at an unusual non B form DNA structure in bcl2. These B cells undergo an epigenetic reprogramming which, in conjunction with the acquisition of additional events, leads to FL development. The t(14;18)(q32;q21) may also be observed in diffuse large B cell lymphoma (DLBCL) [36] and in non-gastric MALT lymphomas. It brings the MALT1 gene under the control of the IGH enhancer [37].

3. Monoclonal immunoglobulins charateristics

3.1. Ig synthesis, secretion and metabolism

The IgH locus contains a region of 40-50 functional variable (VH), 27 diversity (DH) and 6 joining (JH) gene segments which is flanked by exons encoding the Ig constant regions (Cμ, Cδ, Cγ3, Cγ1, Cα1, Cγ2, Cγ4, Cε and Cα2). The Igκ locus contains 34-38 functional Vκ and 5 Jκ gene segments and one exon encoding the constant region of Igκ (Cκ). The Igλ locus comprises 29-30 functional Vλ and 4 functional Jλ-Cλ combinations [16]. Consequently, one of about fifty functional V_H, another of thirty D, and one of six J_H genes and, in the same way, one of thirty V_L and one of four J_L genes will be used. It appears that there are nearly 200 functional heavy and light chain gene segments that give rise to combinations of gene products, allowing the production of more than 5×10^7 antibodies with different unique variable end antigen combining sites [15;38;39]. Independently of the initiating stimulus, partly due to the aberrant Ig locus translocations and the putative activation or silencing of genes in monoclonal diseases, the cell starts to synthesize Ig following the variable domain rearrangement. On the coding DNA strand, the gene segments for the formation of the variable and the constant domains of the heavy chain are in order 5′ VDJ-μ-δ-γ_3-γ_1-α_1-γ_2-γ_4-ε-α_2- 3′. The RNA polymerase binds to the template strand of DNA and starts reading in 3′ to 5′ direction adding nucleotides to the 3′end of pre-mRNA transcript. Alternative splicing of the pre- mRNA brings together the VDJ variable domain and constant domain segments leading to the formation of the mRNA heavy Ig chain. As this procedure occurs in order, initially VDJs will get together with μ constant domain leading to the synthesis of heavy IgM component. This will bind with a light chain forming an IgM molecule. Thus, in order, cells make at first IgM, then IgD, IgG_3, IgG_1, IgA_1, IgG_2, IgG_4, IgE and IgA_2 that consist of the same variable domains but different constant domains due to alternative splicing and giving them different specific properties [40].

Light chains are synthesized in parallel to the heavy chain partner. However, an excess of light chains is produced, that if remained unbound to a heavy Ig component, will enter the blood and the extravascular compartment and circulate as free light chains (FLC). In patients with plasma cell dyscasias (PCD) and B-cell lymphoproliferative disorders, homogeneous serum total Ig molecules (intact Ig) and serum FLCs (sFLCs) are secreted by the malignant clone [40].

sFLCs are rapidly cleared (2-6hrs) and metabolized by the kidney although trace quantities (1-10mg/L) can be found in the urine, produced by the lower urinary tract mucosa. With regard to intact Ig, IgA and IgM are cleared by pinocytosis and have constant half lives of 5-6 days while IgG has a concentration dependent variable half life, ranging from days to weeks or even months. Briefly, IgG is ingested by reticulo-endothelial cells by pinocytosis, but inside the endosome, it is bound by a recycling receptor called neonatal (FcRn) receptor and recycled back to the surface to be released. This process can occur many times and extends the half lives of both IgG and albumin, as FcRn binds to both IgG, via the constant domain, and albumin non-competitively [40]. When there is a large amount of IgG (as can be found in diseases such as IgG MM) the receptor becomes saturated and the half life of IgG is shorter.

3.2. Ig structure

Antibodies are the secreted form of the BCR, the simple symmetrical structure is conserved through the 5 immunoglobulin classes which are defined by their heavy chain amino acid sequences (γ, α, μ, δ and ε) although in MM IgM, IgD and IgE monoclonal proteins are rare. There is further subclass division for γ ($\gamma 1$, $\gamma 2$, $\gamma 3$, $\gamma 4$) and α ($\alpha 1$ and $\alpha 2$) immunoglobulin classes. Amino acid sequence analysis of the 5 immunoglobulin classes showed that each was based upon the same repeating structure, 2 identicial light chains (~25kDa in size, 211-217 amino acids) and 2 identical heavy chains (~50kDa in size, 450-550 amino acids depending upon the class of heavy chain). Each of the immunoglobulin constituent proteins are constructed of β pleated sheets, which form the β barrel (Figure 2, A κ FLC molecule showing the constant region (left), and the variable region (right) with its alpha helix (red). (Courtesy of J Hobbs). Whilst there are obvious similarities between the different classes of immunoglobulin these structures are still being resolved and understood. IgG can be divided into 3 subunits, two identical fragment antigen binding arms (Fab) and an crystallizable (Fc) stem. Furthermore, within each subclass the hinge region shows differences both in the number of amino acids and the flexibility of the protein. More elegant electron tomography imaging of this molecule clearly shows its globular nature which perhaps gives a better indication of the protein structure. Serum IgA is predominantly a monomer, but dimeric forms can be found with J chain linkers. Solution scattering modelling of the two subclasses suggests a structure similar to IgG for IgA2 immunoglobulins, however IgA1 proteins appear to have a flattened "T" shaped structure. The traditional 2 dimensional representation of immunoglobulins belies their globular and highly variable nature, which may wrongly support the assumption that such molecules are simply quantified.

http://dx.doi.org/10.5772/55855

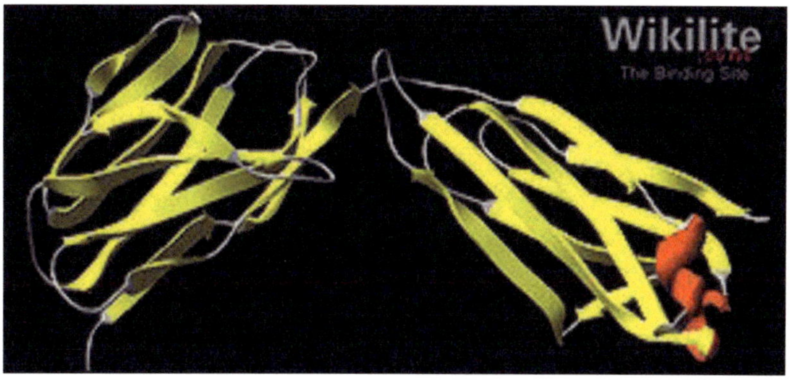

Figure 2. β pleated sheets of the kappa free light chain

3.3. Ig function

In normal conditions, the Ig or Ab (antibody) recognizes a unique part of the foreign target or antigen, called an epitope [40;41]. Each tip of the "Y" of an antibody contains a paratope (a structure analogous to a lock) that is specific for one particular epitope (similarly analogous to a key) on an antigen, allowing these two structures to bind together with precision. Using this binding mechanism, an antibody can tag a microbe or an infected cell for attack by other parts of the immune system, or can neutralize its target directly. Antibodies contribute to immunity in three ways: they prevent pathogens from entering or damaging cells by binding to them; they stimulate removal of pathogens by macrophages and other cells by coating the pathogens; and they trigger their destruction by stimulating other immune responses such as the complement pathway [42-44].

The five major Ab classes present complementary functions are shown in Table 2.

Immunoglobulin	Major Function
IgM	Main Ig during Primary Response (Early antibody). Fixes Complement (most effectively).
IgG	Main Ig during Secondary Response (late antibody). Opsonization. Fixes Complement. Neutralizes Toxins, Viruses.
IgA	Secretory mucosal Ig Prevents invasion from gut mucosa.
IgE	Immediate Hypersensitivity. Mast cell and Basophil reactions. Activates Eosinophils in helminth infection.
IgD	Function Unknown. Mostly on the Surface of B cells (B cell receptor).

Table 2. Major Functions of Antibodies Classes

Monoclonal Igs are not secreted after antigen exposure and do not contribute to combat pathogens; in fact humoral immunity is impaired because monoclonal plasma cells proliferate in detriment of normal Igs. Thus, in B-cell lymphoproliferative disorders, profound polyclonal hypogammaglobulinaemia can be observed leading to the inability to fight infections.

In some cases, the monoclonal Ig can have other effects, such as the ability to agglutinate red cells (cold agglutinin disease), to act as auto-antibody (autoimmune haemolytic anaemia), to aggregate at low temperatures (cryoglobulinemia), cause increased viscosity (Waldenstrom's macroglobulinemia), to deposit in tissues with resulting organ dysfunction (AL amyloidosis or immunoglobulin deposition diseases), and to cause peripheral neuropathy (MGUS, WM, AL amyloidosis, POEMS syndrome) [45].

3.4. Monoclonal immunoglobulin detection and quantification

Monoclonal intact immunoglobulin is routinely detected by serum protein electrophoresis (SPEP), the heavy chain class identified by immunofixation (IF) and quantified by SPEP-densitometry or nephelometry. Guidelines recommend SPEP to monitor monoclonal immunoglobulin concentrations as markers of response and relapse. However, SPEP quantification can be inaccurate at low concentrations (10g/L), can be difficult when the M-Ig co-migrates with other serum proteins (commonly IgA and IgM isotypes), when monoclonal immunoglobulins are produced by multiple small clones and is not suitable for sFLC quantification. Furthermore, poor linearity of SPEP at high concentrations and the variable catabolism of monoclonal IgG can make assessment of the serum load inaccurate. To aid patient monitoring international guidelines (IMWG 2011 concensus) recommend the use of total Ig nephelometric assays. At gross concentrations these assay are suitable tools to monitor patients; however, as they are unable to distinguish between the monoclonal and polyclonal Igs they will be insensitive as the Ig concentration approaches the normal range. One potentially useful addition to the laboratorian's armatorarium to overcome these issues are the newly developed heavy / light chain (HLC) immunoassays targeting the unique junctional epitope between the light chain (CL) and heavy chain (CH1) constant region of immunoglobulin, enabling the separate quantification of the different immunoglobulin classes i.e. HLC-IgGκ, -IgGλ, -IgAκ, -IgAλ, -IgMκ and -IgMλ. Measuring the molecules in pairs with this method enables the calculation of a ratio of the involved/uninvolved-polyclonal Igs (HLCR) [46-48] in the same manner as sFLC κ/λ ratios (FLCR).

SPEP quantification of sFLC is inaccurate and for more than 150 years monoclonal FLC measurements relied upon urinalysis. Collection, handling, renal function and variable light chain biochemistries make this a less than ideal medium for analysis. In the last 10 years the introduction of sheep based, polyclonal immunoassays for the quatification of sFLC κ and λ have changed the paradigm for FLC measurement. Briefly, polyclonal sheep antisera target κ and λ epitopes that are not available when the light chains are bound to their heavy chain partners [49]. As previously discussed FLCs are not homogeneous proteins and have significant genetic differences, particularly in the case of λ FLC, making the use of polyclonal antibodies (rather than monoclonal) necessary to ensure recognition of all FLC clones. The paired tests enable quantification of sFLC within and below the normal range which leads to the identification of subtle monoclonal clones [87], below the sensitivity of SPEP and the qualitative IFE methods.

Intact Ig molecules, due to their size, are not filtered and excreted in the urine. Their presence in urine indicates glomerular damage and is usually part of the nephrotic syndrome that can accompany some monoclonal diseases (amyloidosis). If a simple urinalysis to identify protein in the urine gives a positive result, a 24-hour urine collection is required for urine IF. On the contrary, sFLCs that are much smaller, are freely filtered, excreted in the urine and metabolized in the urinary tract. During the initial stages of a plasma cell disorder, they are produced in small amounts that are entirely filtered by the urinary system; the majority is metabolized while small amounts may be excreted in the urine. Consequently, a negative serum IF may result while urine protein electrophoresis and IF may be positive. Urine test is not required for follow up due to the "paralogue phenomenon "of the sFLC. As the disease progresses the sFLC cause renal damage and decreased excretion from the kidneys leading eventually to decreased levels in the urine. If only urines are tested for follow up, low levels of sFLC could be found leading, in case of relapse, to wrongly consider disease improvement. In addition, during treatment, the reversal of renal damage will cause more excretion of sFLC to the urine, finding that should not be interpreted as disease progression.

3.5. Implications of monoclonal Ig in diseases

Monoclonal Ig, as measured by total Ig quantification, or more recently FLC or HLC, may contribute to diagnosis, response evaluation, disease monitoring or prognostication in plasma cell dyscrasias and B-cell lymphoproliferative disorders (Table 3).

3.5.1. Monoclonal gammopathy of undetermined significance

Monoclonal gammopathy of undetermined significance (MGUS) is an asymptomatic plasma cell dyscrasia that is present in more than 3% of the general white population older than age 50. It has an average multiple myeloma progression risk of about 1% per year [51]. The entity was first described by Waldenstrom in 1960 after abnormal narrow hypergammaglobulinemia bands were noted in the serum of healthy individuals on SPEP [52]. In 1978, Kyle introduced the term "monoclonal gammopathy of undetermined significance" after observing that asymptomatic patients with monoclonal protein have a higher risk of developing multiple myeloma, Waldenstrom macroglobulinemia, light-chain amyloidosis or related disorders [53]. Since then definition of MGUS has undergone several adaptations but always, paraprotein presence represented the backbone of its characterization.

In the updated 2010 IMWG diagnostic criteria, the definition of MGUS includes the presence of a serum monoclonal protein <3 g/dL, <10% clonal BM plasma cells infiltration and absence of end-organ damage (CRAB criteria of multiple myeloma) [54].

Over the last years, 3 distinct clinical subtypes of MGUS have been recognized: non-IgM MGUS, IgM MGUS and light-chain MGUS [55;56]. The best characterized MGUS subtype is non-IgM MGUS. Paraprotein isotypes of non-IgM MGUS patients can be further categorized into IgG (69%), IgA (11%) and biclonal (3%) [57]. Furthermore, IgD and IgE consist just a small

	Diagnostic Purposes	Prognosis	Staging	Response Evaluation	Monitoring
			Total Ig		
MGUS	√	√		-	√
MM					
1. smoldering	√	-	√$^{D-S}$	-	√
2. LC	-	-	-	-	-
3. non-secretory	-	-	-	-	-
4. intact Ig MM	√	-	√$^{D-S}$	√	√
Solitary Bone Plasmacytoma	-	-	-	√*	-
AL Amyloidosis	-	-	-	√*	-
WM	√	-	√**	√	√
CLL	-	-	-	-	-
B-NHL	-	-	-	-	-
			sFLC/sFLCR		
MGUS	√	√	√	-	√
MM					
5. smalldering	√	√	-	-	√
6. LC	√	√	-	√	√
7. non-secretory	√***	√***	-	√***	√***
8. intact Ig MM	-	√	-	√	√
Solitary Bone Plasmacytoma	-	√***	-	-	-
AL Amyloidosis	√	√	√	√	√
WM	-	√	-	?	?
CLL	-	√	√$^{\perp}$	-	-
B-NHL	?	?	-	-	-
			HLC/HLCR		
MGUS	-	√	-	-	?
Intact Ig MM	-	√	-	√	√
WM	-	√	-	?	√
AL Amyloidosis	-	?	-	-	-

√:useful, -: not useful, ?: unknown, √$^{D-S}$: for Durie and Salmon Staging, *If present at diagnosis,** IgM level is included in the IPSS-WM, ***when abnormal sFLCR is observed, its evaluation is useful; $^{\perp}$included in recently proposed CLL staging [50].

Table 3. Contribution of Total Ig, sFLC/sFLCR and HLC/HLCR Measurements In Plasma Cell Dyscrasias and B-cell Lymphoproliferatiive Disorders.

portion of all non-IgM MGUS cases [51]. Malignant transformation of non-IgM MGUS approximates 1% per year and typically develops into multiple myeloma rather than lymphoproliferative disorders [57]. IgM MGUS accounts for about 17% of all MGUS cases. It tends to progress to Waldenstrom macroglobulinemia or other lymphomas [58]. Finally, light-chain MGUS is characterized by the absence of intact IgM protein and the presence of monoclonal FLC characterized by a skewed FLC ratio, due to the increased levels of the monoclonal FLC

[59]. This last type is not frequently identified because asymptomatic patients are rarely tested with FLC assays; light chain MGUS' frequency is estimated at about 20% of cases.

Based on available clinical markers, two major predictive risk models of MGUS progression have been established by the Mayo clinic and the Spanish study group [55]. The Mayo clinic model indentifies 3 major risk factors: abnormal sFLC ratio, presence of non-IgG monoclonal Ig and monoclonal protein ≥ 15 g/l [59]. At 20 years of follow-up, the absolute risk of progression for MGUS patients with 0, 1, 2, and 3 risk factors is 5%, 21%, 37% and 58% respectively [59]. The Spanish study group proposes multiparametric flow cytometry as a tool to indentify aberrant plasma cell populations [60]. In addition, a recent study [61] showed that suppression of uninvolved immunoglobulin in MGUS, as detected by suppression of the isotype-specific heavy and light chain (HLC-pair suppression), is an independent risk factor for progression to malignancy. Uninvolved Ig suppression, occurring several years before malignant transformation takes place, offers a new perspective in early detection or even prediction of MGUS progression.

Monoclonal Ig is also the central marker used for MGUS patients follow-up. Moreover, patients should be followed performing SPEP, Ig and FLC quantification, at a frequency that depends on their risk-group.

Finally, special attention should be given to associations between MGUS and numerous diseases that are commonly encountered in clinical practice, because these may be related to underlying mechanisms with relevance in disease pathogenesis. In a retrospective cohort study of more than 4 million individuals, elevated risks of MGUS and MM were associated with broad categories of autoimmune, infectious, and inflammatory disorders but not allergies [62]. Systemic lupus erythematosus (SLE), a multisystem autoimmune disease characterized by profound B cell hyperactivity, autoantibody formation, and hypergammaglobulinemia, has been associated with MGUS, although the latter is not clearly a manifestation of disease activity and its significance remains to be elucidated [63]. Two possible mechanisms have been proposed for the aforementioned correlation of the two nosological entities. The first hypothesis claims that B cell hyperactivity in SLE favours the escape of B cell clones from the normal regulatory mechanisms. An alternative hypothesis is that defective immunological surveillance, predisposing to malignancies in general, promotes the development of MM and/or its precursor state MGUS. Concerning rheumatoid arthritis (RA), several studies have indicated a direct correlation of the disease with MGUS presence. More specifically, 1.7% of patients with classical RA and high-titre rheumatoid factor present with MGUS [64].

3.5.2. *Multiple myeloma*

Multiple myeloma (MM) is an heterogeneous PCD with a wide range of clinical manifestations and outcomes, affecting terminally differentiated B-cells and characterized by bone marrow infiltration by monoclonal plasma cells secreting a monoclonal Ig. The disease might be asymptomatic, requiring only follow-up, or symptomatic and accompanied by fatigue, bone pains or spontaneous fractures, renal failure, recurrent infections or other morbid symptoms. In such cases treatment is immediately needed to prevent if possible irreversible organ damage. Paraprotein presence and amount are included into the diagnostic criteria [65-67]. The diagnostic criteria for smoldering (asymptomatic) multiple myeloma is a serum M protein level of ≥3g/dL, ≥10% BM plasma cells infiltration, and no related organ or tissue impairment (including bone lesions) or symptoms and the diagnostic criteria for symptomatic multiple myeloma is M protein (serum or urine) presence, BM plasma cell infiltration of ≥10% or histologically proven plasmacytoma, and myeloma-related organ or tissue impairment [68], further characterized by the CRAB criteria of multiple myeloma for end-organ damage, consisting of hypercalcemia (calcium level>11.5 mg/dL), renal failure (serum creatinine>2.0 mg/dL or estimated creatinine clearance <40 mL/min), anemia (hemoglobin level <10 g/dL or hemoglobulin level at least 2g/dL below the lower normal limit) and bone lesions (lytic lesions, severe osteopenia or pathologic fractures) [54]. sFLC measurements also are useful for diagnostic purposes, especially in light chain myeloma (LCM) and oligosecretory disease [69].

The evaluation of response to treatment is largely based on Ig decrease with complete response (CR) identified as negative IFE on both serum and urine, maintained for a minimum of 6 weeks [70]. In an attempt to improve response criteria, sFLCR was incorporated to the MM uniform response criteria [71] and its normalization along with immunohistological or immunophenotype confirmation of clonal disease absence, defined a deeper response, the stringent complete response (sCR). A better evaluation of the depth of response is important as the quality of response is correlated with treatment free and overall survival after treatment [72]. In the same way, relapse is established by an Ig increase on SPEP, total Ig quantification, sFLCs and more recently HLCs; all the aforementioned methods can therefore be used for disease monitoring [73]. An additional contribution of sFLC mesurements for disease monitoring during follow-up of patients is that light chain only relapses may be observed, with the improvement of treatment modalities resulting in prolonged survival. Disease transformation characterized by light chain escape may occur, characterized by a shift in secretion from intact Ig to LC only in a subset of patients [74;75] that could be otherwise considered in plateau.

With regard to prognosis, although serum monoclonal Ig quantification was one of Durie and Salmon staging system's risk factors [76] and was included in older prognostic algorithms [77], it was subsequently not shown to be linked with MM aggressiveness and was not retained as a prognostic risk parameter [78]. However, paraprotein type was shown to influence survival; IgG patients being most favourable, followed by IgA while light chain MM patients had the worst prognosis [79]. The introduction of the new Ig-based biomarkers (sFLC/HLC) rehabilitate monoclonal Igs prognostic potential in MM. Thus, sFLC and sFLCR were shown predictive of outcome in all MM subcategories. Patients with smoldering myeloma and abnormal sFLCR were shown to have an increased progression risk while an adverse outcome was observed in patients with overt MM and increased sFLCR [80;81]. In addition, the combination of sFLCR and other markers of disease activity (LDH, β2-microglobulin, genetic abnormalities) or the International Score System (ISS) for MM, were reported to produce powerful prognostic models [78;82], although this is yet to be proven in the ear of novel therapies [83]. Furthermore three groups showed simultaneously that HLC-IgG and –IgA ratios (HLCR) were predictive of a shorter overall survival [73;84] and progression-free survival [85].

3.5.3. AL amyloidosis

Systemic AL amyloidosis is characterised by the deposition of misfolded monoclonal light chains or their fragments in tissues or organs, leading to visceral dysfunction [86]. Symptomatology depends on the organ(s) involved and includes nephrotic syndrome, skin lesions, cardiomyopathy, demyelinating peripheral neuropathy, hepatomegaly, malabsorption syndrome, etc. Diagnosis is frequently difficult, in the (usual) absence of characteristic signs such as macroglossia or periorbital purpura. Physicians should be aware of the possible diagnosis of AL amyloidosis in patients with unexplained fatigue, and FLCR can aid in the differential diagnosis. In such a context sFLC measurements are useful and will be found increased in up to 94-98% of patients, even in the absence of any Ig monoclonal peak on serum electrophoresis or immunoelectrophoresis. However, diagnosis should be proven by involved tissue biopsy. Kidney is the most frequently involved organ while cardiac deposits are the most deleterious and related to shorter survival. AL amyloidosis may complicate MM or other PCD in less than 10% of cases.

sFLC levels concentrations at diagnosis are by themselves an adverse marker of survival in AL amyloidosis [88]. The addition of cardiac biomarkers to sFLC levels at diagnosis was shown highly predictive of patients survival [89] and a new prognostic staging system was built [90]; a score of 1 for each of three prognostic variables, namely cardiac troponin T (cTnT) (> 0.025 ng/mL, N-terminal pro–B-type natriuretic peptide (NT-ProBNP) (>1,800 pg/mL), and FLC difference (FLC-diff) (>18 mg/dL), was used to divide patients into four stages (I, II, III, and IV) with scores of 0, 1, 2, and 3, respectively. The 5-year survival estimates produced for patients in stage I, II, III, and IV were 59%, 42%, 20%, and 14% respectively ($p<0.001$).

Preliminary data on HLC measurements in AL amyloidosis appear promising. In a subset of AL amyloidosis patients with no detectable serum or urinary monoclonal bands and a normal sFLC ratio, the HLC ratio was abnormal in 19% of cases, identifying 2 IgAκ, 3 IgAλ, and 4 IgGκ clones [91].

3.5.4. Waldenstroms Macroglobulinemia

Waldenstroms Macroglobulinemia (WM) is a lymphoplasmacytic lymphoma (LPL) [22] characterized by lymphoplasmacytic infiltration of BM and eventually other organs, and by the presence of a serum IgM monoclonal component. IgM paraprotein is mandatory to establish the diagnosis. In case of a biology proven LPL without IgM, the disease will be called just LPL, not WM.

WM is a rare disease entity that presents a wide range of clinical signs and symptoms including those due to the lymphoma (lymph nodes' swelling, organomegaly, bone marrow failure) and those due to the presence of the IgM paraprotein. IgM-related symptoms are hyperviscosity, autoimmune phenomena (peripheral neuropathy, haemolytic anaemia, thrombocytopenic purpura), cryoglobulinaemia, amyloidosis. Asymptomatic patients do not require treatment and usually enjoy a prolonged survival, while patients with aggressive symptomatic disease should be immediately treated with chemotherapy [92;93]. Evaluation of response is based on changes in serum IgM concentrations and other factors. Complete response (CR) is characterized by the disappearance of symptoms, of monoclonal serum IgM (by IF), and of monoclonal lymphoplasmacytes from all infiltrated sites, partial response by a serum IgM decrease by 50% or more while progressive disease (PD) by IgM increase; likewise, relapse after response is characterized by IgM increase [94]. With regard to staging and prognosis, serum IgM levels were included into currently used international prognostic staging system for WM (IPSS-WM) that co-evaluated 5 parameters: age above 65 years, haemoglobin below 11,5 g/dL, platelet counts below or equal to 100×10^9/L, β2-microglobulin above 3mg/L and IgM above 7 g/dL [95].

There are so far only preliminary results on the contribution of the new Ig-based biomarkers (sFLC and HLC) levels in WM patients at diagnosis. It was shown that sFLC may be increased and, in such cases, correlate with markers of disease activity, such as increased β2M, anemia [96] and low serum albumin levels. Patients with elevated sFLC presented shorter time to treatment [97] and adverse outcome [98]. Increased HLC-IgM were also found correlated with markers of disease activity such as bone marrow infiltration of more than 50% and low serum albumin levels while high HLCR correlated with shorter time to treatment [98;99].

3.5.5. Chronic llymphocytic leukemia

Chronic lymphocytic leukemia (CLL) is the most common type of leukemia in the Western world and presents a large range of clinical manifestations and a variable outcome. More than two thirds of the patients are asymptomatic at the time of diagnosis and may not require treatment for months or even years. For prognostic purposes, traditional Rai and Binet clinical staging systems are still in use but they do not apply perfectly in modern years. For patients needing treatment, underlying molecular alterations are important predictors of response; however, for the majority of CLL patients, life expectancy largely depends on time to first treatment [100], so reliable markers for time to treatment are needed.

It was shown that increased sFLC is the most common paraprotein observed in CLL, being found in almost half of the cases and that sFLCR abnormalities are present in a significant proportion of patients and identify those at risk of progressive disease [101;102].

More recently, increased polyclonal sFLC were also found to constitute an adverse marker for time to first treatment in CLL [103]. This finding was confirmed by Morabito et al that evaluated the sum of κ and λ sFLC levels and found that the prognostic impact of sFLC (κ + λ) value above 60.6 mg/mL was superior compared to FLCR and built a model based on four variables, namely sFLC (κ + λ) more than 60.6 mg/mL, Binet staging, ZAP-70, and cytogenetics and separated 4 patients' groups with different time to treatment [50].

3.5.6. Other plasma cell dyscrasias & B-cell non Hodgkin's llymphomas

In the other PCD, Ig contribution to diagnosis, prognosis and monitoring is restricted to bone solitary plasmacytoma and mainly concerns sFLC quantification that was shown predictive of evolution to MM [104]. With regards to B-cell non Hodgkin's lymphomas, abnormal Ig secretion, as observed mostly by the new Ig-based biomarkers (sFLC and HLC) levels, the clinical significance of which remains for the time being, under investigation [105], although increasing evidence of sFLCs prognostic role are emerging in these diseases [106;107].

4. Conclusions

Paraprotein presence is the hallmark of monoclonality. Knowledge of biologic mechanisms that lead to monoclonality has allowed understanding of malignant B-cell origin and B-cell neoplasms pathophysiology. New methods for the precise detection and quantification of monoclonal Ig have opened interesting clinical applications concerning patients diagnosis, monitoring and prognostication.

Acknowledgements

We warmly thank Irini Rissakis for technical support and editing.

Author details

Marie-Christine Kyrtsonis[1*], Efstathios Koulieris[1], Vassiliki Bartzis[1], Ilias Pessah[1], Eftychia Nikolaou[1], Vassiliki Karalis[1], Dimitrios Maltezas[1], Panayiotis Panayiotidis[1] and Stephen J. Harding[2*]

*Address all correspondence to: mck@ath.forthnet.gr; Stephen.harding@bindingsite.co.uk

1 Haematology Section of 1st Department of Propaedeutic Internal Medicine, Athens Medical School, Athens, Greece

2 The Binding Site Group Ltd, Birmingham, UK

References

[1] Bird J, Behrens J, Westin J et al. UK Myeloma Forum (UKMF) and Nordic Myeloma Study Group (NMSG): guidelines for the investigation of newly detected M-proteins and the management of monoclonal gammopathy of undetermined significance (MGUS). Br J Haematol 2009;147(1) 22-42.

[2] Pangalis GA, Tzenou T, Kalpadakis C, et al. Biologic and clinical overlap of IgM-secreting lymphomas; focus on Waldenstrom's macroglobulinemia. Haematologica/The Hematology Journal 2007;92 (6, Suppl 2) 74-77.

[3] Nemazee DA, Burki K. Clonal deletion of B lymphocytes in a transgenic mouse bearing anti-MHC class I antibody genes. Nature 1989;337 562-566.

[4] Gay D, Saunders T, Camper S, Weigert M. Receptor editing: an approach by autoreactive B cells to escape tolerance. J.Exp.Med 1993;177 999-1008.

[5] Monroe JG, Dorshkind K. Fate decisions regulating bone marrow and peripheral B lymphocyte development. Adv.Immunol 2007;95 1-50.

[6] Sims GP, Enger R, Shirota Y, et al. Identification and characterization of circulating human transitional B cells. Blood 2005;105 4390-4398.

[7] Bende RJ. B-cell biology and the development of mature B cell lymphomas. PhD Thesis. Faculty of Medicine Amsterdam; 2010.

[8] Schettino EW, Chai SK, Kasaian MT, et al. VHDJH gene sequences and an_gen reactivity of monoclonal antibodies produced by human B-1 cells, evidence for somatic selection. J.Immunol 1997;158 2477-2489.

[9] Bikah G, Carey J, Ciallella JR, Tarakhovsky A, Bondada S. CD5-mediated negative regulation of antigenreceptor-induced growth signals in B-1 B-cells. Science 1996;274 1906-1909.

[10] Chen ZJ., Wheeler CL, Shi W, Wu AJ, Yarboro CH, Gallagher M, Notkins AL. Polyreactive antigen-binding B cells are the predominant cell type in the newborn B cell repertoire. Eur.J.Immunol 1998;28 989-994.

[11] Tsuiji M, Yurasov S, Velinzon K, et al. A checkpoint for autoreactivity in human IgM + memory B cell development. J.Exp.Med 2006;203 393-400.

[12] Berek C, Berger A, Apel M. Maturation of the immune response in germinal centers. Cell 1991;67(6) 1121-1129.

[13] Lindhout E, Koopman G, Pals ST, de Groot C. Triple check for antigen specificity of B cells during germinal centre reactions. Immunol.Today 1997;18 573-577.

[14] Liu YJ, Malisan F, de Bouteiller O, et al. Within germinal centers, isotype switching of immunoglobulin genes occurs after the onset of somatic mutation. Immunity 1996;4 241-250.

[15] Schwartz RS. Jumping genes and the immunoglobulin gene system. N Engl J Med 1995;333 42-44.

[16] Küppers R, Klein U, Hansmann ML, Rajewsky K. Cellular origin of human B-cell lymphomas. N Engl J Med 1999;341(20) 1520-1529.

[17] Muramatsu M, Kinoshita K, Fagarasan S, et al. Class switch recombination and hypermutation require activation-induced cytidine deaminase (AID), a potential RNA editing enzyme. Cell 2000;102 553-563.

[18] MacLennan ICM. Germinal centers. Annu.Rev.Immunol 1994;12 117-139.

[19] Liu Y-J, de Bouteiller O, Arpin C, et al. Normal human IgD+IgM- germinal center B cells can express up to 80 mutations in the variable region of their IgD transcripts. Immunity 1996;4 603-613.

[20] Seifert M, Steimle-Grauer SA, Goossens T, et al. A model for the development of human IgD-only B cells: Genotypic analyses suggest their generation in superantigen driven immune responses. Mol. Immunol 2009;46(4) 630-639.

[21] Tangye SG, Avery DT, Deenick EK, Hodgkin PD. Intrinsic differences in the proliferation of naive and memory human B cells as a mechanism for enhanced secondary immune responses. J.Immunol 2003;170 686-694.

[22] Swerdlow SH, Campo E, Harris NL, et al, editors. WHO classification of tumours of haematopoietic and lymphoid tissues. IARC Press, Geneva, Switzerland; 2008.

[23] Rajkumar SV, Kyle RA, Buadi FK. Advances in the diagnosis, classification, risk stratification and management of monoclonal gammopathy of undetermined significance: Implications for recategorizing disease entities in the presence of evolving scientific evidence. Mayo Clin Proc 2010;85(10) 945-948.

[24] Kyrtsonis M-C, Bartzis V, Papanikolaou X, et al. Genetic and Molecular Advances in Multiple Multiple Myeloma: A Route to Better Understand Disease Heterogeneity. The Application Of Clinical Genetics 2010;3 41-51.

[25] Bergsagel PL, Kuehl WM. Chromosome translocations in multiple myeloma. Oncogene 2001;20(40) 5611-5622.

[26] Bosch F, Jares P, Campo E, et al. PRAD1/cyclinD1 gene overexpression in chronic lymphoproliferative disorders: a high specific marker of mantle cell lymphoma. Blood 1994;84 2726-2732.

[27] Santra M, Zhan F, Tian E et al. A subset of multiple myeloma harbouring the t(4;14) (p16;q32) translocation lacks FGFR3 expression but maintains an IGH/MMSET fusion transcript. Blood 2003;101(6) 2374-2376.

[28] Walker BA, Wardell CP, Melchor L, et al. Intraclonal heterogeneity and distinct molecular mechanisms characterize the development of t(4;14) and t(11;14) myeloma. Blood 2012;120(5) 1077-86.

[29] Keats JJ, Chesi M, Egan JB, et al. Clonal competition with alternating dominance in multiple myeloma. Blood 2012;120(5) 1067-1076.

[30] Dang CV. c-Myc Target Genes Involved in Cell Growth, Apoptosis, and Metabolism. Mol Cell Biol 1999;19(1) 1-11.

[31] Guikema JE, de Boer C, Haralambieva E. IGH switch breakpoints in Burkitt lymphoma: exclusive involvement of non-canonical class switch recombination. Genes chromosomes Cancer 2006;45 808-819.

[32] Williams ME, Whitefield M, Swerdlow SH. Analysis of the cyclin-dependent kinase inhibitors p18 and p19 in the Mantle cell lymphoma and chronic lymphocytic leukemia. Ann Oncol 1997;8;Suppl 2 71-73.

[33] Fu K, Weisenburger DD, Greiner TC, et al. Cyclin D1–negative mantle cell lymphoma: a clinicopathologic study based on gene expression profiling. Blood 2005;106 4315-4321.

[34] Potter M. Pathogenetic mechanisms in B-cell non-Hodgkin's lymphomas in humans. Cancer Research 1992;52 5522-5528.

[35] Tomita N, Tokunaka M, Nakamura N, et al. Clinicopathological features of lymphoma/leukemia patients carrying both bcl2 and myc translocations. Haematologica 2009;94(7) 935-943.

[36] Iqbal J, Neppalli T, Wright G, et al. BCL2 expression is a prognostic marker for the activated B-cell-like type of diffuse large B-cell lymphoma. Journal of Clinical Oncology 2006;24(6) 961-968.

[37] Du M-Q. MALT Lymphoma: Recent Advances in Aetiology and Molecular Genetics. J Clin Exp Hematopathol 2007;47(2) 31-42.

[38] Attaelmannan M, Levinson SS. Understanding and Identifying Monoclonal Gammopathies. Clin Chem. 2000;46(8 Pt 2) 1230-1238.

[39] Matsuda F, Ishii K, Bourvagnet P, et al. The complete nucleotide sequence of the human immunoglobulin heavy chain variable region locus. J Exp Med 1998;188 2151-2162.

[40] Janeway C. Immunobiology, 5th edition. The Immune System in Health and Disease. Garland Publishing, New York, USA; 2001

[41] Litman GW, Rast JP, Shamblott MJ, Haire RN, Hulst M, Roess W et al. Phylogenetic diversification of immunoglobulin genes and the antibody repertoire. Mol. Biol. Evol 1993;10(1) 60–72.

[42] Ravetch J, Bolland S. IgG Fc receptors. Annu Rev Immunol 2001;19(1) 275–290.

[43] Pier GB, Lyczak JB, Wetzler LM. Immunology, Infection and Immunity. ASM Press, Washington DC, USA; 2004

[44] Rus H, Cudrici C, Niculescu F. The role of the complement system in innate immunity. Immunol Res 2005;33(2) 103–112.

[45] Merlini G, Stone MJ. Dangerous small B-cell clones. Blood 2006;108 2520.

[46] Harding SJ, Mead GP, Bradwell AR, Berard AM. Serum free light chain immunoassay as an adjunct to serum protein electrophoresis and immunofixation electrophoresis in the detection of multiple myeloma and other B-cell malignancies. Clin Chem Lab Med 2009;47(3) 302-304 doi:10.1515/CCLM.2009.084

[47] Keren DF. Heavy/Light-Chain Analysis of monoclonal gammopathies. Clin Chem 2009;55 1606–1608.

[48] Bradwell AR. Serum free light chain analysis (plus Hevylite). 5th ed. 2008.

[49] Bradwell AR, Carr-Smith HD, Mead GP, et al. Highly sensitive, automated immune-assay for immunoglobulin free light chains in serum and urine. Clin Chem 2001;47: 4 673-80.

[50] Morabito F, De Filippi R, Laurenti L, et al. The cumulative amount of serum-free light chain is a strong prognosticator in chronic lymphocytic leukemia. Blood 2011;118(24) 6353-6361 doi:10.1182/blood-2011-04-345587

[51] Kyle RA, Therneau TM, Rajkumar SV et al. Prevalence of monoclonal gammopathy of undetermined significance. N Eng J Med 2006;354(13) 1362-1369.

[52] Waldenstrom J. Studies on conditions associated with disturbed gamma globulin formation (gammopathies). Harvey Lect 1960;56 211–231.

[53] Kyle RA. Monoclonal gammopathy of undetermined significance: natural history in 241 cases. Am J Med 1978;64(5) 814–826.

[54] Kyle RA, Durie BG, Rajkumar SV, et al; International Myeloma Working Group. Monoclonal gammopathy of undetermined significance (MGUS) and smoldering (asymptomatic) multiple myeloma: IMWG consensus perspectives risk factors for progression and guidelines for monitoring and management. Leukemia 2010;24(6) 1121-1127. doi:10.1038/leu.2010.60

[55] Korde N, Kristinsson SY, Landgren O. Monoclonal gammopathy of undetermined significance (MGUS) and smoldering multiple myeloma (SMM): novel biological insights and development of early treatment strategies. Blood 2011;117(21) 5573–5581.

[56] Kyle RA, Therneau TM, Rajkumar SV et al. A long-term study of prognosis in monoclonal gammopathy of undetermined significance. N Engl J Med 2002;346(8) 564–569.

[57] Kyle RA, Therneau TM, Rajkumar SV et al. Long-term follow-up of IgM monoclonal gammopathy of undetermined significance. Semin Oncol 2003;30(2) 169–171.

[58] Dispenzieri A, Katzmann JA, Kyle RA et al. Prevalence and risk of progression of light-chain monoclonal gammopathy of undetermined significance: a retrospective population-based cohort study. Lancet 2010;375(9727) 1721–1728.

[59] Rajkumar SV, Kyle RA, Therneau TM et al. Serum free light chain ratio is an independent risk factor for progression in monoclonal gammopathy of undetermined significance. Blood 2005;106(3) 812–817.

[60] Perez-Persona E. Vidriales MB, Mateo G et al. New criteria to identify risk of progression in monoclonal gammopathy of uncertain significance and smoldering multiple myeloma based on multiparameter flow cytometry analysis of bone marrow plasma cells. Blood 2007;110(7) 2586–2592.

[61] Katzmann JA, Clark R, Kyle RA et al. Suppression of uninvolved immunoglobulins defined by heavy/light chain pair suppression is a risk factor for progression of MGUS. Leukemia 2012. doi:10.1038/leu.2012.189

[62] Brown LM, Gridley G, Check D, Landgren O. Risk of multiple myeloma and monoclonal gammopathy of undetermined significance among white and black male United States veterans with prior autoimmune, infectious, inflammatory, and allergic disorders. Blood 2008;111(7) 3388-3394.

[63] Rubin L, Urowitz MB, Pruzanski W. Systemic lupus erythematosus with paraproteinemia. Arthritis Rheum. 1984;27(6) 638-644.

[64] Garton MJ, Keir G, Dickie A, Steven M, Rennie JA. Prevalence and long-term significance of paraproteinaemia in rheumatoid arthritis. Rheumatology 2006;45(3) 355-356.

[65] Durie BG. Staging and kinetics of multiple myeloma. Semin Oncol. 1986;13(3) 300-309.

[66] Nau K, Lewis W. Multiple Myeloma: Diagnosis and Treatment. Am Fam Physician 2008;78 853-859.

[67] Rajkumar SV, Kyle RA. Multiple myeloma: diagnosis and treatment. Mayo Clin Proc 2005;80(10) 1371–1382.

[68] International Myeloma Working Group. Criteria for the classification of monoclonal gammopathies, multiple myeloma and related disorders: a report of the International Myeloma Working Group. Br J Haematol 2003;121(5) 749–757.

[69] Drayson M, Tang LX, Drew R, Mead GP, Carr-Smith H, Bradwell AR. Serum free light-chain measurements for identifying and monitoring patients with nonsecretory multiple myeloma. Blood 2001;97(9) 2900-2902. doi:10.1182/blood.V97.9.2900

[70] Blade J, Samson D, Reece D, et al. Criteria for evaluating disease response and progression in patients with multiple myeloma treated by high-dose therapy and hemopoietic stem cell transplantation. Myeloma Subcommittee of the EBMT. European Group for Blood and Marrow Transplant. Br J Haematol 1998;102(5) 1115–1123. doi: 10.1046/j.1365-2141.1998.00930

[71] Durie BG, Harousseau JL, Miguel JS, et al. International Myeloma Working Group. International uniform response criteria for multiple myeloma. Leukemia 2006;20(9) 1467-1473.

[72] Gay F, Larocca A, Wijermans P, et al. Complete response correlates with long-term progression-free and overall survival in elderly myeloma treated with novel agents: analysis of 1175 patients. Blood 2010;117 3025-3031.

[73] Ludwig H, Milosavljevic D, Zojer N, edt al. Immunoglobulin heavy/light chain ratios improve paraprotein detection and monitoring, identify residual disease and correlate with survival in multiple myeloma patients. Leukemia 2012 ;27 : 213-219.

[74] Koulieris E, Bartzis V, Tzenou T, Kafasi N, Efthymiou A, Mpitsanis C et al. Free light chain clonal escape reflects relapse in intact immunoglobulin multiple myeloma. Haematologica 2011;96(s1) P-414

[75] Kühnemund A, Liebisch P, Bauchmüller K, et al. 'Light-chain escape-multiple myeloma'-an escape phenomenon from plateau phase: report of the largest patient series using LC-monitoring. J Cancer Res Clin Oncol. 2009;135(3) 477-84.

[76] Durie BG, & Salmon SE. A clinical staging system for multiple myeloma. Correlation of measured myeloma cell mass with presenting clinical features, response to treatment, and survival. Cancer 1975;36(3) 842–854.

[77] Kyrtsonis M-C, Maltezas D, Koulieris E, et al. The Contribution of Prognostic Factors to the Better Management of Multiple Myeloma Patients. Book Chapter In "Multiple Myeloma". InTech - Open Access Publisher 2012.

[78] Kyrtsonis M-C, Maltezas D, Tzenou T, Koulieris E, & Bradwell AR. Staging Systems and Prognostic factors as a Guide to Therapeutic Decisions in Multiple Myeloma. Semin Hematol; 2009;46(2) 110–117.

[79] Drayson M, Begum G, Basu S, et al. Effects of paraprotein heavy and light chain type and free light chain load on survival in myeloma: An analysis of patients receiving conventional dose chemotherapy in Medical Research Council UK Multiple Myeloma trials. Blood 2006;108(6) 2013-2019.

[80] Kyrtsonis M-C, Vassilakopoulos TP, Kafasi N, et al. Prognostic value of serum free light chain ratio at diagnosis in multiple myeloma. Br J of Haematol 2007;137(3), 240-243.

[81] Snozek CL, Katzmann JA, Kyle RA, et al. Prognostic value of the serum free light chain ratio in newly diagnosed myeloma: proposed incorporation into the international staging system. Leukemia. 2008;22(10) 1933-1937.

[82] Kumar S, Zhang L, Dispenzieri A, et al. Relationship between elevated immunoglobulin free light chain and the presence of IgH translocations in multiple myeloma. Leukemia 2010;24(8) 1498-1505.

[83] Maltezas D, Dimopoulos MA, Katodritou I, et al. Re-evaluation of prognostic markers including staging, serum free light chains or their ratio and serum lactate dehydrogenase in multiple myeloma patients receiving novel agents. Hematol Oncol 2012

[84] Koulieris E, Panayiotidis P, Harding SJ, et al. Ratio of involved/uninvolved immunoglobulin quantification by Hevylite™ assay: Clinical and prognostic impact in multiple myeloma. Experimental Hematology & Oncology 2012;1(9)

[85] Bradwell A, Harding S, Fourrier N, et al. Prognostic utility of intact immunoglobulin Ig'κ/Ig'λ ratios in multiple myeloma patients. Leukemia 2012;27 :202-7

[86] Dingli D, Kyle RA, Rajkumar SV et al. Immunoglobulin free light chains and solitary plasmacytoma of bone. Blood 2006;108(6) 1979-1983

[87] Lachmann HJ, Gallimore R, Gillmore JD, Carr-Smith HD, Bradwell AR, Pepys MB, Hawkins PN. Outcome in systemic AL amyloidosis in relation to changes in concentration of circulating free immunoglobulin light chains following chemotherapy. Br J Haematol 2003;122 78-84 doi:10.1046/j.1365-2141.2003.04433.x

[88] Dispenzieri A, Lacy MQ, Katzmann JA, et al. Absolute values of immunoglobulin free light chains are prognostic in patients with primary systemic amyloidosis undergoing peripheral blood stem cell transplantation. Blood 2006;107 3378-3383.

[89] Palladini G, Foli A, Milani P, et al. Best use of cardiac biomarkers in patients with AL amyloidosis and renal failure. Am J Hematol 2012;87(5) 465-471 doi: 10.1002/ajh.23141

[90] Kumar S, Dispenzieri A, Lacy MQ, et al. Revised prognostic staging system for light chain amyloidosis incorporating cardiac biomarkers and serum free light chain measurements. J Clin Oncol 2012;30(9) 989-995. doi:10.1200/JCO.2011.38.5724

[91] Wechalekar AD, Harding S, Lachmann HJ, et al. Serum immunoglobulin heavy/light chain ratios (Hevylite) in patients with systemic AL amyloidosis. Amyloid 2010;17 186a.

[92] Kyrtsonis M-C, Vassilakopoulos TP, Angelopoulou et al. Waldenstrom's macroglobulinemia: Clinical course and prognostic factors in 60 patients. Experience From a Single Haematology Unit. Annals of Haematology 2001;80 722-727.

[93] Pangalis GA, Kyrtsonis M-C, Kontopidou FN, et al. Differential Diagnosis Of Waldenstrom's Macroglobulinemia And Other B-Cell Disorders. Clin Lymphoma 2005;5 235-240.

[94] Weber D, Treon SP, Emmanuilides C, et al. Uniform response criteria in Waldenstrom's macroglobulinemia: Consensus Panel Recommendations from the Second International Workshop on Waldenstrom's Macroglobulinemia. Seminars in Oncology 2003;30 127-131.

[95] Morel P, Duhamel A, Gobbi P et al. International prognostic scoring system for Waldenström macroglobulinemia. Blood 2009;113 4163–4170.

[96] Leleu X, Koulieris E, Maltezas D. et al. Novel M-component based biomarkers in Waldenstrom Macroglobulinemia (WM). Clin Lymphoma Myeloma Leukemia 2011;11 164-167.

[97] Itzykson R, Le Garff-Tavernier M, Katsahian S, Diemert MC, Musset L, Leblond V. Serum-free light chain elevation is associated with a shorter time to treatment in Waldenstrom's macroglobulinemia. Haematologica 2008;93 793-794

[98] Maltezas D, Tzenou T, Kafassi N, et al. Clinical Impact of Increased Serum Free Light Chains (sFLCs) or Their Ratio (FLCR) on WM at Diagnosis and During Disease

Course. Sixth International Workshop On Waldenstrom's Macroglobulinemia. 2010, October 6-10, Venice, Italy

[99] Koulieris E, Kyrtsonis M-C, Maltezas D, et al. Quantification of serum IgM kappa and IgM lambda in Patients with Waldenstrom's Macroglobulinemia. Hematology Reports 2010;2: F63a.

[100] Hallek M, Cheson BD, Catovsky D, et al. Guidelines for the diagnosis and treatment of chronic lymphocytic leukemia: a report from the International Workshop on Chronic Lymphocytic Leukemia updating the National Cancer Institute-Working Group 1996 guidelines. Blood 2008;111(12) 5446-5456

[101] Pratt G, Harding S, Holder Ret al. Abnormal serum free light chain ratios are associated with poor survival and may reflect biological subgroups in patients with chronic lymphocytic leukaemia. Br J Haematol 2009;144(2) 217-22

[102] Yegin ZA, Ozkurt ZN, Yağci M. Free light chain: a novel predictor of adverse outcome in chronic lymphocytic leukemia. Eur J Haematol 2010;84(5) 406-411 doi: 10.1111/j.1600-0609.2010.01412.x

[103] Maurer MJ, Cerhan JR, Katzmann JA, et al. Monoclonal and polyclonal serum free light chains and clinical outcome in chronic lymphocytic leukemia. Blood 2011;118(10) 2821-2826.

[104] Leleu X, Moreau AS, Hennache B, et al. Serum Free Light Chain Immunoassays Measurements for Monitoring Solitary Bone Plasmacytoma. Haematologica 2005; 90(1): 110

[105] Charafeddine KM, Jabbour MN, Kadi RH, Daher RT. Extended use of serum free light chain as a biomarker in lymphoproliferative disorders: a comprehensive review. Am J Clin Pathol 2012;137 890-897.

[106] Landgren O, Goedert JJ, Rabkin CS, et al. Circulating serum free light chains as predictive markers of AIDS-related lymphoma. J Clin Oncol 2010;28(5) 773-779

[107] Maurer MJ, Micallef IN, Cerhan JR, et al. Elevated serum free light chains are associated with event-free and overall survival in two independent cohorts of patients with diffuse large B-cell lymphoma. J Clin Oncol 2011;29

Chapter 3

Innovative Models to Assess Multiple Myeloma Biology and the Impact of Drugs

Marina Ferrarini, Giovanna Mazzoleni,
Nathalie Steimberg, Daniela Belloni and
Elisabetta Ferrero

Additional information is available at the end of the chapter

http://dx.doi.org/10.5772/54312

1. Introduction

Tumor and its embedding microenvironment form a unique, dynamic system, largely orchestrated by cellular players, including fibroblasts and endothelial cells (EC), and surrounding extracellular matrix (ECM) with its distinctive physical, biochemical, and biomechanical properties. There is a general consensus that, beyond genetic mutations and epigenetic modifications, the dialogue that occurs between tumor and its microenvironment, through soluble factors and molecular interactions, may affect tumor cells survival, growth, proliferation, response to chemical/physical factors, and lies the basis for metastatization to distant, specific organs. This theory was proposed by Paget in the 1880s [1], who underlined the need, for investigating and targeting tumor, to focus not only on the cancer cell, "the seed", but also on the "soil" where tumor homes and in which it derives its nutrients, oxygen and signals [2, 3]. Accordingly, tight links between tumor and surrounding microenvironment could determine the overall sensitivity to anti-cancer drugs and therefore represent an attractive therapeutic target [4].

Tumor microenvironment plays a critical role also in development and progression of haematological malignancies [5,6]. In this regard, Multiple Myeloma (MM) represents a paradigmatic condition [5,6]. Indeed, MM plasma cells almost exclusively home and thrive inside Bone Marrow (BM) microenvironment, which confers anti-apoptotic and pro-survival signals and resistance to drugs. In turn, tumor cell interactions with BM cells and matrix result in re-shaping of microenvironment, and architectural changes involve in particular the vascular compartment [7].

The establishment of tight links between MM plasma cells and their microenvironment underlines the need for appropriate models for studying MM biology and predicting the impact of drugs.

In the present paper, we briefly summarize the role of BM microenvironment and, particularly, of MM associated angiogenesis, in MM pathogenesis, progression and prognosis. We then provide an overview of the currently available MM models, including animal models and a new three-dimensional (3D), gel-based, *in vitro* model of human MM microenvironment. Finally, we discuss the potential of RCCS™ bioreactor-based, dynamic 3D model systems (cell and tissue culture) to investigate critical aspects of human MM pathobiology and possible clinical applications. Advantages and limitations of each model, relative to MM investigation and assessment of drug sensitivity, are also considered.

2. Role of BM microenvironment and angiogenesis in MM progression and prognosis

MM is a B-cell tumor, characterized by clonal proliferation of malignant plasma cells inside the BM, production of a monoclonal paraprotein, and associated clinical features, including lytic bone lesions, renal insufficiency, hypercalcemia and anemia. It accounts for approximately 1% of neoplastic diseases and 13% of hematologic cancers. Albeit significant advances have been recently achieved in the treatment of MM, the disease still remains incurable, prompting the development of new therapeutic strategies [8].

MM is thought to evolve from a pre-malignant syndrome known as Monoclonal Gammopathy of Uncertain Significance (MGUS), that progresses to smoldering (asymptomatic) myeloma and, finally, to symptomatic myeloma. In addition to genetic abnormalities accumulating in MM cells, BM microenvironment actively participates to the pathogenesis and progression of the disease. Indeed, host stromal components profoundly influence many steps of tumor progression, such as tumor proliferation, invasion, angiogenesis, metastasis, and even malignant transformation [9]. The BM, where MM cells specifically home, provides a highly specialized microenvironment, which optimally "soils" neoplastic plasma cells, and, in turn, is shaped by the interactions with MM cells [5,6,10].

BM microenvironment consists of a series of cellular components, including hematopoietic cells, immune cells, BM stromal cells (BMSC), osteoclasts, osteoblasts and endothelial cells (EC), all embedded in an extracellular matrix (ECM) (Fig.1).

MM cells specifically localize inside the BM milieu through the CXCR4/CXCL12-SDF1-alpha axis [11] and then interact with ECM and BM cellular components by means of adhesion molecules, including integrins. The complex interplay between MM cells and BM milieu, together with the ensuing pathogenetic events, are depicted in Fig. 2 (upper panel).

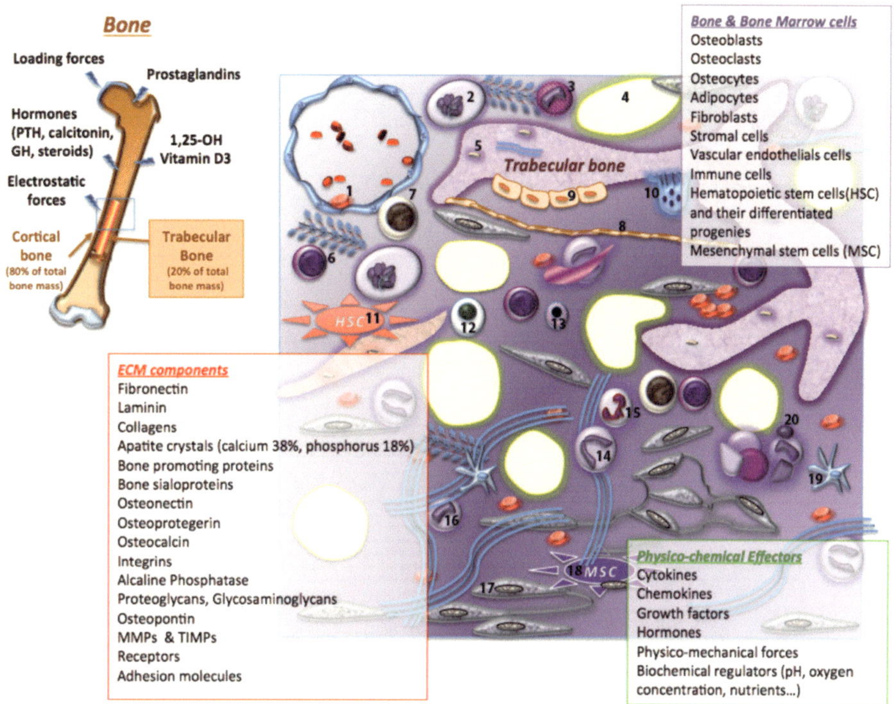

1: erythrocytes; 2: megacaryocytes; 3: basophils; 4: adipocytes; 5: osteocytes; 6: B lymphocytes; 7: monocytes; 8: lining osteoblasts; 9: osteoblasts; 10: osteoclasts; 11: hematopoietic stem cells "niche"; 12: T lymphocytes; 13: NK cells; 14: eosinophils; 15: neutrophils; 16: monocytes; 17: stromal cells; 18: mesenchymal stem cells "niche"; 19: dendritic cells; 20: thrombocytes (platelets).

Figure 1. Bone Marrow microenvironment. Bone homeostasis is the result of a complex network of stimuli, including hormones, vitamins and physico-mechanical forces. In addition to osteoblats and osteoclasts, which are responsible for bone deposition/resorption, BM microenvironment encompasses several cell types, like hematopoietic cells, endothelial cells and mesenchimal cells, all embedded in a complex extra-cellular-matrix (ECM).

Interactions between MM cells and ECM and cellular components (Fig. 2, lower panel) trigger the release of soluble factors, which, in turn, determine autocrine/paracrine loops of MM survival/proliferation and also promote osteoclastogenesis, defective immune functions and the "angiogenic switch", overall leading to MM cells growth, survival, and resistance to chemotherapeutic agents [10]. In particular, adhesion of MM cells to BMSC and to ECM components triggers anti-apoptotic signals and also the release of the pro-survival factor Interleukin (IL)-6. Moreover, MM plasma cells and BM stroma release osteoclast-acivating factors, including IL-1, IL-6, tumor necrosis factor (TNF)-α, RANK-L(Ligand) and Macrophage Inflammatory Protein (MIP)-1α. MM cells have also a unique ability to evade immune surveillance through several mechanisms, including impairment of cytotoxic activity and induction of dendritic cells dysfunction (Fig. 2).

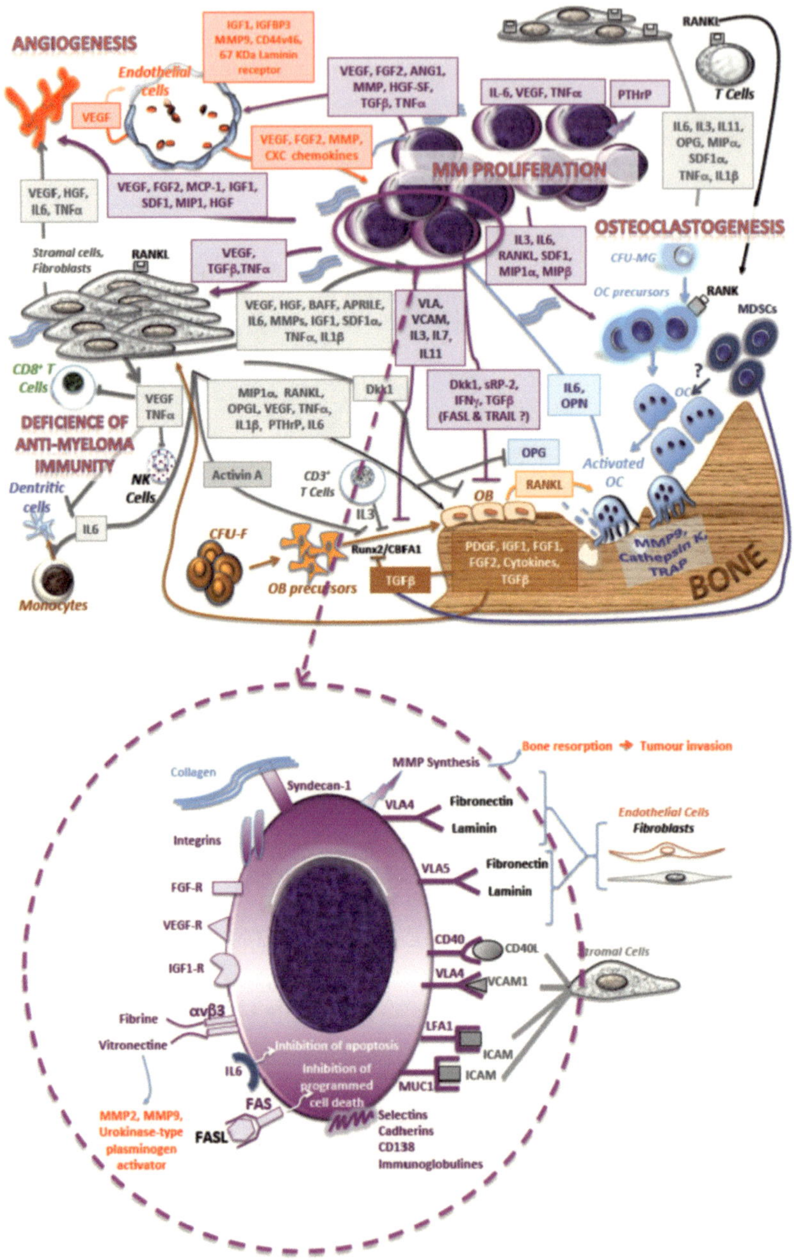

Figure 2. Interactions between MM cellsand BM microenviroment. Upper panel: schematic representation of MM cells inside BM microenvironment; the soluble factors involved in the major pathogenetic events, including tumor proliferation/survival, angiogenesis, osteoclastogenesis and defective immune function are depicted. Lower panel illustrates the major growth factor receptors and adhesion molecules used by MM plasma cells to interact with ECM and cellular components of BM microenvironment

Angiogenesis, the sprouting of capillaries from existing blood-vessels, is a complex, dynamic and tightly regulated process, that occurs physiologically during normal growth, wound repair after injury and regeneration [12,13]. Angiogenesis is controlled by the balance between positive and negative regulators. In a tumor microenvironment, the exaggerate expression of pro-angiogenic cyto-chemokines starts the ''angiogenic switch'', leading to increased micro vessel density (MVD) [14]. The occurrence of an "angiogenic switch", responsible for the transition from the avascular "dormant" phase to the vascular phase of exponential tumor growth [15,16], has also been proposed for MM. Pro- and anti-angiogenic soluble molecules are produced and released by myeloma cells and components of microenvironment, including MMEC, stromal cells and inflammatory cells [17-19] (Fig.2 A, upper panel). Major angiogenic cytokines are VEGF-A, fibroblast growth factor (FGF) and hepatocyte growth factor (HGF). Both EC in general, and in particular MMEC, and MM cells secrete VEGF and express its receptors, thereby contributing to autocrine/paracrine pathways of tumor growth, survival and angiogenesis [19]. Finally, Angiopoietins (Angs, Ang-1 and-2) are important mediators in vasculature homeostasis and their circulating levels are considered of prognostic significance in MM [20].

Overall, BM angiogenesis in MM contributes to disease progression; accordingly, new anti-myeloma agents target not only MM cells, but also the microenvironment, and in particular vessels [21]. This notion is exemplified by the proteasome inhibitor Bortezomib (PS-341, Velcade), which has been approved for treatment of patients with relapsed and refractory MM and more recently used in front-line therapy for the disease. *In vitro*, proteasome inhibition by bortezomib causes apoptosis in both solid tumor and haematological malignancies, particularly MM [22]. More recently, Bortezomib has also been reported to affect viability of angiogenic EC, as shown in *in vitro* experimental conditions as well in animal models [23,24]. Notably, neither reliable biomarkers measurable *in vivo* nor *ex vivo* models of human BM microenvironment are currently available to assess the anti-angiogenic effect of drugs in MM patients.

3. Advantages of models which mimic tumor microenvironment exploiting the third dimension

Since BM microenvironment is of most importance in supporting myeloma cell growth and survival, experimental models of MM should provide insights into the mechanisms that, at molecular level, regulate the complex interplay between MM cells and biochemical and physical cues coming from BM ECM and cell components.

Traditional two-dimensional (2D) *in vitro* models (static culture of single cells kept as monolayer on flat, artificial surfaces) still represent the most popular models for *in vitro* studies, even if they present severe limitations, being unable to reproduce the behaviour and physiological responses of various normal and pathological cell types/tissues. It is now generally accepted that any attempt aimed at the generation of reliable and physiologically relevant *in vitro* tissue analogues, tumors included, should take into account the need of reproducing (or preserving) the specific characteristics of their original microenvironment, which include, in addition to tissue-specific multiple cellularity, biochemical and mechanical properties, also the three-dimensionality [25,26]. Since the pioneering studies of Bissell and colleagues [27], different groups, including ours, have demonstrated that significant differences exist between the biological behaviour and gene expression profiles of normal and transformed/tumor-derived cells maintained in culture with traditional (2D) culture methods, and that of cells kept in 3D culture (see, for example, 28-31), proving that 3D models can mimic *in vivo* conditions better than 2D systems [26,32,33].

Table 1 illustrates the principal characteristics of 3D *versus* conventional 2D *in vitro* models of differentiated and tumoral tissues, and their relevance to the *in vivo* situation.

Characteristics of the *in vitro* models	**2D conformation (on flat glass or plastic substrates)**	**3D conformation (cell spheroids, 3D artificial supports)**	**References**
In vitro models of differentiated tissues			
Architecture	Monolayer Lack of 3D physical cues	Multilayer Nano- and micro-topographies are recreated	34-37
Cell-milieu interaction	Unidirectional, passive fluid diffusion Lack of chemical gradients and reduced gas supply high ECM stiffness (more than 1 GPa)	Pluri-directional active fluid diffusion Gradients of nutrient and gas can be generated Efficient waste removal in dynamic bioreactors ECM stiffness lower than in 2D (variable from 1 to 100 kPa)	26, 38-41
Cell-cell interactions	Reduced interactions between neighbouring cells	Increased interactions between neighbouring cells	25
Cell morphology/ viability	Flat: geometrically-constrained baso-apical polarity Limited spatial distribution of adhesions to ECM Limited cell survival rate	Spheroid: free cell polarity guided by ECM Whole cell surface distribution of adhesions to ECM High cell survival rate	3142-44
Ability to mimic the physiological behaviour of cells in vivo	Lack the major physiological cues (biochemical, chemical, physical, mechanical) of the original tissue Low cell differentiation state and function	3D models are closer to the *in vivo* condition and number of *in vivo* cell/tissue features can be reproduced High differentiation state and functional competence ECM characteristics may vary, according to the culture model,	41, 45,46, 47

Characteristics of the *in vitro* models	2D conformation (on flat glass or plastic substrates)	3D conformation (cell spheroids, 3D artificial supports)	References
	Absent or abnormal neo-synthesized ECM (qualitatively and quantitatively)	from synthetic, natural and de-cellularized ECM, but 3D models are closer to the physiological context	
In vitro models of tumor tissues			
ECM-related cell motility and mechanobiology, compared to the in vivo situation	-	++	48 49
Cell organization	Organized	Disruption of tissue organization, as in *in vivo* tumours	50
Gene expression	Higher growth-/ metabolic-related gene expression Activation of mitochondrial and ribosomal gene clusters Gene expression is, generally, quite different from *in vivo* tumours	Growth-arrest related genes are activated Closer to tumour tissue *in vivo*	51-53
Capability to reproduce specific morphological and behavioural characteristics of in vivo malignant cells	+/-	++	54,55
Responsiveness to surviving signal from ECM	+	++	55
Drug resistance (sensitivity)	Low (high)	High (low)	56-58
Capability to reproduce the complexity of tumour microenvironment	-	+/ +++	56 59,60

Table 1.

In an effort to reproduce *in vitro* the 3D specific microenvironment of the parental tissue, taking advantage of the rapid development of new technologies and tissue engineering techniques, an extremely wide variety of tissue models have been produced. The latter have already been successfully applied for investigating critical aspects of *in vivo* behaviour of a number of normal and tumoral cells (reviewed and discussed in 26). On this basis, 3D culture systems have been proposed as the most physiologically relevant *in vitro* models to investigate tumor development and behaviour [60-62]. Recently, this experimental approach has been also exploited for the study of MM-cell biology and sensitivity to therapeutic agents [63].

Within this context, 3D *in vitro* (cell-based)/*ex-vivo* (tissue-based) human-derived culture systems represent important tools to generate new approaches to the understanding of the molecular mechanisms of MM progression, essential prerequisites for the development of more effective interventional, diagnostic and prognostic strategies.

4. Murine models of MM

4.1. Subcutaneous xenograft models

The simplest way to generate an animal model of cancer consists in the injection of tumor cells into an immune-deficient mouse. This approach, known as the xenograft model, has been extensively employed for solid tumors [64,65] and then extended to MM. The xenograft model of MM consists in the subcutaneous injection of 1-2 x 10^7 human myeloma cells (from RPMI-8226, U266, ARH-77 or OPM-2 cell lines) into the flanks of Severe Combined Immune-Deficient (SCID), nonobese diabetic (NOD), SCID/NOD and SCID/beige, mice [66,67] (Fig.3A). The resulting plasmacytoma is palpable, and tumor burden measurable with a pair of caliper or, when lines are transduced with the eGFP-luc fusion gene, by bioluminescence imaging [68]. After harvesting, tumor mass is suitable for histological examination, allowing identification of vasculature and determination of cell proliferation/apoptosis. The model is currently used to assess the activity of new drugs on MM tumor growth and to establish the effective, minimally toxic, dose. As an example, this model has been employed to investigate the *in vivo* anti-myeloma effect induced by the mTOR inhibitor CCI-779 [69]. More recently, the efficacy of new inhibitors of the CXCR4/CXCL12 axis (AMD3100 and BKT140) [70], and of stressors of the endoplasmic reticulum (spicamycin analogue, KRN5500) [71], which inflict death of MM cells, have been demonstrated using the xenograft model. Besides mono-therapies, the model is suitable to evaluate the maximal effect, in terms of tumor volume reduction, obtainable with combined molecules [72].

While the xenograft model is extremely practical, particularly for drug testing, it still suffers from several limitations. In fact, it does not accurately mimic human disease, since myeloma cell lines do not behave as primary myeloma cells, more closely resembling the aggressive stage of plasma cell leukemia. More importantly, it fails to recapitulate the reciprocal interactions between MM cells and their microenvironment, which follow MM cell localization and retention inside the BM. As a result, drug efficacy can be over-estimated, lacking implanted MM cells the specific, proper human context of ECM and non-malignant accessory cells.

Murine models of MM, including the 5TMM model, contribute to overcome this latter limitation.

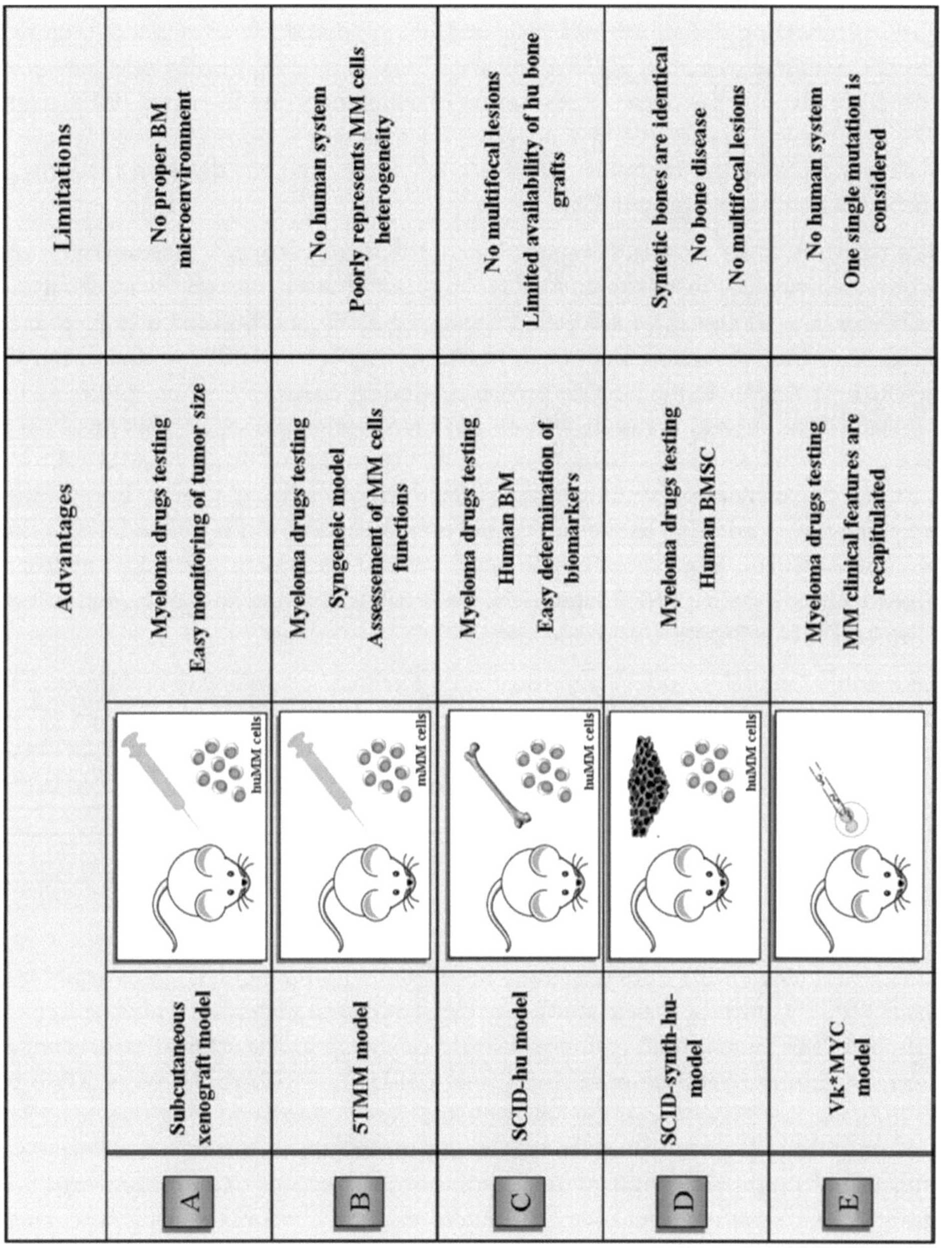

Figure 3. Schematic representation of currently available MM animal models. The major murine (m) and murine-human(hu) models together with their main advantages and limitations are depicted. Synth = synthetic polymeric scaffold; BMSC= Bone Marrow Stromal Cells; SCID=severe combined immune deficient.

4.2. 5TMM models

The 5T model has been developed in the late seventies upon injection of mice with syngeneic murine MM cells, spontaneously arising in elderly C57BL/KaLwRij mice [73,74]. The group of MM murine models collectively indicated as 5TMM mice comprises different types of mice, each bearing different tumor cells and having distinct characteristics (Figure 3B). The most commonly used, the 5T2MM and the 5T33MM models, display selective localization of cells in the BM, the presence of a serum M component and increased BM angiogenesis. The first one is characterized by moderate growth and development of osteolytic lesions more closely reproducing the human disease, while the second one displays a more aggressive behaviour with rapid growth [75].

Studies based on these models, substantially contributed by Karin Vanderkerken's group, have provided valuable insights into MM biology, and in particular on the mechanisms responsible for bone disease, MM-associated neoangiogenesis, and MM cell homing to the BM [75]. Indeed, taking advantage from these models, it has been possible to dissect the single steps which participate to the homing process, including chemo-attraction, adhesion, trans-endothelial migration and invasion, and also to identify the molecular pairs involved [75]. Moreover, these models allow the assessment of the impact of drugs on MM cells inside their proper microenvironment. In particular, the 5T2MM model allowed to unravel the anti-tumor activity, in addition to prevention of bone resorption, of the amino-biphosphonate zolendronic acid [76]. More recently, the novel 'second-generation' pyrimidyl-hydroxamic acid-based histone deacetylase inhibitor JNJ-26481585 was found to reduce tumor burden and also to affect angiogenesis and osteolysis [77].

A major limitation of the model is represented by the limited availability of different 5T cell lines, which fails to recapitulate the high variability both in terms of genetics and of tumor behaviour which characterize MM developing in humans. Moreover, the results obtained with 5T models should be interpreted with caution, given the potential differences in the biology of human vs murine myeloma.

4.3. SCID-hu and SCID-synth-hu models

In an attempt to "humanize" murine models, in 1997 Urashima established an *in vivo* model of human MM using SCID mice bilaterally implanted with human fetal bone grafts (SCID-hu mice) [78]. The purpose was to study the role of adhesion molecules which participate to human MM-BMSC interactions and regulate MM cell homing. The original experimental design consisted in the injection of MM cell lines (ARH-77, OCI-My5, U-266 or RPMI-8226) ($1x10^4$-10^5) into the BM cavity of the left bone implants in irradiated mice (Fig.3C). Human monoclonal MM cells grew within the human BM replacing the stroma and metastatized to the controlateral right bone implant, but not to murine bones or other murine organs [79], suggesting the existence of species-specific interactions. In myeloma-bearing mice, circulating human Ig were detectable and mice developed tubular nephropathy, due to light chains deposition, closely mirroring MM clinical manifestations and physiopathology [79]. The model was successfully employed to study the efficacy of thalidomide as an anti-myeloma drug, disclosing its anti-angiogenic properties [80]. The engraftment of IL-6-dependent

INA-6 cells in SCID-hu mice, but not in SCID mice, as well as their sensitivity to anti-myeloma agents, has also been documented [81].

More recently, Pierfrancesco Tassone and Filippo Causa developed the so-called "SCID-synth-hu" model (Figure 3D), based on the implantation of artificial bone scaffolds repopulated with human BMSC into SCID mice, followed by injection of purified MM cells from patients [82] (Fig. 3D). This model represents a further advancement over the previously described SCID-hu mouse (Fig. 3C). In fact, the use of 3D poly-β-caprolactone polymeric scaffolds, closely reproducing the micro-architecture of a human bone, overcomes the restricted availability of human fetal bones for implant, and also allows to perform studies in the context of an autologous setting [82].

As for SCID-hu models, in SCID-synth-hu mice injected human MM cells were found to optimally engraft the implanted "niche" and to interact with the human bone milieu, as demonstrated not only by histological and immunohistochemical analyses of the retrieved implants, but also by demonstration of immungloglobulin production *in vivo* [82].

Both systems thereby offer the possibility to investigate human MM cells-BM microenvironment interactions and to perform pre-clinical testing of anti-MM drugs in a clinically relevant context.

4.4. Transgenic models

MM cells accumulate a series of somatic mutations in the initiating and progressing phases of the disease [10], thus justifying development of genetically modified MM murine models, which recapitulate and explore the genetics of MM [83]. Recently, a model has been developed based on the enforced B cell lineage-directed transgene expression of XBP-1s [84]. XBP-1 is a major regulator of the Unfolded Protein Response (UPR) and plasma cell differentiation. Moreover, XBP-1 over-expression has been implicated in human carcinogenesis and tumor growth in solid tumors and also in MM [84]. XBP-1 transgenic mice spontaneously develop MGUS which progresses to MM, exhibiting remarkable clinical features common to human MM. In particular, BM involvement with clonal MM cells, serum M spike, bone lytic lesions and renal Ig deposition could be demonstrated [84].

Another model exploited the deregulated expression of Myc. Myc activation occurs in post-germinal center malignancies, including Burkitt's lymphoma, and is a common feature in MM; in particular its over-expression is generally considered of prognostic significance [85]. Mice engineered to express c-Myc under the control of mouse immunoglobulin kappa (IgK) light-chain gene–regulatory elements (Vk-Myc mice) were developed [86]. Myc is a strong oncogene, and its constitutive expression in early B cells of Vk-Myc mice led to a very aggressive lymphoma, with extra-medullary localization [86].

To create a transgenic mouse model more closely resembling human MM, in their elegant work Chesi and co-workers selected the C57Bl6 strain, genetically predisposed to develop MGUS, and generated a vector (Vk*Myc) containing a stop codon insertion in the human c-myc oncogene, which prevented its expression [87] (Fig. 3E). Myc could be then sporadically activated in post-germinal B cells as a result of somatic hypermutation, leading to the transition from the spontaneous monoclonal gammopathy to a disease that fully recapitulate the biological and clinical features of human MM. In fact, Vk*Myc mice are characterized by the accumulation of slowly proliferating plasma cells exclusively inside the BM. Moreover, high levels of monoclonal antibody are detectable and end-organ damage develops, including anemia, kidney failure and lytic bone disease [87]. The model was found to be highly predictive of the activity of anti-myeloma drugs [88], including those that target microenvironment, and may potentially help to select new agents for evaluation in clinical trials.

5. Human-derived models of MM

5.1. 3D *in vitro* /*ex-vivo* human-derived models of MM

Due to inter-species differences, animal models have incomplete predictive value for human MM disease and drug response. New models are, therefore, needed that more closely resemble the *in vivo* situation in patients. Reliable, human-derived *in vitro* models, able to reproduce myelomagenesis within the specificity of BM microenvironment, are therefore of extreme value.

Kirshner and her group have reconstructed, *in vitro,* human BM microenvironment, through the proper overlay of matrix components, on which isolated cells from BM aspirate of MM patients were seeded [63]. Cells spontaneously redistributed throughout the gel-matrix 3D substrate, mimicking human BM architecture and BM-MM interactions, thus providing a powerful tool for understanding the biology of MM [89]. Strikingly, reconstructed BM allowed the expansion of primary myeloma cells, including the putative stem cell fraction. Moreover, the model allowed the assessment of the impact of anti-MM drugs on distinct cellular compartments inside a 3D architecture [63].

5.2. 3D culture of human MM isolated cells and tissue explants in the microgravity-based RCCS™ bioreactor

It is well known that the metabolic requirements of complex 3D cell constructs are substantially higher than those needed for the maintenance of traditional cell monolayers (2D culture) kept in liquid media under static conditions. Dynamic bioreactors were primarily developed to modulate mass transfer, a crucial element for guaranteeing gas/nutrient supply and waste elimination, essential factors for maintaining cell viability within large 3D cell/tissue masses. Despite a wide array of fluid-dynamic bioreactors has been devised [47,90], the low-shear environment and optimal mass transfer, needed for the long-term culture of functional 3D tissue constructs and explants, were attained only with the introduction of the microgravity-based *Rotary Cell Culture System* (RCCS™, Synthecon Inc., USA) bioreactors (91,92; a vast literature is also available at http://www.synthecon.com). The relevance of this technology in enabling the long-term culture of complex tissue-like engineered 3D bio-constructs and tissue explants of various origin has been demonstrated also by our group, and, namely, in the case of bone [31,47.93].

On this basis, we successfully employed the microgravity-based RCCS™ technology for the generation (and long-term maintenance) of viable human-derived MM tissue explants and 3D cell constructs. Fig. 4 shows the culture chamber of the RCCS™ microgravity-based bioreactor, and histo-morphological images of the *ex-vivo* models of human MM developed by our group. Isolated cells from the RPMI myeloma cell line, kept in Bioreactor, spontaneously self–aggregated forming spheroid-like structures which retained viability and were identifiable with the specific anti-CD38 monoclonal antibody (Fig.4B).

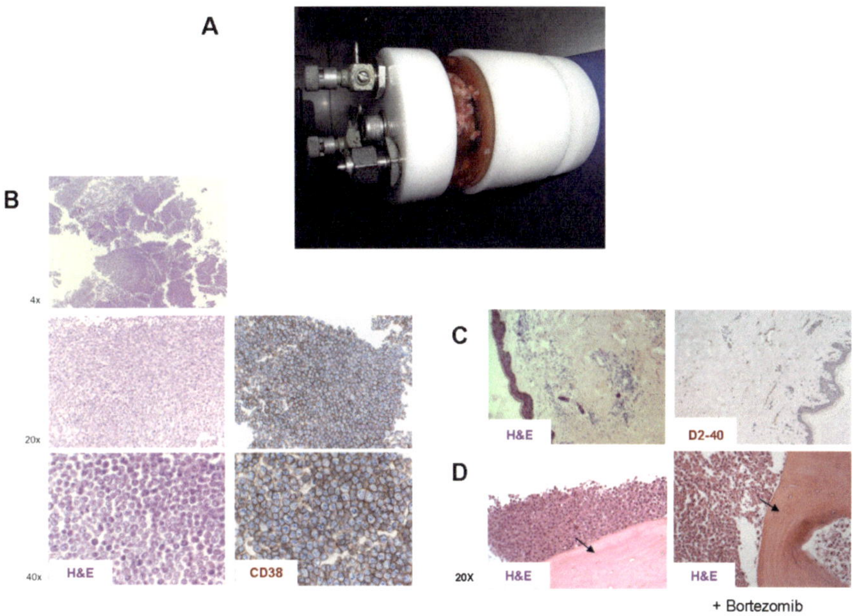

Figure 4. RCCS ™-based 3D *ex-vivo* models of MM developed by our group. A: Detail of the culture chamber of the RCCS™ microgravity-based bioreactor; **B**: Monotypic 3D multi-cellular spheroids (RPMI cell line) cultured for 1 week in the RCCS™ bioreactor (H&E staining, left panels; CD38 staining, right panels); **C:** 3D tissue culture of skin biopsies (1 week) showing intact architecture and identifiable blood and lymphatic (D2-40+) vessels **D**: MM tissue explants cultured for 3 days in the RCCS™ bioreactor (H&E staining), in the absence or presence of Bortezomib, the latter showing plasma cells death. Arrows indicate bone lamellae.

The suitability of our method for the culture of human tissue samples was, firstly, proved by using skin biopsies, which retained intact epidermal and dermal architecture, including keratin stratum and skin annexes. Moreover, both blood and lymphatic vasculature was identifiable and exhibited normal morphology, in particular patent lumen and complete endothelial lining (Fig.4C). The 3D culture of thick sections of human MM tissue explants fully preserved tissue architecture and microenvironment integrity (Fig.4D) for extended periods of time. Moreover, the system was suitable for the assessment of drug sensitivity, not only of tumor compartment, but also of angiogenic vessels (Fig.4D). Indeed, quantification of MVD in treated specimens could represent a unique method to assess the anti-angiogenic effect of a drug in human samples *ex vivo*. Finally, specialized functions of both MM cells and their microenvironment, including beta-2 microglobulin and cytokine release and metalloproteases activities, could be also assessed (M. Ferrarini *et al., submitted*). Overall, these observations suggest that the 3D culture model in Bioreactor can be exploited as a novel translational tool, allowing prospective pre-clinical toxicity and drug efficacy testing in individual patients.

6. Conclusions

A major challenge in cancer biology and cancer therapy relies in the availability of suitable models that recapitulate the complex tumor-host interplay and responsiveness to drugs. This is especially true for MM, where the existence of tight links between MM cells and BM microenvironment has hampered for long the development of adequate animals and *in vitro* models. Recently, innovative murine and chimeric *in vivo* models have been developed, which allowed both to investigate MM physiopathology and to perform drugs testing. On the other hand, the exploitation of novel technologies for *ex-vivo* 3D culturing of human MM samples is emerging as a tool to properly investigate its pathogenetic mechanisms (and interactions) within a human context, and also to predict response to drugs in individual patients.

The availability of more and more sophisticated systems is expected to pave the way to a deeper understanding of pathogenetic events and also to development of novel patients-tailored therapeutic strategies.

Acknowledgements

This work was partially supported by the Italian Association for Cancer Research (AIRC)-Special Program Molecular Clinical Oncology AIRC 5x1000 project N° 9965 (to Prof. Federico Caligaris-Cappio) and by local funds of the University of Brescia (to GM). We wish to thank Prof. F. Caligaris-Cappio (Università Vita-Salute San Raffaele, Milano) for helpful discussion and dr. Maurilio Ponzoni (Department of Pathology, San Raffaele Scientific Institute, Milan) for the precious contribution to histochemical analyses.

Author details

Marina Ferrarini[1,2], Giovanna Mazzoleni[3], Nathalie Steimberg[3], Daniela Belloni[1,2] and Elisabetta Ferrero[1,2]

1 Department of Oncology, San Raffaele Scientific Institute, Milan, Italy

2 Myeloma Unit, San Raffaele Scientific Institute, Milan, Italy

3 Laboratory of Tissue Engineering, Department of Clinical and Experimental Sciences, Faculty of Medicine and Surgery, University of Brescia, Brescia, Italy

http://dx.doi.org/10.5772/54312

References

[1] Paget S. The distribution of secondary growths in cancer of the breast. The Lancet 1889;1: 571–573.

[2] Witz IP. The tumor microenvironment: the making of a paradigm. Cancer Microenvironment 2009;2(Suppl. 1):9-17.

[3] Weber CE, Kuo PC. The tumor microenvironment. Journal of Surgical Oncology 2012;21(3): 172-177.

[4] Correia AL, Bissell MJ. The tumor microenvironment is a dominant force in multidrug resistance. Drug Resistance Update 2012;15(1-2):39-49.

[5] Tripodo C, Sangaletti S, Piccaluga PP, Prakash S, Franco G, Borrello I, Orazi A, Colombo MP, Pileri SA.The bone marrow stroma in hematological neoplasms: a guilty bystander. Nature Reviews Clinical Oncology 2011;8(8):456-466.

[6] Burger JA, Ghia P, Rosenwald A, Caligaris-Cappio F. The microenvironment in mature B-cell malignancies: a target for new treatment strategies Blood 2009;114:3367-375.

[7] Vacca A, Ribatti D. Bone Marrow angiogenesis in Multiple Myeloma. Leukemia 2006;20:193-199.

[8] Palumbo A; Anderson K. Multiple Myeloma. New. English Journal of Medicine 2011;364:1046-1060.

[9] Dvorak HF, Weaver VM, Tlsty TD, Bergers G. Tumor microenvironment and progression. Journal of Surgical Oncology 2011;103:468-474.

[10] Hideshima T, Mitsiades C, Tonon G, Richardson PG, Anderson KC. Understanding multiple myeloma pathogenesis in the bone marrow to identify new therapeutic targets. Nature Reviews Cancer 2007;7:585-598.

[11] Alsayed Y, Ngo H, Runnels J, Leleu X, Singha UK, Pitsillides CM, Spencer JA, Kimlinger T, Ghobrial JM, Jia X, Lu G, Timm M, Kumar A, Côté D, Veilleux I, Hedin KE, Roodman GD, Witzig TE, Kung AL, Hideshima T, Anderson KC, Lin CP, Ghobrial IM. Mechanisms of regulation of CXCR4/SDF-1 (CXCL12)-dependent migration and homing in multiple myeloma. Blood. 2007;109(7):2708-17.

[12] Semenza GL. Angiogenesis in ischemic and neoplastic disorders. Annual Review of Medicine2003;54:17-28

[13] Carmeliet P, Jain RK. Angiogenesis in cancer and other diseases. Nature 2000;407:249-257.

[14] Moserle L, Amadori A, Indraccolo S. The angiogenic switch: implications in the regulation of tumor dormancy. Current Molecular Medicine 2009;9:935-941.

[15] Ramanujan S, Koenig GC, Padera TP, Stoll BR, Jain RK. Local imbalance of proangiogenic and antiangiogenic factors: a potential mechanism of focal necrosis and dormancy in tumors. Cancer Research 2000; 60:1442–1448.

[16] Bergers G, Benjamin LE. Tumorigenesis and the angiogenic switch. Nature Reviews Cancer 2003;3:401-410.

[17] Di Raimondo F. Angiogenesis in hematology: a field of active research. Leukemia Research 2003;27:571-573.

[18] Vacca A, Ribatti D. Bone marrow angiogenesis in multiple myeloma. Leukemia 2006;20:193-199.

[19] Pour L, Svachova H, Adam Z, Almasi M, Buresova L, Buchler T, Kovarova L, Nemec P, Penka M, Vorlicek J, Hajek R. Levels of angiogenic factors in patients with multiple myeloma correlate with treatment response. Annals of Hematology 2010; 89:385-389.

[20] Terpos E, Anargyrou K, Katodritou E, Kastritis E, Papatheodorou A, Christoulas D, Pouli A, Michalis E, Delimpasi S, Gkotzamanidou M, Nikitas N, Koumoustiotis V, Margaritis D, Tsionos K, Stefanoudaki E, Meletis J, Zervas K, Dimopoulos MA, Greek Myeloma Study Group, Greece. Circulating angiopoietin-1 to angiopoietin-2 ratio is an independent prognostic factor for survival in newly diagnosed patients with multiple myeloma who received therapy with novel antimyeloma agents. International Journal of Cancer 2012;130(3):735-742.

[21] Ferrarini M, Ferrero E. Proteasome inhibitors and modulators of angiogenesis in multiple myeloma. Current Medicinal Chemistry 2011;18(34):5185-5195.

[22] Hideshima T, Richardson P, Chauhan D, Palombella VJ, Elliott PJ, Adams J, Anderson KC. The proteasome inhibitor PS-341 inhibits growth, induces apoptosis, and overcomes drug resistance in human multiple myeloma cells. Cancer Research 2001;61(7):3071-3076.

[23] Roccaro AM, Hideshima T, Raje N, Kumar S, Ishitsuka K, Yasui H, Shiraishi N, Ribatti D, Nico B, Vacca A, Dammacco F, Richardson PG, Anderson KC. Bortezomib mediates antiangiogenesis in multiple myeloma via direct and indirect effects on endothelial cells. Cancer Research 2006;66(1):184-191.

[24] Belloni D, Veschini L, Foglieni C, Dell'Antonio G, Caligaris-Cappio F, Ferrarini M, Ferrero E. Bortezomib induces autophagic death in proliferating human endothelial cells. Experimental Cell Research 2010;316(6):1010-1018.

[25] Pampaloni, F., Reynaud, EG. & Stelzer, EH. (2007). The third dimension bridges the gap between cell culture and live tissue. Nature Reviews. Molecular Cell Biology, Vol. 8, No. 10, (October 2007), pp. 839-845, ISSN 1471-0080

[26] Mazzoleni, G., Di Lorenzo, D. & Steimberg, N. (2009) Modelling tissues in 3D: the next future of pharmaco-toxicology and food research? Genes and Nutrition, Vol. 4, No. 1 (March 2009), pp. 13-22, ISSN 1555-8932

[27] Roskelley CD, Desprez PY, Bissell MJ (1994) Extracellular matrix-dependent tissue-specific gene expression in mammary epithelial cells requires both physical and biochemical signal transduction. Proc Natl Acad Sci USA 91:12378–12382.

[28] Lee GY, Kenny PA, Lee EH, Bissel MJ, (2007) Three-dimensional culture models of normal and malignant breast epithelial cells. Nat Methods 4:359-365.

[29] Chang, TT. & Hughes-Fulford, M. (2009). Monolayer and Spheroid Culture of Human Liver Hepatocellular Carcinoma Cell Line Cells Demonstrate Distinct Global Gene Expression Patterns and Functional Phenotypes. Tissue Engineering: Part A, Vol. 15, No. 3, pp. 559-567, ISSN 1557-8690

[30] Pickl M & CH Ries (2009) Comparison of 3D and 2D tumor models reveals enhanced HER2 activation in 3D associated with an increased response to trastuzumab. Oncogene 28:461-468.

[31] Steimberg, N., Boniotti, J. & Mazzoleni, G. (2010). 3D culture of primary chondrocytes, cartilage, and Bone/cartilage explants in simulated microgravity. In: Methods in Bioengineering: Alternative Technologies to Animal Testing, Maguire and Novak, pp. 205- 212, ISBN 978-1-60807-011-4, Boston, USA

[32] Birgersdotter A, Sandberg R, Ernberg I (2005) Gene expression perturbation in vitro - a growing case for three-dimensional (3D) culture systems. Semin Cancer Biol 15:405–412.

[33] Fischbach C, Chen R, Matsumoto T, Schmelzle T, Brugge JS, Polverini PJ, Mooney DJ (2007) Engineering tumors with 3D scaffolds. Nat Methods 4:855–860.

[34] Yim EK, Darling EM, Kulangara K, Guilak F, Leong KW. Nanotopography-induced changes in focal adhesions, cytoskeletal organization, and mechanical properties of human mesenchymal stem cells. Biomaterials. 2010;31(6):1299-1306.

[35] Bierwolf J, Lutgehetmann M, Feng K, Erbes J, Deichmann S, Toronyi E, Stieglitz C, Nashan B, Ma PX, Pollok JM. Primary rat hepatocyte culture on 3D nanofibrous polymer scaffolds for toxicology and pharmaceutical research. Biotechnology and bioengineering 2011;108(1):141-150.

[36] Yoshii Y, Waki A, Yoshida K, Kakezuka A, Kobayashi M, Namiki H, Kuroda Y, Kiyono Y, Yoshii H, Furukawa T, Asai T, Okazawa H, Gelovani JG, Fujibayashi Y. The use of nanoimprinted scaffolds as 3D culture models to facilitate spontaneous tumor cell migration and well-regulated spheroid formation. Biomaterials. 2011; 32(26): 6052-6058.

[37] Kuo SM, Chiang MY, Lan CW, Niu GC-C, Chang SJ. Evaluation of nanoarchitectured collagen type II molecules on cartilage engineering. 2012; Journal of biomedical materials research. Part A. 2012:00A:000–000.

[38] Lo CM, Wang HB, Dembo M, Wang YL. Cell movement is guided by the rigidity of the substrate. Biophysical journal. 2000; 79(1):144-152.

[39] Paszek MJ, Zahir N, Johnson KR, Lakins JN, Rozenberg GI, Gefen A, Reinhart-King CA, Margulies SS, Dembo M, Boettiger D, Hammer DA, Weaver VM. (2005) Tensional homeostasis and the malignant phenotype. Cancer Cell 8: 241–254.

[40] Schindler M, Nur-E-Kamal A, Ahmed I, Kamal J, Liu HY, Amor N, Ponery AS, Crockett DP, Grafe TH, Chung HY, Weik T, Jones E, Meiners S. Living in three dimensions: 3D nanostructured environments for cell culture and regenerative medicine. Cell Biochemistry and Biophysics. 2006;45(2):215-227.

[41] Mazzoleni, G., Boukhechba, F., Steimberg, N., Boniotti, J., Bouler, JM. & Rochet, N. (2011). Impact of the dynamic culture condition in the RCCS™ bioreactor on a three-dimensional model of bone formation. Procedia Engineering, Vol. 10, pp. 3662-3667, ISSN 1877-7058

[42] Gruber HE, Hanley EN Jr. Human disc cells in monolayer vs 3D culture: cell shape, division and matrix formation. BMC musculoskeletal disorders. 2000;1:1.

[43] Lin RZ, and Chang HY. Recent advances in three-dimensional multicellular spheroid culture for biomedical research. Biotechnol J. 2008;3(9-10):1172-1184.

[44] Ortinau S, Schmich J, Block S, Liedmann A, Jonas L, Weiss DG, Helm CA, Rolfs A, Frech MJ. Effect of 3D-scaffold formation on differentiation and survival in human neural progenitor cells. Biomed Eng Online. 2010 Nov 11;9:70.

[45] Campbell JJ, and Watson CJ. Three-dimensional culture models of mammary gland. Organogenesis. 2009; 5(2): 43-49.

[46] Ross AM, Jiang Z, Bastmeyer M, Lahann J. Physical aspects of cell culture substrates: topography, roughness, and elasticity. Small. 2012;8(3):336-355.

[47] Mazzoleni, G. & Steimberg, N. (2012) New models for the in vitro study of liver toxicity: 3D culture systems and the role of bioreactors. In"The continuum of Health Risk Assessment", edited by Dr. M.G. Tyshenko; Intech Open Access Publisher, Rijeka, Croatia; chapter 8, pp. 161-194; ISBN 978-953-51-0212-0.

[48] Ulrich TA, de Juan Pardo EM, Kumar S. The mechanical rigidity of the extracellular matrix regulates the structure, motility, and proliferation of glioma cells. Cancer Research; 2009; 69: 4167–4174.

[49] Pathak A. and Kumar S. Independent regulation of tumor cell migration by matrix stiffness and confinement. Proceedings of the National Academy of Sciences (PNAS) (2012); 109 (26): 10334-10339

[50] Bissell MJ, Radisky DC, Rizki A, Weaver VM, Petersen OW. The organizing principle: microenvironmental influences in the normal and malignant breast. Differentiation. 2002;70(9-10):537-546.

[51] Debnath J, and Brugge JS. Modelling glandular epithelial cancers in three-dimensional cultures. Nature Review Cancer. 2005;5(9):675-688

[52] Sandberg R, and Ernberg I. The molecular portrait of in vitro growth by meta-analysis of gene-expression profiles. Genome Biol. 2005; 6(8):R65

[53] Härmä V, Virtanen J, Mäkelä R, Happonen A, Mpindi J-P, Knuuttila M, Kohonen P, Lötjönen j, Kallioniemi O, Nees M. A Comprehensive Panel of Three-Dimensional Models for Studies of Prostate Cancer Growth, Invasion and Drug Responses. 2010, PLoS ONE 5(5): e10431

[54] Petersen OW, R.nnov-Jessen L, Howlett AR, Bissell MJ: Interaction with basement membrane serves to rapidly distinguish growth and differentiation pattern of normal and malignant human breast epithelial cells. Proceedings of the National Academy of Sciences USA 1992, 89:9064-9068.

[55] Smalley KS, Lioni M, Herlyn M. Life isn't flat: taking cancer biology to the next dimension In vitro Cellular & Developmental Biology 2006a; 42(8-9): 242-247.

[56] Fischbach C, Kong HJ, Hsiong SX, Evangelista MB, Yuen W, Mooney DJ. Cancer cell angiogenic capability is regulated by 3D culture and integrin engagement. Proc Natl Acad Sci U S A. 2009 Jan 13;106(2):399-404.

[57] Horning JL, Sahoo SK, Vijayaraghavalu S, Dimitrijevic S, Vasir JK, Jain TK, Panda AK, Labhasetwar V. 3-D tumor model for in vitro evaluation of anticancer drugs. Mol Pharm. 2008;5:849-862

[58] Chitcholtan K, Sykes PH and Evans JJ. The resistance of intracellular mediators to doxorubicin and cisplatin are distinct in 3D and 2D endometrial cancer. Journal of Translational Medicine 2012, 10:38

[59] Sasser AK, Mundy BL, Smith KM, Studebaker AW, Axel AE, Haidet AM, Fernandez SA, Hall BM. Human bone marrow stromal cells enhance breast cancer cell growth rates in a cell line-dependent manner when evaluated in 3D tumor environments. Cancer Lett. 2007 Sep 8;254(2):255-264.

[60] Yamada KM & Cukierman E (2007) Modeling tissue morphogenesis and cancer in 3D. Cell, 130:601-610.

[61] Kim JB. Three-dimensional tissue culture models in cancer biology. Seminars in Cancer Biology (2005)15: 365–377

[62] Hutmacher DW, Loessner D, Rizzi S, Kaplan DL, Mooney DJ, Clements JA (2010). Can tissue engineering concepts advance tumor biology research? Trends in Biotechnology, Vol.28 No.3, pp. 125-133

[63] Kirshner J, Thulien KJ, Martin LD, Debes Marun C, Reiman T, Belch AR, Pilarski LM. (2008) A unique three-dimensional model for evaluating the impact of therapy on multiple myeloma. Blood Vol. 112(7):2935-2945.

[64] Sausville EA, Burger AM. Contributions of human tumor xenografts to anticancer drug development. Cancer Research 2006;66(7):3351-3354.

[65] Teicher BA. Tumor models for efficacy determination. Molecular Cancer Therapeutics 2006;5(10):2435-2443.

[66] Tong AW, Huang YW, Zhang BQ, Netto G, Vitetta ES, Stone MJ. Heterotransplantation of human multiple myeloma cell lines in severe combined immunodeficiency (SCID) mice. Anticancer Research 1993;13(3):593-597.

[67] Mitsiades CS, Anderson KC, Carrasco DR. Mouse models of human myeloma. Hematology/Oncology Clinics of North America 2007;21(6):1051-1069.

[68] Wu KD, Zhou L, Burtrum D, Ludwig DL, Moore MA. Antibody targeting of the insulin-like growth factor I receptor enhances the anti-tumor response of multiple myeloma to chemotherapy through inhibition of tumor proliferation and angiogenesis. Cancer Immunology, Immunotherapy 2007;56(3):343-57

[69] Frost P, Moatamed F, Hoang B, Shi Y, Gera J, Yan H, Frost P, Gibbons J, Lichtenstein A. In vivo antitumor effects of the mTOR inhibitor CCI-779 against human multiple myeloma cells in a xenograft model. Blood 2004;104(13):4181-4187.

[70] Beider K, Begin M, Abraham M, Wald H, Weiss ID, Wald O, Pikarsky E, Zeira E, Eizenberg O, Galun E, Hardan I, Engelhard D, Nagler A, Peled A. CXCR4 antagonist 4F-benzoyl-TN14003 inhibits leukemia and multiple myeloma tumor growth. Experimental Hematology 2011;39(3):282-292.

[71] Miki H, Ozaki S, Nakamura S, Oda A, Amou H, Ikegame A, Watanabe K, Hiasa M, Cui Q, Harada T, Fujii S, Nakano A, Kagawa K, Takeuchi K, Yata K, Sakai A, Abe M, Matsumoto T. KRN5500, a spicamycin derivative, exerts anti-myeloma effects through impairing both myeloma cells and osteoclasts. British Journal of Haematology 2011;155(3):328-39.

[72] Mirandola L, Yu Y, Chui K, Jenkins MR, Cabos E, John CM, Chiriva-Internati M. Galectin-3C inhibits tumor growth and increases the anticancer activity of bortezomib in a murine model of human multiple myeloma. PLoS One 2011;6(7):e21811.

[73] Radl J, Hollander CF, Van den Berg P, De Glopper E. Idiopathic paraproteinaemia I. Studies in an animal model--the ageing C57BL/KaLwRij mouse. Clinical & Experimental Immunology 1978;33(3):395-402.

[74] Radl J. Age-related monoclonal gammapathies: clinical lessons from the aging C57BL mouse. Immunology Today 1990;11(7):234-236.

[75] Menu E, Asosingh K, Van Riet I, Croucher P, Van Camp B, Vanderkerken K. Myeloma cells (5TMM) and their interactions with the marrow microenvironment. Blood Cells, Molecule and Disease 2004;33(2):111-119.

[76] Croucher PI, De Hendrik R, Perry MJ, Hijzen A, Shipman CM, Lippitt J, Green J, Van Marck E, Van Camp B, Vanderkerken K. Zoledronic acid treatment of 5T2MM-bearing mice inhibits the development of myeloma bone disease: evidence for decreased osteolysis, tumor burden and angiogenesis, and increased survival, Journal of Bone and Mineral Research 2003;18(3):482–492.

[77] Deleu S, Lemaire M, Arts J, Menu E, Van Valckenborgh E, King P, Vande Broek I, De Raeve H, Van Camp B, Croucher P, Vanderkerken K. The effects of JNJ-26481585, a novel hydroxamate-based histone deacetylase inhibitor, on the development of multiple myeloma in the 5T2MM and 5T33MM murine models. Leukemia 2009;23(10): 1894-1903.

[78] Urashima M, Chen BP, Chen S, Pinkus GS, Bronson RT, Dedera DA, Hoshi Y, Teoh G, Ogata A, Treon SP, Chauhan D, Anderson KC. The development of a model for the homing of multiple myeloma cells to human bone marrow. Blood 1997;90(2): 754-765

[79] Yaccoby S, Barlogie B, Epstein J. Primary myeloma cells growing in SCID-hu mice: a model for studying the biology and treatment of myeloma and its manifestations. Blood 1998;92(8):2908-2913.

[80] Yaccoby S, Johnson CL, Mahaffey SC, Wezeman MJ, Barlogie B, Epstein J. Antimyeloma efficacy of thalidomide in the SCID-hu model. Blood 2002;100(12):4162-4168.

[81] Tassone P, Neri P, Carrasco DR, Burger R, Goldmacher VS, Fram R, Munshi V, Shammas MA, Catley L, Jacob GS, Venuta S, Anderson KC, Munshi NC. A clinically relevant SCID-hu in vivo model of human multiple myeloma. Blood 2005;106(2): 713-716.

[82] Calimeri T, Battista E, Conforti F, Neri P, Di Martino MT, Rossi M, Foresta U, Piro E, Ferrara F, Amorosi A, Bahlis N, Anderson KC, Munshi N, Tagliaferri P, Causa F, Tassone P. A unique three-dimensional SCID-polymeric scaffold (SCID-synth-hu) model for in vivo expansion of human primary multiple myeloma cells. Leukemia 2011;25(4):707-711.

[83] DeWeerdt S. Animal models: Towards a myeloma mouse. Nature 2011;480(7377):S38-9

[84] Carrasco DR, Sukhdeo K, Protopopova M, Sinha R, Enos M, Carrasco DE, Zheng M, Mani M, Henderson J, Pinkus GS, Munshi N, Horner J, Ivanova EV, Protopopov A, Anderson KC, Tonon G, DePinho RA. The differentiation and stress response factor XBP-1 drives multiple myeloma pathogenesis. Cancer Cell 2007;11(4):349-360

[85] Zhan F, Tian E, Bumm K, Smith R, Barlogie B, Shaughnessy J Jr. Gene expression profiling of human plasma cell differentiation and classification of multiple myeloma based on similarities to distinct stages of late-stage B-cell development. Blood 2003;101(3):1128-1140

[86] Robbiani DF, Colon K, Affer M, Chesi M, Bergsagel PL. Maintained rules of development in a mouse B-cell tumor. Leukemia 2005;19(7):1278-1280

[87] Chesi M, Robbiani DF, Sebag M, Chng WJ, Affer M, Tiedemann R, Valdez R, Palmer SE, Haas SS, Stewart AK, Fonseca R, Kremer R, Cattoretti G, Bergsagel PL. AID-dependent activation of a MYC transgene induces multiple myeloma in a conditional mouse model of post-germinal center malignancies. Cancer Cell 2008;13(2):167-180.

[88] Chesi M, Matthews GM, Garbitt VM, Palmer SE, Shortt J, Lefebure M, Stewart AK, Johnston RW, Bergsagel PL. Drug response in a genetically engineered mouse model of multiple myeloma is predictive of clinical efficacy. Blood. 2012;120(2):376-85.

[89] Jelinek DF. Myeloma research goes 3D. Blood 2008;112(7):2600-2601.

[90] Martin Y. & Vermette P. (2005) Bioreactors for tissue mass culture: design, characterization, and recent advances. Biomaterials; 26:7481-503.

[91] Mazzoleni, G. & Steimberg, N. (2010) 3D culture in microgravity: a realistic alternative to experimental animal use. Alternatives to Animal Experimentation (ALTEX), Vol. 27, special issue, pp. 321-324, ISSN 0946-7785

[92] Barzegaru A, & Saei AA (2012) An update to space biomedical research: tissue engineering in microgravity bioreactors. Bioimpacts, Vol.2(1), pp. 23-32

[93] Cosmi, F., Steimberg, N., Dreossi, D. & Mazzoleni, G. (2009). Structural analysis of rat bone explants kept in vitro in simulated microgravity conditions. Journal of the Mechanical Behavior of Biomedical Materials, Vol. 2, No. 2, (April 2009), pp. 164-172

Chapter 4

Heterogeneity and Plasticity of Multiple Myeloma

Hana Šváchová, Sabina Sevcikova and Roman Hájek

Additional information is available at the end of the chapter

http://dx.doi.org/10.5772/55365

1. Introduction

Modern molecular and cytogenetic approaches have furthered progress in our understanding of MM biology and have led to the development of targeted therapy that has improved management of this incurable disease. Novel agents such as bortezomib, lenalidomide or thalidomide, have increased median survival rates and improved prospects for MM patients resistant to conventional therapy [1, 2]. Despite these therapeutic advances, MM remains a very difficult disease to treat still accompanied by the threat of repeated relapses with a fatal ending. These observations indicate that at least some of the MM cells are not targeted efficiently by current drug therapies. The existence of such persistent populations, called myeloma stem cells (MSC) or myeloma-initiating cells (MIC) has been suspected for more than two decades. However, the cells of origin remain elusive [3-9]. Timeline of growing knowledge about putative MSC is displayed in **Figure 1**. Discrepancies among myeloma stem cell concepts have arisen in parallel with the high phenotypic heterogeneity of clonal PCs that might be another factor contributing to the failure of therapies and identification of the population responsible for relapse. Myeloma PCs strongly depends on the supportive role of the bone marrow (BM) microenvironment (MEV) – it is a source of essential growth factors, supports survival and dissemination of pathological PCs [10-14]. Furthermore, hypoxic conditions of tumor microenvironments support tumor progression by inducing angiogenesis, maintaining the malignant phenotype and stimulating osteoclastogenesis [15-18]. There is growing evidence that signals from pathological microenvironments can (reversibly) alter the phenotype of PCs. Such plasticity of PCs might result in obvious heterogeneity of MM and generate inconsistencies among myeloma stem cell concepts.

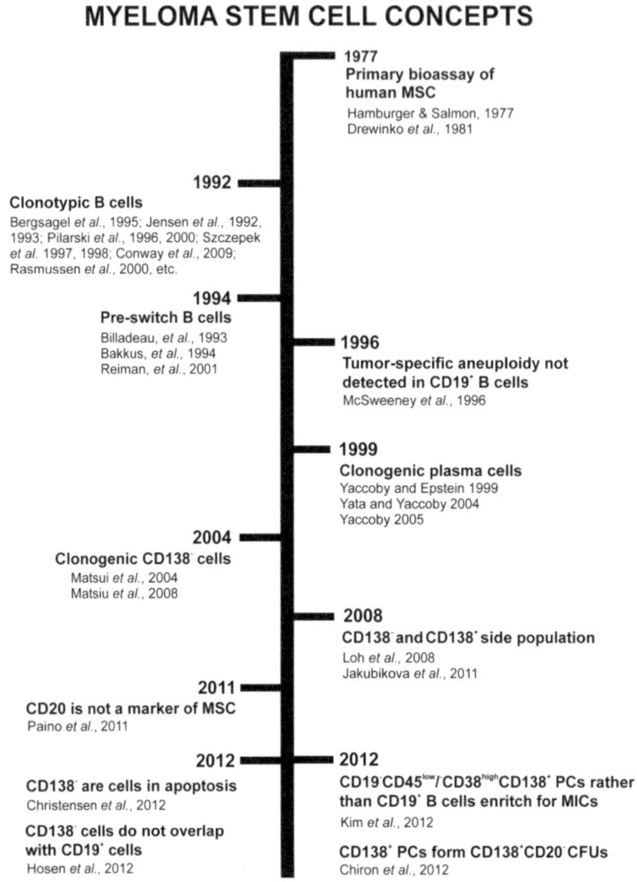

Figure 1. Timeline of myeloma stem cell concepts

2. Myeloma stem cell concepts

A number of laboratories have tried to identify a biologically distinct population of so called myeloma precursors or myeloma stem cells (MSC) which are responsible for the incurability of MM (see **Table 1**). However, none of these concepts have been unambiguously proven until now. With regards to the fact that abnormal PCs of MM show features of advanced differentiation and mature morphology, the population responsible for the origin and sustainability of tumor mass has been suspected in the minor population of clonotypic or clonogenic CD138$^-$ cells retaining key stem cell properties, tumor-initiating potential, self-renewal and resistance to chemotherapy [6, 19-25]. However, it was demonstrated that even the dominant population of human CD138$^+$ PCs contained clonogenic cells; these cells show plasticity potential that might be responsible for dedifferentiation and acquiring of stem cell properties [8, 26-30].

	Characteristics of the cells	Citation
Clonotypic B cells	PB CD19, CD38, CD10, CD11b, CD34 (HPCA-1), variable CD20, PCA-1, CD45RO, variable CD45, and CD56	[19-23, 31-34]
	PB $CD34^{\pm}$, $CD38^{+}$, $CD184^{+}$, $CD31^{\pm}$, $CD50^{\pm}$, $CD138^{-}$, $CD19^{-}$, $CD20^{-}$	[35]
	PB $CD19^{+}CD27^{+}CD38^{-}$ memory B-like cells	[24]
Clonotypic pre-switch B cells	pre-switch somatically hypermutated clonotypic cells (VDJ sequence still joined to Cμ gene) PB and BM CD19, HLA class II or surface IgM	[36-38]
Clonogenic $CD138^{-}$ cells	BM $CD20^{+}CD27^{+}CD34^{-}CD138^{-}$ clonogenic myeloma stem cells	[6, 39-41]
Side population	capacity to exclude dyes sideways from the diagonal in FACS analysis plots $CD138^{-}$ and $CD138^{+}$	[42, 43]
Clonogenic plasma cells	BM $CD38^{+}CD45^{-}$ PC (SCID-hu model) BM clonogenic $CD38^{+}CD138^{-}CD45^{-}$ PC (SCID-rab model)	[7, 26, 28]
	BM $CD38^{+}CD138^{-}CD45^{-}CD19^{-}CD34^{-}$ PC (osteoclast coculture)	[27]
	$CD19^{-}CD45^{low/-}CD38^{high}/CD138^{+}$ PCs	[30]
Intermediate PC precursors	CD138+CD44+ give rise to short-lived PC CD138+CD44-/CD138-CD44+ give rise to long-lived PC in murine model candidates for the normal counterpart of transformed MM cells	[44-46]

Table 1. Candidates for putative neoplastic PC precursors/MSC.

2.1. Clonotypic B cells

Myeloma precursors that share identical variable diversity joining (VDJ) regions, rearrangements of immunoglobulin heavy chain gene (*IgH*) with patient's tumor PCs and show a pre-plasma cell phenotype are referred to as clonotypic B cells (CBL). They have been identified in peripheral blood, lymph nodes and bone marrow [32, 36, 37, 47-49]. An extensive accumulation of somatic mutations in *IgH* gene and an absence of intraclonal variation suggest that CBLs originate from post-germinal center B cells [37, 50]. Although the concept of clonotypic B lymphocytes as neoplastic PC precursors is widely accepted, other studies suggest the existence of MM precursors in other compartments (see Table 1). Additionally, phenotypic profile and amount of CBLs vary among studies – e.g., it is not clear if these cells resemble $CD19^{+}CD27^{+}CD38^{-}$ memory B-cells or carry a marker of hematopoietic stem cells, CD34 with or without expression of the CD19 surface marker [21, 23, 35]. Furthermore, McSweeney *et al.* (1996) did not find bone marrow $CD19^{+}$ cells to be clonally restricted to kappa/lambda or revealed any deviations of expression patterns of B-cell maturation markers from normal B-cell components [51]. His results do not support a hypothesis of disturbed B-cell maturation and development of the disease from early stages of B-cell ontogeny. Moreover, DNA analysis proved that $CD38^{++}CD19^{-}$ cells were aneuploid in most cases with a typical cell cycle profile indicating the presence of a proliferating population, while cells expressing CD19 were diploid. This suggests the existence of self-replicating plasma cell compartments that have a capacity to replenish the tumor without the involvement of early B lymphocyte progenitors.

A number of studies that confirmed the presence of clonotypic B cells have been based mainly on the detection of the same IgH rearrangements by PCR-based methods. The percentage of MM patients with IgH-positive clonotypic B-cells ranged from 40% and 87% [36, 48, 52]. Limited dilution PCR assays detected the abundance of CBLs in 0.24% - 25% of peripheral blood mononuclear cells (PBMC) and 66% of all peripheral B cells [32, 36, 52, 53]. This wide range of occurrence may result from methodological errors of the PCR technique or expression of atypical, non-clinical Ig transcripts [53]. The major disadvantage of the PCR method is that this approach does not allow the morphological identification of cells of interest or sort cells for subsequent functional analyses. In addition, it is important to take into account that the presence of the same IgH rearrangements is reliable marker of clonality; it does not confirm the malignity of cells *per se*. Therefore, the detection of IgH rearrangements in $CD19^{+}$ cells could also indicate that a small clone of premalignant or premyelomatous B cells persists despite the transformation of other cells into malignant clones but this population does not actively contribute to myeloma clones [51]. Rasmussen *et al.* (2010) suggests that peripheral blood memory B cells represent pre-malignant, partially transformed remnants that could have some proliferative advantage over normal memory B cells. They questioned the involvement of CBLs in MM maintenance due to the fact these cells expressed specific 'early' oncogenes (*FGFR3, MMSET, CCND1*) that were deregulated by an IgH translocation but lacked 'late' oncogene (*KRAS*) mutations [54].

A large interpatient and interstudy variability led Trepel *et al.,* (2012) to establish patient-individual ligands mimicking the epitope recognized by the myeloma immunoglobulin to specifically target clonotypic surface IgH-positive B cells of MM patients [53]. In a cohort of 15

MM patients, semi-nested PCR using HCDR3-specific patient-individual primers detected CBLs in 50% of peripheral blood and/or bone marrow samples. This frequency is line with published data. However, a new flow cytometric protocol detected clonotypic B cells only in one patient with a sensitivity of 10^{-3}, ie. less than one clonotypic B cell per 1000 PBMCs. These cells accounted for about 0.15% of PBMCs and 5% of B cells in this patient. Surprising discrepancies between these two approaches could indicate nonspecific annealing of the CDR3-primer leading to false positive PCR results. Conclusions of this study suggest that the abundance of CBLs is exceedingly low and has been enormously overestimated in previous studies. Similarly to findings of Rasmussen *et al.* (2010), authors consider that unlike those CBLs they are true "feeder" cells for malignant PC compartments and an essential prerequisite of myeloma maintenance and progression [54]. In regard to the rare occurrence of CBLs in MM, it is more likely that these cells are non-malignant remnants, which may be a part of the malignant plasma cell clone but do not participate in tumor maintenance [53].

2.2. Clonotypic pre-switch B cells

An identical rearrangement of the IgH VDJ region with a consistent pattern of hypermutations within the clone is a signature of CBLs. MM plasma cell clones generally express monoclonal Igs of these isotypes: IgG, IgA, IgD, IgM, in rare cases kappa or lambda light chains and non-secretory myeloma is detected [55]. Clonotypic isotypes with identical Vh gene sequences and patterns of hypermutations linked to different classes of Ig heavy-chain constant region genes (including Cμ gene) compared to clinical isotypes have been identified in some MM patients [36-38, 56]. B cells with "non-clinical" isotype have been called pre-switch (IgM^+) clonotypic B cells. Particular classes of Ig are generated by mechanism of class switch recombination (CSR) resulting in the formation of a hybrid switch region composed of switch region Sμ and a respective isotype switch region (Cδ, Cγ3, Cγ1, Cα1, Cγ2, Cγ4, Cε and Cα2). Consequently, immunoglobulin production is 'switched' from IgM to IgG and IgA (occasionally to IgD or IgE). Sequences between the switch regions are cut out as a deletion loop after double-stranded breaks without changing the VDJ sequence [57-59]. The presence of CSR is a hallmark of "post-switch" B cells. However, pre-switch B cells do not seem to undergo CSR because IgH transcript is composed of the clonotypic VDJ sequence still joined to Cμ gene [56].

Preswitch (IgM^+) CBLs have been identified in BM and PB of most MM patients; however their frequency is very low. Palumbo *et al.* (1992) have already suggested that MM may originate from pre-switch cells [60]. Billadeau *et al.* (1993), using the allele-specific oligonucleotide PCR, demonstrated the existence of the pre-switch isotype species that were clonally related to the myeloma tumor. Another study also proved the evidence of pre-switch cells with somatically hypermutated clonotypic VDJ region [37]. These cells exhibited expression of CD19 and HLA class II or surface bound IgM. Reiman *et al.* (2001) described the presence of clinical and nonclinical clonotypic isotypes in PB, BM and G-CSF – mobilized blood autografts of MM patients. Expression of preswitch clonotypic transcripts persisted in the blood despite high-dose chemotherapy with stem cell support suggesting drug resistance of this pre-switch population. The persistence of preswitch clonotypic isotypes was associated with reduced survival and with a more advanced disease at the time of diagnosis. Moreover, both pre-switched and postswitched cells were able to engraft in the NOD/SCID mice indicating their potential clinical relevance. Authors considered the fact that MM is the disease of post-switch cells, IgH isotype switching in MM may accompany worsening disease [38]. Despite these facts, Taylor *et al.* (2008) questioned the role of preswitch (IgM^+) clonotypic cells as a progenitor pool for postswitch MM-PCs. They hypothesized that if they are progenitors for MM-PCs, multiple clonotypic switch junctions, or changes in the switch junction, are expected in the postswitch progeny. However, results of specific clonotypic-switch PCR determined the presence of a single, unchanged clonotypic switch junction. Thus, postswitch MM-PCs most likely originate from a single CSR event and pre-switch IgM^+ cells do not represent MM-PC progenitors [52].

Interestingly, pre-switch (non-clonotypic) IgM^+ $CD27^+$ cells with mutated IgH V region have been detected in various immunodeficiencies and autoimmune diseases but also in healthy donors [61, 62]. Expression of surface marker CD27 suggests that these cells maybe IgM^+ $CD27^+$ memory B cells. On the other hand, considering the occurrence of IgM^+ $CD27^+$ cells in humans who cannot form germinal centers (GC), it was presumed that these cells: 1) are generated independently of germinal centers and therefore cannot represent a subset of memory B cells; 2) undergo SHM during generation of the preimmune repertoire; and 3) they mediate responses to T cell-independent antigen. The evidence for these presumptions came from the studies of patients with hyper-IgM syndrome, X-linked lymphoproliferative disease or common variable immunodeficiency that are characterized by some type of defect in GC formation. However, quantification of IgM^+ $CD27^+$ cells in these diseases showed that their numbers reached approximately 20–40% of the number observed in normal individuals. These results indicate that germinal centers may play a role in the development of IgM^+ $CD27^+$ cells. IgM^+ memory B cells may be generated at the centroblast stage and undergo SHM but leave GC before the onset of isotype switching. Whether IgM^+ $CD27^+$ cells with mutated IgH V region might be a source of preswitch (IgM^+) CBLs, it remains a matter of further debate and research.

2.3. Clonogenic $CD138^-$ cells

Matsui *et al.*, (2004) suggested that the source of MSC responsible for the initiation and maintenance of MM might be due to a minor population of less differentiated cells reminiscent of memory B-lymphocytes with surface markers $CD20^+CD27^+CD34^-CD138^-$. They showed that $CD138^-/CD34^-$ cells derived from MM cell lines RPMI 8226, NCI-H929 and primary clinical samples were clonogenic *in vitro.* Cloning efficiency correlated with the disease stage [6]. The depletion of either $CD20^+$ or $CD27^+$ cells from the $CD138^-/CD34^-$ population significantly limited clonogenic growth of MM, therefore the phenotype of MM cells with *in vitro* clonogenic potential were suggested to be characterized by a pattern of surface markers $CD20^+CD27^+CD138^-$ [39]. Clonogenic potential of $CD138^-/CD34^-$ cells was evaluated by successful engraftment of non-obese diabetic/severe combined immunodeficiency (NOD/SCID) mice during both primary and secondary transplantation. $CD138^+/CD34^-$ were unable to form colonies *in vitro* and human engraftment was not detected in any of the mice injected with $CD138^+$ cells. A chimeric anti-CD20 monoclonal antibody, rituximab, was showed to inhibit clonogenic growth of $CD138^-$ cells *in vitro* [6,39]. However, clinical trials failed to confirm an effect of rituximab as a useful maintenance therapy for MM [63, 64].

Paino *et al.*, (2011) reevaluated the presence and function of $CD20^+$ putative MSC in a panel of myeloma cell lines [65]. Although, Matsui *et al.* (2004) described a small population (2-5%) of $CD138^-20^+$ cells in NCI-H929 and RPMI-8226 cell lines, Paino *et al.* (2011) were not able to detect CD20 by flow cytometry in the majority of tested MM cell lines [6, 65]. Only RPMI-8226 cell lines contained a small population of $CD20^{dim+}$ cells (0.3%). These data are consistent with the report of Rossie *et al.* (2010) that showed that U266, NCI-H929 and RPMI-8226 MM cell lines are $CD20^-$ [66]. Despite previous results, memory B-cell phenotype of putative $CD20^+$ MSC was also not confirmed. On the contrary, $CD20^{dim+}$ cells displayed a myelomatous plasma cell phenotype: $CD38^+CD138^+CD19^-CD27^-CD45^-$. Additionally, $CD20^{dim+}$ cells did not exhibit stem cell properties and compared to the $CD20^-$ population they showed a lower level of self-renewal potential. Both populations developed plasmacytomas when they were injected into CD17-SCID mice suggesting that $CD20^{dim+}$ cells are not essential for tumor formation. Furthermore, sorted and plated $CD20^{dim+}$ cells did not differentiate into $CD20^-$ cells. However, $CD20^-$ cells give rise to $CD20^{dim+}$ cells indicating a hierarchical order of differentiation from $CD20^-$ to $CD20^{dim+}$ cells. Overall, these results do not support CD20 as a marker associated with MSC phenotype [65].

Other drugs, such as dexamethasone, lenalidomide, bortezomib, or 4-hydroxycyclophosphamide did not significantly affect $CD138^-$ cells indicating resistance to some conventional or novel therapy, a characteristic feature of CSC [39]. All four agents significantly inhibited the clonogenic growth of $CD138^+$ cells isolated from MM cells. Nevertheless, it could not be evaluated in $CD138^+$ PCs from MM patients because they lack *in vitro* clonogenic activity. Detection of a small $CD138^-$ population of MM cell lines (< 2%) that displayed stem cell properties mediating drug resistance, such as the capacity to efflux the DNA binding dye Hoechst 33342 and higher relative levels of aldehyde dehydrogenase (ALDH) activity further supports the existence of a resistant MSC compartment in MM. Moreover, $CD138^-$ cells of MM cell lines also exhibited cellular quiescence similar to adult stem cells – almost all $CD138^-$ cells were shown to remain in $G_0 – G_1$ phase and less than 1,5 % in S phase, compared to two thirds of $CD138^+$ cells in $G_0 – G_1$ and about 20% in S phase [39]. On the other hand, results of the first study proved that $CD138^-$ cells isolated from the same MM cell lines expressed higher levels of the proliferation marker Ki67 than $CD138^+$ cells [6]. These discrepancies might come from different passages of cell lines or culture conditions but cannot conclusively prove a quiescent state of $CD138^-$ cells.

Besides the clonogenic population of $CD138^-$ cells, Matsui *et al.* (2004) also isolated circulating clonotypic $CD19^+CD27^+$ B cells in peripheral blood of MM patients which were successfully engrafted into NOD/SCID mice. However, it remains unclear whether $CD138^-$ clonogenic cells are identical to clonotypic $CD19^+$ B cells. Hosen *et al.* (2012) examined 16 MM samples and found that only $CD138^-CD19^-CD38^{++}$ cells formed colonies *in vitro* whereas $CD19^+$ B cells did not [67]. Moreover, $CD138^-CD19^-CD38^{++}$ cells engrafted into SCID-rab mouse models in 3 cases out of 9, whilst there was no detection of $CD19^+$ B cell engrafment. Neither $CD19^+$ B cells transplanted into NOD/SCID IL2Rγc(-/-) mice propagated into MM. Surprisingly, $CD138^+$ PCs also give rise of MM, but more slowly than $CD138^-$ cells. Thus, CD138-negative clonogenic cells might represent a population which has the potential to give rise to MM but does not overlap with the population of $CD19^+$ B cells. These results indicate that CD138-negative clonogenic cells are more PCs than B cells but this does not necessarily mean that Matsui's myeloma stem cell concept is wrong. Although, MSCs phenotypically resemble memory B cells, they may be modified PCs and CD138-positive PCs might represent some "transit" population that subsequently lost its mature phenotype (this will be discussed later). However, Christensen *et al.* (2012) reexamined $CD138^-$ population of so called MSC and obtained surprising results which were strongly controversial to both previous mentioned reports [68]. An analysis of primary $CD138^+$ PCs of MM patients showed that the number of $CD138^-$ cells increased in parallel with increasing time from sampling to analysis. In regards to the fact that myeloma PCs loses expression of the surface antigen CD138 in apoptosis, Annexin V was included in all analyses to monitor apoptotic cells [69]. Expectedly, if a $CD138^-$ population was detected, these cells were positive for Annexin V. Similar results were also obtained by Chiron *et al.* (2011). Furthermore, qPCR techniques confirmed similarly high levels of CD138 mRNA in both $CD138^-$ and $CD138^+$ MM cells. $CD138^-$ and $CD138^+$ subpopulations varied neither in expression of CD19 nor in expression of CD20. These contradictory results would imply that the CD138-negative population may represent only cells undergoing apoptosis as a consequence of previous sample handling [68]. Nevertheless, these new findings cannot completely deny results of previous studies that showed the potential of $CD138^-$ cells to form colonies *in vitro* and engraft mouse models.

2.4. Side population

Side population (SP) cells were defined based on their capacity to exclude dyes such as Hoechst 33342 [70]. Hoechst 33342 dye binds to the AT-rich regions found in the minor groove of DNA. Upon UV excitation, cells with this efflux capacity can be identified as the minor population of the positively stained cells sideways from the diagonal in FACS analysis plots. SP cells have been detected in various cancer cell lines as well as primary tumors (rev. in 71). Side population possesses CSC characteristics such as the capacity for regrowth of the tumor, expression of stem cell-like genes and resistance to chemotherapy. This is why SP cells are believed to be the true population responsible for tumor maintenance.

The presence of SP cells were investigated in four MM cell lines, RPMI 8226, U266, OPM2 and KMS-11, and primary MM samples [42]. SP was defined using control cells stained with both Hoechst and verapamil, L-type calcium channel blocker, to establish the SP gate[72]. Reduction of SP cells was demonstrated in all tested cell lines. In 18 of 21 bone marrow samples from MM patients the percentage of SP cells ranged from 0 to 4.9% compared to 0.05% of SP in normal bone marrow. There was neither a significant difference between treated and non-treated MM patients based on the percentage of SP nor a correlation between the percentage of SP and the paraprotein concentration or disease stage. 0.18–0.83% of SP cells express the clonal surface immunoglobulin light chain restriction that matched 89–97% of each patient's PCs. SP cells were also analyzed for the expression of CD138. A mean of 96.1% of SP cells were found to be $CD138^-$. However the $CD138^+$ fraction also contained SP indicating that they are present in both CD138⁻ and CD138⁺ compartments. Jakubikova *et al.* (2011) also demonstrated that the SP fraction of MM cell lines expressed CD138 antigen [43]. Moreover, these results did not prove a correlation between expression of CD19, CD20, or CD27 and the proportion of SP cells. Conversely, SP cells showed more clonogenic potential and proliferation index than the main population. Furthermore, adherence to stromal cells increased percentage, viability and proliferation potential of SP cells. Supportive role of BM microenvironment was attenuated by lenalidomide and thalidome. Lenalidomide itself directly decreased the percentage and clonogenicity of SP cells. This study demonstrated innovative and promising strategies for targeting putative myeloma-initiating cells and prevention of relapse.

Although SPs exhibit stem cell properties and might represent a "feeder" population responsible for the relapse of the disease, others question the method for detection of SP. Hoechst staining binds to DNA resulting in toxicity to live cells, that is why SP cells might represent only a population that survived the lethal effect of Hoechst. SP phenotype might also be affected by staining time, dye concentration or cellular concentration. The problem also lies in cytometric approaches that showed inconsistencies among gating strategies and might lead to contamination of the SP fraction by non-SP cells. Furthermore, usage of verapamil as an inhibitor of efflux was also criticized because verapamil-sensitive cells were detected in the negative or SP gate [73]. These problematic findings require more stringent gating strategies to clear doubts about SP.

2.5. Clonogenic plasma cells

The clonogenic potential of primary MM cells was first demonstrated by Hamburger & Salmon (1977). They showed that freshly explanted human myeloma cells are able to form colonies of monoclonal PCs. Colonies consisted of immature plasmablasts and mature PCs. Drewinko *et al.*, (1981) investigated the growth fraction of MM cells. In untreated and nonresponsive patients the growth fraction represented 4% of MM cells. Patients in relapse had the growth fraction ranging from 14% to 83%. Nonproliferating fraction contained true quiescent cells, some proliferating cells with very long intermitotic times, and some proliferating cell that have entered the maturation phase. Although these two reports demonstrated clonogenic and proliferative capacity of primary MM tumors, these cells were not phenotypically defined as whole mononuclear fraction of BM was used for analyses. Therefore, results of these studies cannot answer what kind of cells represents true growth fraction.

First experiments demonstrating the clonogenic growth of phenotypically defined PCs were carried out by Yaccoby and Epstein (1999). They proved that $CD38^{++}CD45^{-}$ PCs derived from PB and BM are able to engraft severe combined immunodeficiency (SCID)-hu host system with implanted human bone. Circulating clonal PCs grew more rapidly in SCID-hu hosts than those in the BM suggesting that this may represent a subpopulation with a higher growth potential. In contrast to previous reports, PC-depleted blood cells did not give rise to MM in SCID-hu hosts [7]. Yata & Yaccoby, 2004 presented an alternative model for study of myeloma-initiating cells (MIC) that uses rabbit bones implanted subcutaneously in unconditioned SCID mice. The SCID-rab model was also successfully engrafted with CD138⁺ PCs of MM patients. Although, these two models did not show a serial engraftment of the disease, they strongly indicate a critical role of specific bone marrow microenvironments for plasma cell survival and proliferation [28].

A dependence of myeloma PCs on human BM microenvironment was clearly demonstrated in an experiment with NOD/SCID/common cytokine receptor γ chain-deficient (NSG) and recombinase-activating gene 2/common cytokine receptor γ chain-deficient (RAG2-/ γ c-) mice [30]. Results proved that CD138^{+}/CD38^{high} cells from MM patients led to a repopulation of CD19^{+}CD38^{low} or CD138^{+}CD38^{+} B-lineage cells in human bone-bearing mice but no engraftments were detected in human bone-free mice even after orthotropic intrafemoral injection. Moreover, serially xenotransplantated CD19^{-}CD138^{+} cells preferably engrafted from a human bone graft but were not detected in any mouse hematopoietic tissues. All grafts derived from CD138^{+}/CD38^{high} cells were clonally related to myeloma PCs, whereas engraftments of CD19^{+}CD38$^{low/-}$ B cells were polyclonal CD19^{+}CD38^{low} cells. Further fractionation of CD138^{+}/CD38^{high} cells and theirs subsequent xenotransplantation showed that CD45$^{low/-}$ or CD19^{-}CD38^{high}/CD138^{+} cells had a higher engraftment ability than CD45^{high} or CD19^{+} plasmablasts. In line with the above mentioned results, it was concluded that CD19^{-}CD45$^{low/-}$CD38^{high}/CD138^{+} PCs rather than CD19^{+} B cells or plasmablasts enrich for MICs. In addition, analysis of clonogenic potentials of CD138^{+} and CD138^{-} populations derived from plasma cell leukemia patients strongly favored these findings [29]. This study demonstrated that, though, CD138^{+} PCs derived from plasma cell leukemia patients formed colony forming units (CFU) in a very low frequency, no CFU were found when CD138^{-} cells were seeded. Harvested cells of CFUs derived from CD138^{+} PCs were strongly positive for CD138 but negative for CD20. There was no evidence that they can be CD138^{-}CD19^{+}CD20^{-} plasmablasts or CD19^{+}CD20^{+}CD138^{-} B-cells. These findings further underline an important role of CD20^{-}CD138^{+} population as a conceivable reservoir of clonal PCs at least in plasma cell leukemia.

Against the statement that CD138-positive PCs represent a "feeder" population responsible for incurability of MM is the fact that abnormal PCs show a low proliferation potential with a plasma cell labeling index (PCLI) ranging from 0.5% in MGUS to 1% in early MM, PCLI. Therefore, the growth fraction of progenitor cells giving rise to MM has been expected in less differentiated stages of B cell development. Despite low proliferative activity of malignant PCs, PCLI is one of the most important prognostic factor with a strong impact on overall survival [98, 99]. Additionally, limited proliferation potential of PCs could be explained by error reduction during DNA synthesis that was proposed for normal adult stem cells that are highly clonogenic but proliferatively silenced [100].

2.6. Intermediate plasma cell precursors

O'Connor *et al.* (2002) identified post-GC-precursors in a mouse model that might contribute to long-lived humoral immunity. These cells were distinct from splenic B cells, mature or memory B cells as well as mature PCs. Mediate levels of CD138 indicated that PC precursors might represent a transition state of PC development. PC precursors were demonstrated to migrate to the BM where they proliferate and persist for a long period of time and consequently differentiate to mature PCs without antigen stimulation. CD138^{+}CD44^{+} give rise to short-lived PCs, CD138^{+}CD44^{-} or CD138^{-}CD44^{+} differentiated to long-lived PCs. Two roles of PC precursors were suggested; (i) they might either serve as a reservoir of PCs upon PC attrition or (ii) contribute to post-GC affinity maturation of the humoral immune response. Due to similarities of phenotype, proliferative potential, and differential capacity of the PC precursors to putative MM progenitors, authors suggested that these cells are candidates for the normal counterpart of transformed MM progenitors [74].

The true origin of MM remains a matter for further debate. An unanswered question persists whether clonotypic $CD138^-$ cells or side populations represents myeloma precursors or phenotypic variants of the MM tumor cells that have lost some plasma cell markers and gained some B-cell markers as Yaccoby (2005) suggested [27, 54]. He presented a new model for myelomagenesis; that mature $CD45^{low/intermediate}$ $CD38^{high}$ $CD138^{high}$, $CD19^-CD34^-$ PC situated closely with osteoclasts in the lytic bone lesions reverse senescence, acquire a stem cell phenotype, ($CD45^{intermediate/high}$ $CD19^{low}$ and$CD34^{low}$), and become quiescent and apoptosis-resistant. This indicates that myeloma PCs have plasticity that allows them to reprogram, dedifferentiate and acquire autonomous survival properties which are responsible for drug-resistance and relapse of MM patients. Similar results were also obtained by Kukreja *et al.* (2006) when cultured U266 myleoma cell line and primary myeloma PCs with dendritic cells (DC). The coculture of U266 cells and DCs led to an increase in the proportion of cells lacking CD138; a marker of terminally differentiated PCs, and induction of B cell lymphoma 6 (BCL6) expression. It was suggested that BCL6 plays an important role in survival and self-renewal of germinal center B cells and that suppression of BCL6 is a critical feature of normal PC differentiation. Furthermore, a presence of DCs in the culture enhanced clonogenic growth of the myeloma cell line and as well as primary myeloma PCs [75]. Just as in the previous report, this data suggests that the differentiation state of myeloma cells is plastic and can be modified in the presence of DCs. Both reports emphasize an importance of tumor microenvironments for myleoma plasticity. Whether myeloma PCs exhibit plasticity that might be responsible for phenotypic heterogeneity of MMs, and also form inconsistencies among myeloma stem cell concepts, it will be discussed further.

3. Phenotypic heterogeneity of multiple myeloma

The high phenotypic heterogeneity of clonal PCs is a hallmark of MM; abnormal PCs frequently express a wide spectrum of multi-lineage antigens such as myeloid, T-cell and natural killer-associated antigens. Compared to normal polyclonal PCs which show high CD38 and CD138 expression along with the B-lymphocyte marker CD19 abnormal PCs generally lack CD19 expression, show variable expression of CD45, dim expression of CD38 and heterogeneous signals of CD138. Further, they have weaker expression of CD27, increased expression of CD28, CD33 and CD56 and variable expression of CD20 and CD117 (rev. in [76, 77]). Causes of phenotypic heterogeneity remain unclear.

PCs belong to the B-cell lineage that expresses paired box protein 5 (PAX5) and its target, CD19. PAX5 activation and inactivation is essential for early B cell commitment as well as for maintenance of the functional identity of B cells throughout B cell development. PAX5 represses B lineage 'inappropriate' genes and simultaneously activates B lineage-specific genes [78, 79]. Conditional PAX5 reduction in late B lymphocytes promotes development to the mature B cell stage. PAX5 and CD19 expression are considered to be downregulated or lost but it has been reported that expression of PAX5 and CD19 is restored in normal PCs of pleural effusion, ascitic fluid and BM aspirate. In contrast to normal PCs, clonal PCs of MM do not express PAX5 or CD19 (> 95% of cases) [80, 81].

Phenotypic heterogeneity of abnormal PCs might reflect a certain degree of dedifferentiation of these cells. It has been previously shown that elimination of PAX5 shifts B cells to multipotency [82]. Therefore expression of multi lineage markers on clonal PCs might be due to a lack of *PAX5* gene expression but not only as a consequence of malignant transformation. Cell heterogeneity is the phenomenon that is commonly seen in many cancer types. The cause of this variability might be due to the loss of the lineage master gene which can lead to dedifferentiation or transdifferentiation into cells of other lineages [83].

The ability to differentiate into multiple lineages is a characteristic feature of pluripotent embryonic stem cells. However, pluripotency does not necessarily have to be limited to a population of undifferentiated stem cells of the early embryo and lost irreversibly upon terminal differentiation [84]. Fully differentiated somatic cells can be reprogrammed into inducible pluripotent stem cells (iPSC) by 'forced' expression of pluripotency/reprogramming factors: OCT4, SOX2, c-Myc and KLF4 or NANOG, LIN28, c-Myc and KLF4 [85, 86]. Human somatic cells from all three germ layers, including human differentiated mature B lymphocytes, have been successfully reprogrammed [87-93] Reprogramming of mature B cells required additional 'sensitization' by the myeloid transcription factor CCAAT/enhancer-binding protein-α (C/EBPα) that causes a disruption of PAX5 functions, or a specific knock-down of the B cell transcription factor PAX5. This indicates that the loss of PAX5 expression might be associated with gain of stem cell features for mature PCs and represent one of the key events in the pathogenesis of MM.

4. Plasticity of multiple myeloma

There is growing evidence that MM encompasses a certain degree of plasticity that might be responsible for expression of a wide spectrum of multi lineage markers and discrepancies among myeloma stem cell theories. Two facts support this hypothesis:

i. There is a strong link between induction of pluripotency and tumor progression; several human cancers acquire stem cell-like plasticity upon (re)expression of reprogramming factors. It raises the possibility that dedifferentiation is a key mechanism for the generation of tumor-initiating cells in human cancer [84]. The process of dedifferentiation is suggested to be under control of tumor microenvironment. Interaction of tumor cells with their microenvironment might induce altered differentiation; epithelial-mesenchymal transition (EMT) which has been observed in some solid tumors [94, 95]. Similarly to MM, phenotypic plasticity of myeloma PCs were observed in long-term co-culture with osteoclasts; myeloma PCs lost their mature phenotype and dedifferentiated to an immature, resilient, apoptosis-resistant phenotype. In addition, CD138^{+} PCs cocultured with DCs lost expression of CD138 and increased the clonogenic potential [75]. It raises the possibility that signals from the microenvironment can (reversibly) alter the phenotype of PCs and cause obvious heterogeneity of MM. This regulation might keep dynamic equilibrium between CSC and non-CSC compartments [96].

Dynamic state between CSC and non-CSC like compartments were also observed in a subpopulation of differentiated basal-like human mammary epithelial cells that spontaneously converted to stem-like cells *in vitro* and *in vivo*. Moreover, oncogenic transformation enhances this spontaneous conversion. These findings indicate that normal and CSC-like cells can arise *de novo* and indicate the importance of the differentiation state of cells-of-origin as a critical factor determining the phenotype of their transformed derivatives [97]. Whether mature PCs exhibit a plasticity potential responsible for dedifferentiation into cells with stem cell like properties is questionable but highly attractive. Confirmation that mature PCs have the capacity to convert into CSCs could resolve current inconsistencies among myeloma stem cell theories and help to target the population responsible for relapse of the disease.

ii. Despite of mature phenotype, myeloma PCs have been reported to express pluripotency factors (SOX2, c-Myc or KLF4) and stem/progenitor markers, such as germline stem cell markers of the MAGE family, the hematopoietic progenitor marker CD117 or neural stem cell marker nestin [83, 101-105]. Some of these factors provide valuable prognostic information. Currently, the role of c-myc is growing as the key transforming factor in the progression of asymptomatic MGUS to a symptomatic disease [101]. SOX2 and MAGE have been demonstrated to be relevant targets for immunotherapy due to their immunogenicity. Interestingly, MGUS patients frequently mount a humoral and cellular immune response against SOX2 but MM patients lack anti-SOX2 immunity [104, 106]. CD117 (c-kit) is an essential hematopoietic growth factor receptor with tyrosine-kinase activity. Aberrant expression of CD117 is detected on a subset of MGUS and MM and is associated with a favorable outcome for MM patients [107, 108]. KLF4 was described in regulation of apoptosis, proliferation and differentiation of B cells and B-cell malignancies. Strong up-regulation of KLF4 was detected in MM cell lines in the process of apoptosis suggesting a role of KLF4 in MM progression [105]. Nestin is a remarkable protein that is found in rapidly dividing cells of developing and regenerating tissues [109]. Therefore, it is surprising that this gene and protein expression of the stem cell marker nestin has been detected in terminally differentiated PCs of MM patients [83, 110]. Moreover, our recent work proved that nestin protein is a tumor specific marker for CD138^{+}38^{+}PC of MM [110]. Expression of nestin, a marker of stem/progenitor cells in malignant PCs that are considered to be terminally differentiated, is highly controversial and indicates that nestin might play an exceptional role in the pathology of MM. However, biological or clinical implications of nestin have not been determined in monoclonal gammopathies or other hematological malignancies so far.

Summarizing these findings supports the hypothesis that stem cell-like features are not rare in monoclonal gammopathies and might indicate the existence of inducible stem cell properties in more differentiated cells than was initially thought [27, 111] (see **Fig. 2**).

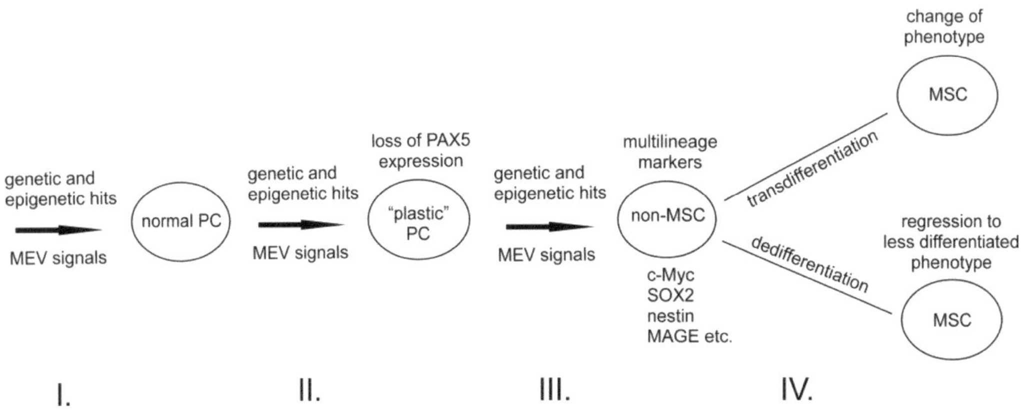

Figure 2. Model of inducible stem cell properties in myeloma

5. Putative role of nestin in myeloma plasticity

Neural stem cell marker nestin was first identified in neuroepithelial stem/progenitor cells of the rat central nervous system (CNS) by Hockfield and McKay in 1985 [112]. Nestin is detected in a wide range of undifferentiated tissues under normal and pathological conditions [113-116]. Expression of nestin is a common feature of multipotent proliferative progenitor cells with self-renewal and regeneration potentials. During terminal differentiation, nestin expression is silenced but can be reactivated upon injury or other pathological conditions such neoplastic transformation. The human nestin gene is located at 1q23 locus and is composed of four exons and three introns. Nestin expression is driven by a minimal promoter that is activated by transcriptional factor Sp1 [117]. Moreover, epigenetic regulation was also demonstrated. Results indicated that histone acetylation might be sufficient to mediate activation of nestin transcription [118].

Nestin protein belongs to a large family of intermediate filament (IF) proteins that are encoded by more than 70 genes expressed in a time and site-specific manner in metazoan cells. Members of the IF family are divided into six classes of proteins according to their structure, properties and localization [119]. Nestin, a class VI protein, is characterized by a α-helical central 'rod' domain which is typical for all IF, that contains repeated hydrophobic heptad motifs, a short N-terminus (head) and a very long C-terminus (tail) (**Fig. 3**) C-terminus is suggested to function as a linker or cross-bridge between intermediate filaments, microfilaments and

http://dx.doi.org/10.5772/55365

microtubules [120]. The molecular weight of human nestin protein is ~ 200 – 220 kDa; more often it is found in its glycosylated form with molecular weight of 240kDa [121, 122]. Nestin does not fold by itself most likely because of its very short N-terminus. Therefore, nestin requires the presence of other IF proteins such as type III vimentin, desmin or type IV α-internexin [109, 123, 124].

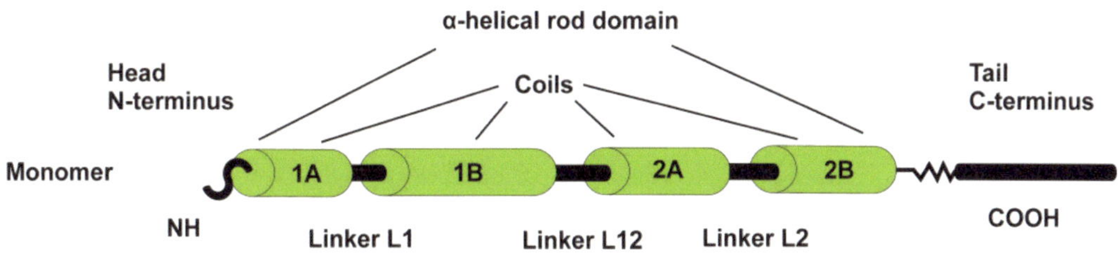

Figure 3. Structure of intermediate filaments (adopted and modified from Michalzyk & Ziman, [2005]

5.1. Cellular roles of nestin

An important regulator of nestin organization and dynamics during mitosis is cdc2-mediated phosphorylation. Phosphorylation/dephosphorylation of nestin may modulate disassembly and assembly of intermediate filaments [125]. These processes might play a role during increased cytoplasmic trafficking in progenitor cells undergoing division or in migrating interphase cells [126-128]. Nestin was shown to participate in asymmetric redistribution of cytoskeletal proteins and other factors to daughter neuroepithelial cells [129]. Nestin structure serves also as a scaffold for cdk5/p35 activity resulting in a cytoprotective effect against stress induced cell death in neural progenitor cells [122, 130]. Moreover, nestin is supposed to be a major determinant in suppression of anti-proliferative activity of glucocorticoid receptors (GR) in undifferentiated tissues by anchoring GRs in cytoplasm but cells lacking nestin accumulate GRs in the nucleus [131]. This mechanism might be responsible for glucocorticoid resistance seen in many cancers.

5.2. Nestin in multiple myeloma

Biological or clinical implications of nestin have not been systematically studied in monoclonal gammopathies or other hematological malignancies so far. The first mention of nestin expression in MM was described in malignant PCs of 5 MM patients and two myeloma cell lines (NOP2 and Liu01) by Liu et al. (2007). Authors referred to the existence of $CD56^{+}$ primary MM cells expressing neuronal markers, such as nestin, neuron-specific enolase and β-tubulin III [83]. Expression of nestin was reported to be stimulated by the Notch signaling pathway in human gliomas [132]. The Notch pathway plays also an important role in survival and proliferation of malignant PCs and negatively affects bone disease in MM [133]. Our recent work proved that nestin protein is a tumor-specific marker for CD138$^+$38$^+$PC of MM patients [110]. Regarding the fact that myeloma PCs appear to be mature, terminally differentiated cells with a low proliferative potential, the presence of nestin is very surprising. Cells expressing nestin may represent a transient population undergoing dedifferentiation into CSC-like phenotype. Providing that PCs possess a truly dedifferentiation potential, the direction of dedifferentiate needs to be elucidated and whether or not this process is reversible.

Unexpectedly, our results showed that nestin was present in one-third of cases in 50% to almost 100% of PCs. Also expression of MAGE genes was found in majority of PCs [102, 134]. Thus, if nestin is expressed in most cells, it means that majority of PCs might gain stem cell features and could repopulate the tumor after therapy. These findings take into question the hierarchical model of myelomagenesis based on the presumption that MM originates from a minor population of MSC. Conversely, stochastic clonal evolution model better describes mechanisms responsible for recurrence of MM. This model suggests that majority of tumor cells have a character of stem cells and may repopulate tumor cells after treatment [135]. Plasticity of PCs better fits the clonal evolution model because weakly proliferating PCs would not be able to quickly repopulate the tumor, therefore we hypothesized that they need to convert into more rapidly dividing cells.

Association of nestin with plasticity of terminally differentiated cell types were demonstrated in the study of metaplastic conversion of mature pancreatic epithelial cells [136] Metaplastic conversion is defined as the replacement of one differentiated cell type by another mature cell type and is frequently associated with an increased risk of subsequent neoplasia. Causes of these changes remains unclear but one possible mechanism may be transdifferantiation of one mature cell type to another one either directly or via an undifferentiated transient cells (rev. in [137]). Means *et al.* (2005) showed that mature acinar cells can convert into ductal epithelia under EGFR signaling. Metaplastic changes were accompanied by occurrence of nestin-positive intermediates similar to nestin-positive precursors observed during early pancreatic development. Results of this study proved a real trans-differentiation potential of mature mammalian cells and indicated that plasticity of mature cell types may play a role in the generation of neoplastic precursors. Whether nestin-positive myeloma PCs might represent particular intermediates undergoing changes leading to the occurrence of cells with a changed (transdifferantiation) or less differentiated phenotype (dedifferentiation), it remains a matter for future research. On the other hand, nestin expression might represent only a byproduct of tumor transformation without any association with myeloma heterogeneity. However, the dynamic character of nestin network plays an important role in the key cell processes such as proliferation, migration and cell survival. Nestin polymerization/ depolymerization influences intracellular signaling, it is likely responsible for rapid redistribution of intracellular proteins, cytoskeletal remodeling and/or might function as a scaffold for protein interactions [122, 125, 129, 130] (**Fig. 4**). All these properties might represent an important prerequisite for myeloma plasticity.

http://dx.doi.org/10.5772/55365

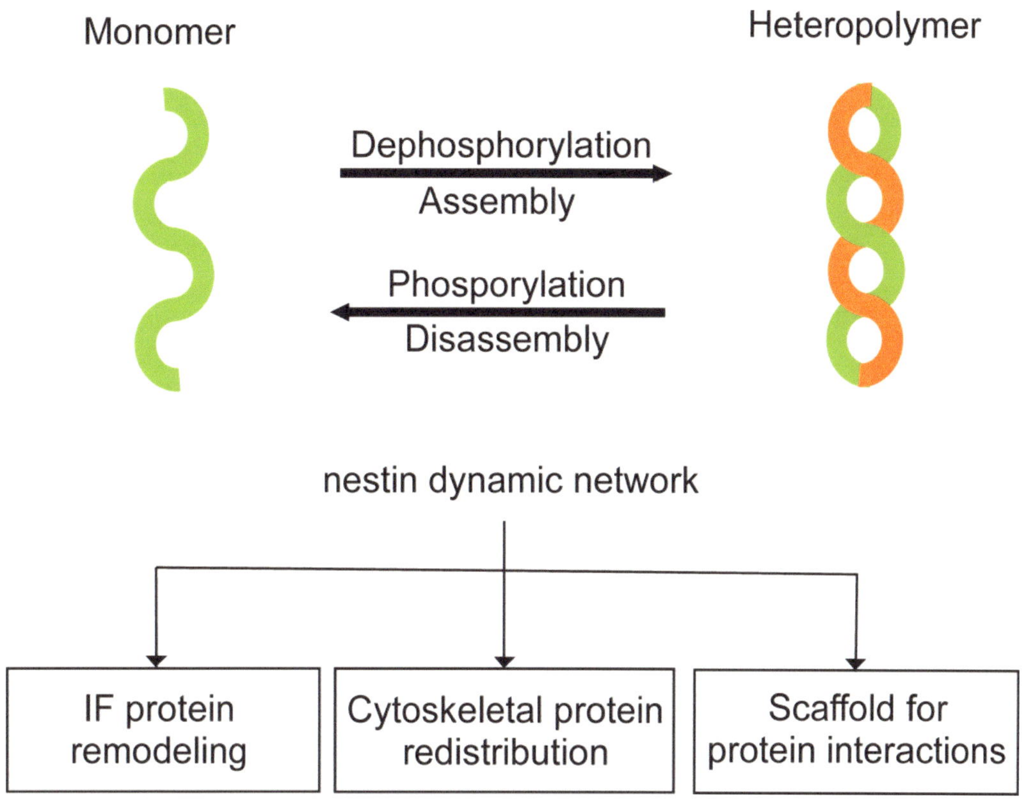

Figure 4. Nestin remodeling and cellular functions

6. Cancer stem cell phenotype and tumor microenvironment

Recent knowledge supports the hypothesis that altered BM microenvironments participate in both mechanisms leading to tumor progression; induction of stem cell features and stimulation of angiogenesis. Cancer stem cell phenotypes may be a plastic state induced in cancer cells depending upon microenvironmental signals, such as hypoxia. Hypoxia has a great impact on the production of angiogenic factors but it is also a crucial regulator of the stem cell phenotype. Several reports have shown that hypoxia and HIFs are involved in maintaining a stem-like state in normal tissues [138]. One example can represent hematopoietic stem cells that reside in regions regulated by oxygen tension. It is hypothesized that undifferentiated phenotypes of these cells relies on HIF activity in hypoxic areas. Hypoxic areas in tumors might be an analog to stem cell niches in normal tissues. Furthermore, Yoshida *et al.* (2009) have shown that hypoxic conditions significantly improve generation of iPSC [139]. Growing knowledge of cancer stem cell biology suggests that hypoxia may act as a critical regulator of the cancer stem cell phenotype.

Series of experiments have demonstrated that hypoxia is responsible for altering the cellular phenotype by causing an increase in proliferation, self-renewal and upregulation of stem cell genes in both CSC and non-CSC. Several groups have shown that hypoxia can regulate histone methylation and thus alter the epigenetic status of cancer cells [140-142]. Tumor hypoxia also correlates with poor outcome of patients. HIFs were shown to induce the embryonal stem cell-like transcriptional program, including *OCT4, NANOG, SOX2, KLF4, MYC,* and microRNA-302 in cancer cell lines of prostate, brain, kidney, cervix, lung, colon, liver and breast tumors [143]. Hypoxic microenvironment potentiates biological effect of Notch signaling in adenocarcinoma of the lung or alters gene expression of neuroblastoma cells to induce more immature phenotype [144, 145]. CD133, a cancer stem cell marker, has been reported by several groups to be upregulated under hypoxic conditions [146, 147]. McCord et al. [2009] showed that hypoxia not only increased the sub-population of glioblastoma cells positive for CD133, but also enhanced expression of other stem cell markers, such as SOX2, OCT4 and nestin [148]. Low oxygen levels induced also HIF-2α expression that can increase the expression of stem cell-associated genes and confer tumorigenic potential to non-CSC [140].

The BM microenvironment of MM is also hypoxic, and myeloma PCs are long term exposed to low oxygen levels. Tumor adaptation to hypoxia is mediated by the production of HIF-1 [149]. Both HIF-1α and HIF-2α have been reported to be activated in MM patients resulting in stimulation of angiogenesis [150]. Although a role of BM microenvironment is generally recognized as a crucial factor affecting myeloma development and support progression, it is surprising that an importance of hypoxic microenvironment for modulation of plasma cell phenotype have never been studied in MM.

7. Conclusion

Despite the achievements of currently used therapy, MM remains difficult to treat. Novel agents such as inhibitors of proteasome or immunomodulatory drugs have prolonged survival of patients with MM and even some patients persist in long term remission. However, there is a little known about mechanisms of myeloma development or the population responsible for the origin and relapse of the disease. Many scientists have tried to explain causes of the relapse but none of their theories have been conclusively confirmed so far. In this review, we explain inconsistencies among particular concepts and the inability to detect cells of origin by the plasticity potential of myeloma PCs. Plasticity of myeloma PCs might be a cause of vast phenotypic heterogeneity of MM and different characteristics of putative myeloma precursors. Under specific signals from aberrant microenvironments, PCs might undergo dedifferentiation/transdifferentiation changing their phenotype profile, and acquire stem cell-like properties to ensure survival. Therefore, an effort to target the specific cell type based only on surface markers is not sufficient. Instead, it is necessary to concentrate on pathologic mechanisms responsible for the transition from non-CSC to CSC like cells. Additional focus on adjacent microenvironments and specific prevention of stem cell-like conversion might increase success of future therapy.

http://dx.doi.org/10.5772/55365

Acknowledgements

This work was supported by grants from The Ministry of Education, Youth and Sports: MSM0021622434 and Czech Science Foundation GAP304/10/1395. The authors would like to thank Andrea Knight for proof reading the manuscript.

Author details

Hana Šváchová[1], Sabina Sevcikova[1] and Roman Hájek[1,2]

*Address all correspondence to: roman.hajek@fno.cz

1 Babak Myeloma Group, Department of Pathological Physiology, Faculty of Medicine, Masaryk University, Czech Republic

2 Faculty of Medicine, University of Ostrava and University Hospital of Ostrava, Czech Republic,, Czech Republic

References

[1] Rajkumar SV, Kyle RA. Multiple myeloma: diagnosis and treatment. Mayo Clin Proc. 2005 Oct;80(10):1371-82.

[2] Richardson P, Anderson K. Thalidomide and dexamethasone: a new standard of care for initial therapy in multiple myeloma. J Clin Oncol. 2006 Jan;24(3):334-6.

[3] Hamburger A, Salmon SE. Primary bioassay of human myeloma stem cells. J Clin Invest. 1977 Oct;60(4):846-54.

[4] Bergsagel DE, Valeriote FA. Growth characteristics of a mouse plasma cell tumor. Cancer Res. 1968 Nov;28(11):2187-96.

[5] Park CH, Bergsagel DE, McCulloch EA. Mouse myeloma tumor stem cells: a primary cell culture assay. J Natl Cancer Inst. 1971 Feb;46(2):411-22.

[6] Matsui W, Huff CA, Wang Q, Malehorn MT, Barber J, Tanhehco Y, et al. Characterization of clonogenic multiple myeloma cells. Blood. 2004 Mar;103(6):2332-6.

[7] Yaccoby S, Epstein J. The proliferative potential of myeloma plasma cells manifest in the SCID-hu host. Blood. 1999 Nov;94(10):3576-82.

[8] Pfeifer S, Perez-Andres M, Ludwig H, Sahota SS, Zojer N. Evaluating the clonal hierarchy in light-chain multiple myeloma: implications against the myeloma stem cell hypothesis. Leukemia. 2011 Jul;25(7):1213-6.

[9] Mellstedt H, Hammarström S, Holm G. Monoclonal lymphocyte population in human plasma cell myeloma. Clin Exp Immunol. 1974 Jul;17(3):371-84.

[10] Vacca A, Ribatti D. Bone marrow angiogenesis in multiple myeloma. Leukemia. 2006 Feb;20(2):193-9.

[11] Laroche M, Brousset P, Ludot I, Mazières B, Thiechart M, Attal M. Increased vascularization in myeloma. Eur J Haematol. 2001 Feb;66(2):89-93.

[12] Sezer O, Niemöller K, Eucker J, Jakob C, Kaufmann O, Zavrski I, et al. Bone marrow microvessel density is a prognostic factor for survival in patients with multiple myeloma. Ann Hematol. 2000 Oct;79(10):574-7.

[13] Rajkumar SV, Leong T, Roche PC, Fonseca R, Dispenzieri A, Lacy MQ, et al. Prognostic value of bone marrow angiogenesis in multiple myeloma. Clin Cancer Res. 2000 Aug;6(8):3111-6.

[14] Rajkumar SV, Mesa RA, Fonseca R, Schroeder G, Plevak MF, Dispenzieri A, et al. Bone marrow angiogenesis in 400 patients with monoclonal gammopathy of undetermined significance, multiple myeloma, and primary amyloidosis. Clin Cancer Res. 2002 Jul;8(7):2210-6.

[15] Liao D, Johnson RS. Hypoxia: a key regulator of angiogenesis in cancer. Cancer Metastasis Rev. 2007 Jun;26(2):281-90.

[16] Brahimi-Horn MC, Chiche J, Pouysségur J. Hypoxia and cancer. J Mol Med (Berl). 2007 Dec;85(12):1301-7.

[17] Colla S, Storti P, Donofrio G, Todoerti K, Bolzoni M, Lazzaretti M, et al. Low bone marrow oxygen tension and hypoxia-inducible factor-1α overexpression characterize patients with multiple myeloma: role on the transcriptional and proangiogenic profiles of CD138(+) cells. Leukemia. 2010 Nov;24(11):1967-70.

[18] Knowles HJ, Athanasou NA. Hypoxia-inducible factor is expressed in giant cell tumour of bone and mediates paracrine effects of hypoxia on monocyte-osteoclast differentiation via induction of VEGF. J Pathol. 2008 May;215(1):56-66.

[19] Bergsagel PL, Masellis Smith A, Belch AR, Pilarski LM. The blood B-cells and bone marrow plasma cells in patients with multiple myeloma share identical IgH rearrangements. Curr Top Microbiol Immunol. 1995;194:17-24.

[20] Bergsagel PL, Smith AM, Szczepek A, Mant MJ, Belch AR, Pilarski LM. In multiple myeloma, clonotypic B lymphocytes are detectable among CD19+ peripheral blood cells expressing CD38, CD56, and monotypic Ig light chain. Blood. 1995 Jan;85(2):436-47.

[21] Szczepek AJ, Bergsagel PL, Axelsson L, Brown CB, Belch AR, Pilarski LM. CD34+ cells in the blood of patients with multiple myeloma express CD19 and IgH mRNA

and have patient-specific IgH VDJ gene rearrangements. Blood. 1997 Mar;89(5): 1824-33.

[22] Jensen GS, Belch AR, Mant MJ, Ruether BA, Yacyshyn BR, Pilarski LM. Expression of multiple beta 1 integrins on circulating monoclonal B cells in patients with multiple myeloma. Am J Hematol. 1993 May;43(1):29-36.

[23] Pilarski LM, Hipperson G, Seeberger K, Pruski E, Coupland RW, Belch AR. Myeloma progenitors in the blood of patients with aggressive or minimal disease: engraftment and self-renewal of primary human myeloma in the bone marrow of NOD SCID mice. Blood. 2000 Feb;95(3):1056-65.

[24] Rasmussen T, Jensen L, Johnsen HE. Levels of circulating CD19+ cells in patients with multiple myeloma. Blood. 2000 Jun;95(12):4020-1.

[25] Kubagawa H, Vogler LB, Capra JD, Conrad ME, Lawton AR, Cooper MD. Studies on the clonal origin of multiple myeloma. Use of individually specific (idiotype) antibodies to trace the oncogenic event to its earliest point of expression in B-cell differentiation. J Exp Med. 1979 Oct;150(4):792-807.

[26] Yaccoby S, Pennisi A, Li X, Dillon SR, Zhan F, Barlogie B, et al. Atacicept (TACI-Ig) inhibits growth of TACI(high) primary myeloma cells in SCID-hu mice and in coculture with osteoclasts. Leukemia. 2008 Feb;22(2):406-13.

[27] Yaccoby S. The phenotypic plasticity of myeloma plasma cells as expressed by dedifferentiation into an immature, resilient, and apoptosis-resistant phenotype. Clin Cancer Res. 2005 Nov;11(21):7599-606.

[28] Yata K, Yaccoby S. The SCID-rab model: a novel in vivo system for primary human myeloma demonstrating growth of CD138-expressing malignant cells. Leukemia. 2004 Nov;18(11):1891-7.

[29] Chiron D, Surget S, Maïga S, Bataille R, Moreau P, Le Gouill S, et al. The peripheral CD138+ population but not the CD138- population contains myeloma clonogenic cells in plasma cell leukaemia patients. Br J Haematol. 2012 Mar;156(5):679-83.

[30] Kim D, Park CY, Medeiros BC, Weissman IL. CD19(-)CD45(low/-)CD38(high)/CD138(+) plasma cells enrich for human tumorigenic myeloma cells. Leukemia. 2012 May.

[31] Pilarski LM, Masellis-Smith A, Szczepek A, Mant MJ, Belch AR. Circulating clonotypic B cells in the biology of multiple myeloma: speculations on the origin of myeloma. Leuk Lymphoma. 1996 Aug;22(5-6):375-83..

[32] Szczepek AJ, Seeberger K, Wizniak J, Mant MJ, Belch AR, Pilarski LM. A high frequency of circulating B cells share clonotypic Ig heavy-chain VDJ rearrangements with autologous bone marrow plasma cells in multiple myeloma, as measured by single-cell and in situ reverse transcriptase-polymerase chain reaction. Blood. 1998 Oct;92(8):2844-55.

[33] Pilarski LM, Jensen GS. Monoclonal circulating B cells in multiple myeloma. A continuously differentiating, possibly invasive, population as defined by expression of CD45 isoforms and adhesion molecules. Hematol Oncol Clin North Am. 1992 Apr; 6(2):297-322.

[34] Jensen GS, Mant MJ, Pilarski LM. Sequential maturation stages of monoclonal B lineage cells from blood, spleen, lymph node, and bone marrow from a terminal myeloma patient. Am J Hematol. 1992 Nov;41(3):199-208.

[35] Conway EJ, Wen J, Feng Y, Mo A, Huang WT, Keever-Taylor CA, et al. Phenotyping studies of clonotypic B lymphocytes from patients with multiple myeloma by flow cytometry. Arch Pathol Lab Med. 2009 Oct;133(10):1594-9.

[36] Billadeau D, Ahmann G, Greipp P, Van Ness B. The bone marrow of multiple myeloma patients contains B cell populations at different stages of differentiation that are clonally related to the malignant plasma cell. J Exp Med. 1993 Sep;178(3):1023-31.

[37] Bakkus MH, Van Riet I, Van Camp B, Thielemans K. Evidence that the clonogenic cell in multiple myeloma originates from a pre-switched but somatically mutated B cell. Br J Haematol. 1994 May;87(1):68-74.

[38] Reiman T, Seeberger K, Taylor BJ, Szczepek AJ, Hanson J, Mant MJ, et al. Persistent preswitch clonotypic myeloma cells correlate with decreased survival: evidence for isotype switching within the myeloma clone. Blood. 2001 Nov;98(9):2791-9.

[39] Matsui W, Wang Q, Barber JP, Brennan S, Smith BD, Borrello I, et al. Clonogenic multiple myeloma progenitors, stem cell properties, and drug resistance. Cancer Res. 2008 Jan;68(1):190-7.

[40] Peacock CD, Wang Q, Gesell GS, Corcoran-Schwartz IM, Jones E, Kim J, et al. Hedgehog signaling maintains a tumor stem cell compartment in multiple myeloma. Proc Natl Acad Sci U S A. 2007 Mar;104(10):4048-53.

[41] Huff CA, Matsui W. Multiple myeloma cancer stem cells. J Clin Oncol. 2008 Jun; 26(17):2895-900.

[42] Loh YS, Mo S, Brown RD, Yamagishi T, Yang S, Joshua DE, et al. Presence of Hoechst low side populations in multiple myeloma. Leuk Lymphoma. 2008 Sep;49(9):1813-6.

[43] Jakubikova J, Adamia S, Kost-Alimova M, Klippel S, Cervi D, Daley JF, et al. Lenalidomide targets clonogenic side population in multiple myeloma: pathophysiologic and clinical implications. Blood. 2011 Apr;117(17):4409-19.

[44] Munshi NC, Anderson KC, Bergsagel PL, Shaughnessy J, Palumbo A, Durie B, et al. Consensus recommendations for risk stratification in multiple myeloma: report of the International Myeloma Workshop Consensus Panel 2. Blood. 2011 May;117(18): 4696-700.

[45] O'Connor BP, Gleeson MW, Noelle RJ, Erickson LD. The rise and fall of long-lived humoral immunity: terminal differentiation of plasma cells in health and disease. Immunol Rev. 2003 Aug;194:61-76.

[46] O'Connor BP, Cascalho M, Noelle RJ. Short-lived and long-lived bone marrow plasma cells are derived from a novel precursor population. J Exp Med. 2002 Mar;195(6):737-45.

[47] Caligaris-Cappio F, Bergui L, Gregoretti MG, Gaidano G, Gaboli M, Schena M, et al. 'Role of bone marrow stromal cells in the growth of human multiple myeloma. Blood. 1991 Jun;77(12):2688-93.

[48] Chen BJ, Epstein J. Circulating clonal lymphocytes in myeloma constitute a minor subpopulation of B cells. Blood. 1996 Mar;87(5):1972-6.

[49] Rasmussen T, Lodahl M, Hancke S, Johnsen HE. In multiple myeloma clonotypic CD38- /CD19+ / CD27+ memory B cells recirculate through bone marrow, peripheral blood and lymph nodes. Leuk Lymphoma. 2004 Jul;45(7):1413-7.

[50] Vescio RA, Cao J, Hong CH, Lee JC, Wu CH, Der Danielian M, et al. Myeloma Ig heavy chain V region sequences reveal prior antigenic selection and marked somatic mutation but no intraclonal diversity. J Immunol. 1995 Sep;155(5):2487-97.

[51] McSweeney PA, Wells DA, Shults KE, Nash RA, Bensinger WI, Buckner CD, et al. Tumor-specific aneuploidy not detected in CD19+ B-lymphoid cells from myeloma patients in a multidimensional flow cytometric analysis. Blood. 1996 Jul;88(2):622-32.

[52] Taylor BJ, Kriangkum J, Pittman JA, Mant MJ, Reiman T, Belch AR, et al. Analysis of clonotypic switch junctions reveals multiple myeloma originates from a single class switch event with ongoing mutation in the isotype-switched progeny. Blood. 2008 Sep;112(5):1894-903.

[53] Trepel M, Martens V, Doll C, Rahlff J, Gösch B, Loges S, et al. Phenotypic detection of clonotypic B cells in multiple myeloma by specific immunoglobulin ligands reveals their rarity in multiple myeloma. PLoS One. 2012;7(2):e31998.

[54] Rasmussen T, Haaber J, Dahl IM, Knudsen LM, Kerndrup GB, Lodahl M, et al. Identification of translocation products but not K-RAS mutations in memory B cells from patients with multiple myeloma. Haematologica. 2010 Oct;95(10):1730-7.

[55] Basak GW, Carrier E. The search for multiple myeloma stem cells: the long and winding road. Biol Blood Marrow Transplant. 2010 May;16(5):587-94.

[56] Corradini P, Voena C, Omedé P, Astolfi M, Boccadoro M, Dalla-Favera R, et al. Detection of circulating tumor cells in multiple myeloma by a PCR-based method. Leukemia. 1993 Nov;7(11):1879-82.

[57] Bergsagel PL, Chesi M, Nardini E, Brents LA, Kirby SL, Kuehl WM. Promiscuous translocations into immunoglobulin heavy chain switch regions in multiple myeloma. Proc Natl Acad Sci U S A. 1996 Nov;93(24):13931-6.

[58] Fenton JA, Pratt G, Rawstron AC, Morgan GJ. Isotype class switching and the pathogenesis of multiple myeloma. Hematol Oncol. 2002 Jun;20(2):75-85.

[59] Nemec P, Kuglík P, Hájek R. (The origin and formation of chromosomal translocations in multiple myeloma). Klin Onkol. 2008;21(2):53-8.

[60] Palumbo A, Battaglio S, Astolfi M, Frieri R, Boccadoro M, Pileri A. Multiple independent immunoglobulin class-switch recombinations occurring within the same clone in myeloma. Br J Haematol. 1992 Dec;82(4):676-80.

[61] Souto-Carneiro MM, Mahadevan V, Takada K, Fritsch-Stork R, Nanki T, Brown M, et al. Alterations in peripheral blood memory B cells in patients with active rheumatoid arthritis are dependent on the action of tumour necrosis factor. Arthritis Res Ther. 2009;11(3):R84.

[62] Tangye SG, Good KL. Human IgM+CD27+ B cells: memory B cells or "memory" B cells? J Immunol. 2007 Jul;179(1):13-9.

[63] Lim SH, Zhang Y, Wang Z, Varadarajan R, Periman P, Esler WV. Rituximab administration following autologous stem cell transplantation for multiple myeloma is associated with severe IgM deficiency. Blood. 2004 Mar;103(5):1971-2.

[64] Musto P, Carella AM, Greco MM, Falcone A, Sanpaolo G, Bodenizza C, et al. Short progression-free survival in myeloma patients receiving rituximab as maintenance therapy after autologous transplantation. Br J Haematol. 2003 Nov;123(4):746-7.

[65] Paíno T, Ocio EM, Paiva B, San-Segundo L, Garayoa M, Gutiérrez NC, et al. CD20 positive cells are undetectable in the majority of multiple myeloma cell lines and are not associated with a cancer stem cell phenotype. Haematologica. 2012 Jul;97(7): 1110-4.

[66] Rossi EA, Rossi DL, Stein R, Goldenberg DM, Chang CH. A bispecific antibody-IFNalpha2b immunocytokine targeting CD20 and HLA-DR is highly toxic to human lymphoma and multiple myeloma cells. Cancer Res. 2010 Oct;70(19):7600-9.

[67] Hosen N, Matsuoka Y, Kishida S, Nakata J, Mizutani Y, Hasegawa K, et al. CD138-negative clonogenic cells are plasma cells but not B cells in some multiple myeloma patients. Leukemia. 2012 Sep;26(9):2135-41.

[68] Christensen JH, Jensen PV, Kristensen IB, Abildgaard N, Lodahl M, Rasmussen T. Characterization of potential CD138 negative myeloma "stem cells". Haematologica. 2012 Jun;97(6):e18-20.

[69] Jourdan M, Ferlin M, Legouffe E, Horvathova M, Liautard J, Rossi JF, et al. The myeloma cell antigen syndecan-1 is lost by apoptotic myeloma cells. Br J Haematol. 1998 Mar;100(4):637-46.

[70] Goodell MA, Brose K, Paradis G, Conner AS, Mulligan RC. Isolation and functional properties of murine hematopoietic stem cells that are replicating in vivo. J Exp Med. 1996 Apr;183(4):1797-806.

[71] Wu C, Alman BA. Side population cells in human cancers. Cancer Lett. 2008 Sep; 268(1):1-9.

[72] Srinivasan V, Sivaramakrishnan H, Karthikeyan B. Detection, isolation and characterization of principal synthetic route indicative impurities in verapamil hydrochloride. Sci Pharm. 2011 Sep;79(3):555-68.

[73] Montanaro F, Liadaki K, Schienda J, Flint A, Gussoni E, Kunkel LM. Demystifying SP cell purification: viability, yield, and phenotype are defined by isolation parameters. Exp Cell Res. 2004 Aug;298(1):144-54.

[74] O'Connor BP, Cascalho M, Noelle RJ. Short-lived and long-lived bone marrow plasma cells are derived from a novel precursor population. J Exp Med. 2002 Mar;195(6): 737-45.

[75] Kukreja A, Hutchinson A, Dhodapkar K, Mazumder A, Vesole D, Angitapalli R, et al. Enhancement of clonogenicity of human multiple myeloma by dendritic cells. J Exp Med. 2006 Aug;203(8):1859-65.

[76] Kumar S, Kimlinger T, Morice W. Immunophenotyping in multiple myeloma and related plasma cell disorders. Best Pract Res Clin Haematol. 2010 Sep;23(3):433-51.

[77] Paiva B, Almeida J, Pérez-Andrés M, Mateo G, López A, Rasillo A, et al. Utility of flow cytometry immunophenotyping in multiple myeloma and other clonal plasma cell-related disorders. Cytometry B Clin Cytom. 2010 Jul;78(4):239-52.

[78] Busslinger M. Transcriptional control of early B cell development. Annu Rev Immunol. 2004;22:55-79.

[79] Calame K. MicroRNA-155 function in B Cells. Immunity. 2007 Dec;27(6):825-7.

[80] Harada H, Kawano MM, Huang N, Harada Y, Iwato K, Tanabe O, et al. Phenotypic difference of normal plasma cells from mature myeloma cells. Blood. 1993 May; 81(10):2658-63.

[81] Mahmoud MS, Huang N, Nobuyoshi M, Lisukov IA, Tanaka H, Kawano MM. Altered expression of Pax-5 gene in human myeloma cells. Blood. 1996 May;87(10): 4311-5.

[82] Nutt SL, Heavey B, Rolink AG, Busslinger M. Commitment to the B-lymphoid lineage depends on the transcription factor Pax5. Nature. 1999 Oct;401(6753):556-62.

[83] Liu S, Otsuyama K, Ma Z, Abroun S, Shamsasenjan K, Amin J, et al. Induction of multilineage markers in human myeloma cells and their down-regulation by interleukin 6. Int J Hematol. 2007 Jan;85(1):49-58.

[84] Allan AL. Cancer Stem Cells in Solid Tumors. Stem Cell Biology and Regenerative Medicine: Springer, 2011; 2011. 475 p.

[85] Takahashi K, Yamanaka S. Induction of pluripotent stem cells from mouse embryonic and adult fibroblast cultures by defined factors. Cell. 2006 Aug;126(4):663-76.

[86] Yu J, Vodyanik MA, Smuga-Otto K, Antosiewicz-Bourget J, Frane JL, Tian S, et al. Induced pluripotent stem cell lines derived from human somatic cells. Science. 2007 Dec;318(5858):1917-20.

[87] Lowry WE, Richter L, Yachechko R, Pyle AD, Tchieu J, Sridharan R, et al. Generation of human induced pluripotent stem cells from dermal fibroblasts. Proc Natl Acad Sci U S A. 2008 Feb;105(8):2883-8.

[88] Park IH, Lerou PH, Zhao R, Huo H, Daley GQ. Generation of human-induced pluripotent stem cells. Nat Protoc. 2008;3(7):1180-6.

[89] Takahashi K, Tanabe K, Ohnuki M, Narita M, Ichisaka T, Tomoda K, et al. Induction of pluripotent stem cells from adult human fibroblasts by defined factors. Cell. 2007 Nov;131(5):861-72.

[90] Hanna J, Markoulaki S, Schorderet P, Carey BW, Beard C, Wernig M, et al. Direct reprogramming of terminally differentiated mature B lymphocytes to pluripotency. Cell. 2008 Apr;133(2):250-64.

[91] Aasen T, Raya A, Barrero MJ, Garreta E, Consiglio A, Gonzalez F, et al. Efficient and rapid generation of induced pluripotent stem cells from human keratinocytes. Nat Biotechnol. 2008 Nov;26(11):1276-84.

[92] Maherali N, Hochedlinger K. Guidelines and techniques for the generation of induced pluripotent stem cells. Cell Stem Cell. 2008 Dec;3(6):595-605.

[93] Aoi T, Yae K, Nakagawa M, Ichisaka T, Okita K, Takahashi K, et al. Generation of pluripotent stem cells from adult mouse liver and stomach cells. Science. 2008 Aug; 321(5889):699-702.

[94] Mani SA, Guo W, Liao MJ, Eaton EN, Ayyanan A, Zhou AY, et al. The epithelial-mesenchymal transition generates cells with properties of stem cells. Cell. 2008 May; 133(4):704-15.

[95] Prindull G, Zipori D. Environmental guidance of normal and tumor cell plasticity: epithelial mesenchymal transitions as a paradigm. Blood. 2004 Apr;103(8):2892-9.

[96] Dhodapkar MV. Immunity to stemness genes in human cancer. Curr Opin Immunol. 2010 Apr;22(2):245-50.

[97] Chaffer CL, Brueckmann I, Scheel C, Kaestli AJ, Wiggins PA, Rodrigues LO, et al. Normal and neoplastic nonstem cells can spontaneously convert to a stem-like state. Proc Natl Acad Sci U S A. 2011 May;108(19):7950-5.

[98] Bergsagel PL, Kuehl WM. Chromosome translocations in multiple myeloma. Oncogene. 2001 Sep;20(40):5611-22.

[99] Greipp PR, San Miguel J, Durie BG, Crowley JJ, Barlogie B, Bladé J, et al. International staging system for multiple myeloma. J Clin Oncol. 2005 May;23(15):3412-20.

[100] Clevers H. Stem cells, asymmetric division and cancer. Nat Genet. 2005 Oct;37(10): 1027-8.

[101] Chesi M, Robbiani DF, Sebag M, Chng WJ, Affer M, Tiedemann R, et al. AID-dependent activation of a MYC transgene induces multiple myeloma in a conditional mouse model of post-germinal center malignancies. Cancer Cell. 2008 Feb;13(2): 167-80.

[102] Jungbluth AA, Ely S, DiLiberto M, Niesvizky R, Williamson B, Frosina D, et al. The cancer-testis antigens CT7 (MAGE-C1) and MAGE-A3/6 are commonly expressed in multiple myeloma and correlate with plasma-cell proliferation. Blood. 2005 Jul; 106(1):167-74.

[103] Schoenhals M, Kassambara A, De Vos J, Hose D, Moreaux J, Klein B. Embryonic stem cell markers expression in cancers. Biochem Biophys Res Commun. 2009 May;383(2): 157-62.

[104] Spisek R, Kukreja A, Chen LC, Matthews P, Mazumder A, Vesole D, et al. Frequent and specific immunity to the embryonal stem cell-associated antigen SOX2 in patients with monoclonal gammopathy. J Exp Med. 2007 Apr;204(4):831-40.

[105] Zhu L, Somlo G, Zhou B, Shao J, Bedell V, Slovak ML, et al. Fibroblast growth factor receptor 3 inhibition by short hairpin RNAs leads to apoptosis in multiple myeloma. Mol Cancer Ther. 2005 May;4(5):787-98.

[106] Dhodapkar MV, Dhodapkar KM. Spontaneous and therapy-induced immunity to pluripotency genes in humans: clinical implications, opportunities and challenges. Cancer Immunol Immunother. 2011 Mar;60(3):413-8.

[107] Bataille R, Pellat-Deceunynck C, Robillard N, Avet-Loiseau H, Harousseau JL, Moreau P. CD117 (c-kit) is aberrantly expressed in a subset of MGUS and multiple myeloma with unexpectedly good prognosis. Leuk Res. 2008 Mar;32(3):379-82..

[108] Schmidt-Hieber M, Pérez-Andrés M, Paiva B, Flores-Montero J, Perez JJ, Gutierrez NC, et al. CD117 expression in gammopathies is associated with an altered maturation of the myeloid and lymphoid hematopoietic cell compartments and favorable disease features. Haematologica. 2011 Feb;96(2):328-32.

[109] Michalczyk K, Ziman M. Nestin structure and predicted function in cellular cytoskeletal organisation. Histol Histopathol. 2005 Apr;20(2):665-71.

[110] Svachova H, Pour L, Sana J, Kovarova L, Raja KR, Hajek R. Stem cell marker nestin is expressed in plasma cells of multiple myeloma patients. Leuk Res. 2011 Aug;35(8): 1008-13.

[111] Blau HM, Brazelton TR, Weimann JM. The evolving concept of a stem cell: entity or function? Cell. 2001 Jun;105(7):829-41.

[112] Hockfield S, McKay RD. Identification of major cell classes in the developing mammalian nervous system. J Neurosci. 1985 Dec;5(12):3310-28.

[113] About I, Laurent-Maquin D, Lendahl U, Mitsiadis TA. Nestin expression in embryonic and adult human teeth under normal and pathological conditions. Am J Pathol. 2000 Jul;157(1):287-95.

[114] Ha Y, Kim TS, Yoon DH, Cho YE, Huh SG, Lee KC. Reinduced expression of developmental proteins (nestin, small heat shock protein) in and around cerebral arteriovenous malformations. Clin Neuropathol. 2003 2003 Sep-Oct;22(5):252-61.

[115] Yamada H, Takano T, Ito Y, Matsuzuka F, Miya A, Kobayashi K, et al. Expression of nestin mRNA is a differentiation marker in thyroid tumors. Cancer Lett. 2009 Jul; 280(1):61-4.

[116] Wiese C, Rolletschek A, Kania G, Blyszczuk P, Tarasov KV, Tarasova Y, et al. Nestin expression--a property of multi-lineage progenitor cells? Cell Mol Life Sci. 2004 Oct; 61(19-20):2510-22.

[117] Cheng L, Jin Z, Liu L, Yan Y, Li T, Zhu X, et al. Characterization and promoter analysis of the mouse nestin gene. FEBS Lett. 2004 May;565(1-3):195-202.

[118] Han DW, Do JT, Araúzo-Bravo MJ, Lee SH, Meissner A, Lee HT, et al. Epigenetic hierarchy governing Nestin expression. Stem Cells. 2009 May;27(5):1088-97.

[119] Guérette D, Khan PA, Savard PE, Vincent M. Molecular evolution of type VI intermediate filament proteins. BMC Evol Biol. 2007;7:164.

[120] Marvin MJ, Dahlstrand J, Lendahl U, McKay RD. A rod end deletion in the intermediate filament protein nestin alters its subcellular localization in neuroepithelial cells of transgenic mice. J Cell Sci. 1998 Jul;111 (Pt 14):1951-61.

[121] Grigelioniené G, Blennow M, Török C, Fried G, Dahlin I, Lendahl U, et al. Cerebrospinal fluid of newborn infants contains a deglycosylated form of the intermediate filament nestin. Pediatr Res. 1996 Dec;40(6):809-14.

[122] Sahlgren CM, Mikhailov A, Hellman J, Chou YH, Lendahl U, Goldman RD, et al. Mitotic reorganization of the intermediate filament protein nestin involves phosphorylation by cdc2 kinase. J Biol Chem. 2001 May;276(19):16456-63.

[123] Sjöberg G, Jiang WQ, Ringertz NR, Lendahl U, Sejersen T. Colocalization of nestin and vimentin/desmin in skeletal muscle cells demonstrated by three-dimensional fluorescence digital imaging microscopy. Exp Cell Res. 1994 Oct;214(2):447-58.

[124] Coulombe PA, Wong P. Cytoplasmic intermediate filaments revealed as dynamic and multipurpose scaffolds. Nat Cell Biol. 2004 Aug;6(8):699-706.

[125] Steinert PM, Chou YH, Prahlad V, Parry DA, Marekov LN, Wu KC, et al. A high molecular weight intermediate filament-associated protein in BHK-21 cells is nestin, a type VI intermediate filament protein. Limited co-assembly in vitro to form heteropolymers with type III vimentin and type IV alpha-internexin. J Biol Chem. 1999 Apr; 274(14):9881-90.

[126] Lendahl U, Zimmerman LB, McKay RD. CNS stem cells express a new class of intermediate filament protein. Cell. 1990 Feb;60(4):585-95.

[127] Kachinsky AM, Dominov JA, Miller JB. Intermediate filaments in cardiac myogenesis: nestin in the developing mouse heart. J Histochem Cytochem. 1995 Aug;43(8): 843-7.

[128] Vaittinen S, Lukka R, Sahlgren C, Hurme T, Rantanen J, Lendahl U, et al. The expression of intermediate filament protein nestin as related to vimentin and desmin in regenerating skeletal muscle. J Neuropathol Exp Neurol. 2001 Jun;60(6):588-97.

[129] Chou YH, Khuon S, Herrmann H, Goldman RD. Nestin promotes the phosphorylation-dependent disassembly of vimentin intermediate filaments during mitosis. Mol Biol Cell. 2003 Apr;14(4):1468-78.

[130] Sahlgren CM, Pallari HM, He T, Chou YH, Goldman RD, Eriksson JE. A nestin scaffold links Cdk5/p35 signaling to oxidant-induced cell death. EMBO J. 2006 Oct; 25(20):4808-19.

[131] Reimer R, Helmbold H, Szalay B, Hagel C, Hohenberg H, Deppert W, et al. Nestin modulates glucocorticoid receptor function by cytoplasmic anchoring. PLoS One. 2009;4(6):e6084.

[132] Shih AH, Holland EC. Notch signaling enhances nestin expression in gliomas. Neoplasia. 2006 Dec;8(12):1072-82.

[133] Schwarzer R, Kaiser M, Acikgoez O, Heider U, Mathas S, Preissner R, et al. Notch inhibition blocks multiple myeloma cell-induced osteoclast activation. Leukemia. 2008 Dec;22(12):2273-7.

[134] Atanackovic D, Hildebrandt Y, Jadczak A, Cao Y, Luetkens T, Meyer S, et al. Cancer-testis antigens MAGE-C1/CT7 and MAGE-A3 promote the survival of multiple myeloma cells. Haematologica. 2010 May;95(5):785-93.

[135] Adams JM, Strasser A. Is tumor growth sustained by rare cancer stem cells or dominant clones? Cancer Res. 2008 Jun;68(11):4018-21.

[136] Means AL, Meszoely IM, Suzuki K, Miyamoto Y, Rustgi AK, Coffey RJ, et al. Pancreatic epithelial plasticity mediated by acinar cell transdifferentiation and generation of nestin-positive intermediates. Development. 2005 Aug;132(16):3767-76.

[137] Tosh D, Slack JM. How cells change their phenotype. Nat Rev Mol Cell Biol. 2002 Mar;3(3):187-94.

[138] Heddleston JM, Li Z, Lathia JD, Bao S, Hjelmeland AB, Rich JN. Hypoxia inducible factors in cancer stem cells. Br J Cancer. 2010 Mar;102(5):789-95.

[139] Yoshida Y, Takahashi K, Okita K, Ichisaka T, Yamanaka S. Hypoxia enhances the generation of induced pluripotent stem cells. Cell Stem Cell. 2009 Sep;5(3):237-41.

[140] Heddleston JM, Li Z, McLendon RE, Hjelmeland AB, Rich JN. The hypoxic microenvironment maintains glioblastoma stem cells and promotes reprogramming towards a cancer stem cell phenotype. Cell Cycle. 2009 Oct;8(20):3274-84.

[141] Pan ZH, Chen ZD. (Hypoxia-inducible factor 1 and prostate cancer). Zhonghua Nan Ke Xue. 2007 Apr;13(4):356-9.

[142] Xia X, Lemieux ME, Li W, Carroll JS, Brown M, Liu XS, et al. Integrative analysis of HIF binding and transactivation reveals its role in maintaining histone methylation homeostasis. Proc Natl Acad Sci U S A. 2009 Mar;106(11):4260-5.

[143] Mathieu J, Zhang Z, Zhou W, Wang AJ, Heddleston JM, Pinna CM, et al. HIF induces human embryonic stem cell markers in cancer cells. Cancer Res. 2011 Jul;71(13): 4640-52.

[144] Chen YQ, Zhao CL, Li W. Effect of hypoxia-inducible factor-1alpha on transcription of survivin in non-small cell lung cancer. J Exp Clin Cancer Res. 2009;28:29.

[145] Jögi A, Øra I, Nilsson H, Lindeheim A, Makino Y, Poellinger L, et al. Hypoxia alters gene expression in human neuroblastoma cells toward an immature and neural crest-like phenotype. Proc Natl Acad Sci U S A. 2002 May;99(10):7021-6.

[146] Seidel S, Garvalov BK, Wirta V, von Stechow L, Schänzer A, Meletis K, et al. A hypoxic niche regulates glioblastoma stem cells through hypoxia inducible factor 2 alpha. Brain. 2010 Apr;133(Pt 4):983-95.

[147] Soeda A, Park M, Lee D, Mintz A, Androutsellis-Theotokis A, McKay RD, et al. Hypoxia promotes expansion of the CD133-positive glioma stem cells through activation of HIF-1alpha. Oncogene. 2009 Nov;28(45):3949-59.

[148] McCord AM, Jamal M, Shankavaram UT, Shankavarum UT, Lang FF, Camphausen K, et al. Physiologic oxygen concentration enhances the stem-like properties of CD133+ human glioblastoma cells in vitro. Mol Cancer Res. 2009 Apr;7(4):489-97.

[149] Hickey MM, Simon MC. Regulation of angiogenesis by hypoxia and hypoxia-inducible factors. Curr Top Dev Biol. 2006;76:217-57.

[150] Martin SK, Diamond P, Williams SA, To LB, Peet DJ, Fujii N, et al. Hypoxia-inducible factor-2 is a novel regulator of aberrant CXCL12 expression in multiple myeloma plasma cells. Haematologica. 2010 May;95(5):776-84.

Chapter 5

Immunophenotyping in Multiple Myeloma and Others Monoclonal Gammopathies

Lucie Rihova, Karthick Raja Muthu Raja,
Luiz Arthur Calheiros Leite, Pavla Vsianska and
Roman Hajek

Additional information is available at the end of the chapter

http://dx.doi.org/10.5772/55938

1. Introduction

Clonal plasma cell disorders (PCD) including mostly monoclonal gammopathy of undetermined significance (MGUS) and multiple myeloma (MM) are characterised by expansion of abnormal (clonal) plasma cells (PCs) producing monoclonal protein (M-protein, MIG). Although multiparametric flow cytometry (MFC) allows identification and characterisation of these neoplastic PCs, this approach is used in routine diagnostics of monoclonal gammopathies (MGs) complementarily, mostly in unusual cases [4-6]. The technological development of flow cytometry (FC) in connection with new findings reveal the need for MFC in clinical analysis of MGs. The main applications of immunophenotypisation in MGs are (1) differential diagnosis, (2) determining the risk of progression in MGUS and asymptomatic MM (aMM), (3) detection of minimal residual disease in treated patients with MM, and (4) analysis of prognostic and/or predictive markers. MFC is also very useful also for research analyses focused on different aspects of B and plasma cell (PC) pathophysiology in term of MG development as well as in looking for potential myeloma-initiating cells. MFC thus should be included as a routine assay in monoclonal gammopathy patients. Clinical significance, usefulness and examples of MFC analyses in MGs are reviewed in this chapter.

2. Flow Cytometry in MGs — Past, present and future

The basic principle of flow cytometry has not changed from the past, it is used for identification of cell subtypes according to their functional and structural properties. Flow cytometers are usually equipped with 2-3 lasers allowing excitation of 6 or more standard fluorochromes and the term multiparametric and/or polychromatic flow cytometry is used for this approach [7]. The classical immunophenotypisation identifies cells based on their size and granularity/ complexity as well as by the "visualization" of antigen-antibody binding. More than 360 antigens are currently known and commercial monoclonal antibodies conjugated with different fluorochromes are widely available.

Flow cytometry has been used in diagnostics of MM since 90th years of the 20th century. Mostly ploidy and proliferative characteristics were analysed, but also the combination of DNA analysis with cytoplasmic immunoglobulin detection was done [8-10]. Discovery of new monoclonal antibodies (MoAb) against PCs helped in the development of immunophenotypisation in MGs [11,12].

It is well known that MFC underestimate the number of PCs when compared to routine morphological evaluation. However, the sensitivity of MFC is similar to light microscopy, results obtained using both approaches correlate and the percentage of PCs provided by MFC is also an independent prognostic factor affecting the overall survival of patients [13]. MFC is precise in detecting even a small number of PCs and together with analysis of expression of selected markers, normal and abnormal PCs could be easily discriminated [4]. So MFC is helpful method for clinical analyses of MGs.

Development of flow cytometry, including powerful instruments with the possibility to analyze many fluorochromes, availability of new dyes and antibodies, together with accessible specific software for complex phenotype analysis, require reviewing of current settings in MG analyses. The shift towards polychromatic analyses should be associated with standardisation and validation of this method as it is necessary to be consistent in providing analyses and reporting results. Recently, the European Myeloma Network (EMN) started to use the Euroflow settings which led to the development of a uniform protocol for the analysis of biological material of MG cases [14].

3. Development and differentiation of B cells as PC precursors

B cells and PCs as their terminally differentiated stage play an essential role in humoral immune response. The antigen-dependent phase of B cell differentiation has been extensively studied for many years. Mature naive B cell ($CD19^{+}CD38^{+/-}CD20^{+}CD27^{-}IgM^{+}IgD^{+}$) pass from the circulation into lymph nodes. Recognition of antigen presented on a follicular dendritic cell together with a costimulatory signal from a specific T lymphocyte causes B cell activation [15,16]. The activated B cell either migrates to extrafolicullar areas where it differentiates into a short term plasma cell or moves into a lymphoid follicle to establish a germinal centre (GC) [17,18]. Massive proliferation of B cell, somatic hypermutation of variable region of Ig chains, isotype switch and subsequent affinity maturation occur in GC [19,20,18,16]. The aim of these processes is to generate B cells able to bind the appropriate antigen with a high affinity. Part of these cells then differentiate into plasmablasts ($CD19^{+}CD38^{++}CD20^{-}$ $CD138^{-}CD27^{+}$) migrating into the bone marrow where they mature into long-lived PCs ($CD38^{+}CD138^{+}$) producing high-

http://dx.doi.org/10.5772/55938

affinity antibodies. The second group differentiate into long-lived memory B cells ($CD19^{+}CD38^{+/-}CD20^{+}CD27^{+}IgM^{-/+}IgD^{-/+}$) [21-23]. Besides these GC derived memory B cells also exist memory B cells lacking their typical marker CD27 ($CD19^{+}CD38^{+/-}CD20^{+}CD27^{-}IgM^{+/-}IgD^{-}$) [24], which likely arise independently from the germinal center reaction [25].

Different maturation stages of B cells give a rise to a variety of B cell lymphoproliferations including post-germinal centre (post-GC) neoplasms [26-28]. Knowledge of B and PC phenotype is thus important for determination of PCD diagnosis and its discrimination from other haematological malignancies (Fig 1).

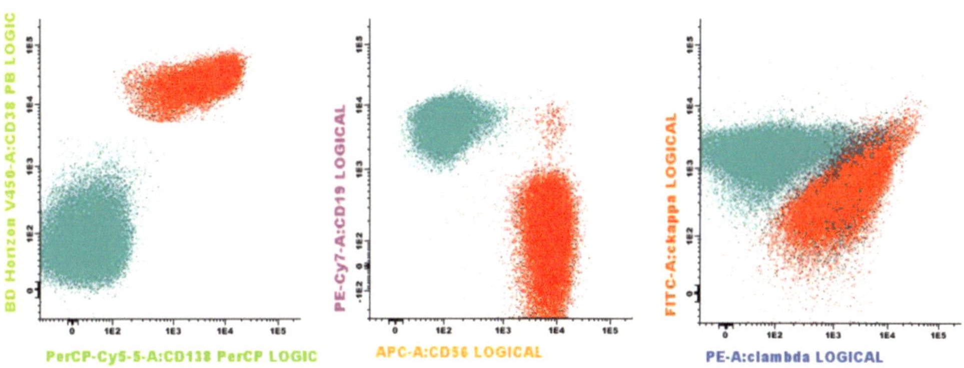

Figure 1. Coexistence of B-CLL and MM. Clone of B-CLL is represented by $CD19^{+}CD38^{-}CD138^{-}$ B cells (turquoise dots) with cytoplasmic κ expression; clone of myeloma cells (red dots) are typical $CD38^{+}CD138^{+}CD56^{+}$ PCs with cytoplasmic λ expression.

4. Identification and immunophenotype of PCs

Syndecan-1 (CD138) is a specific marker of PCs expressed on the surface of both, normal and malignant PCs from their early stages [29]. Expression of CD138 is usually missing and/or is not very intensive on circulating PCs and/or plasmablasts in peripheral blood as well as on immature PCs and/or lymphoplasmacytic cells in bone marrow. Another important marker is CD38, a non-specific marker, whose bright expression (brighter on normal than on abnormal PCs) was used to identify PCs for a long time period. Together with CD138 helps in precise identification of PCs. An important marker for pathological PCs identification is also CD45 which is usually missing on PCs. These surface antigens are still used in analyses, but adding of other antigens is necessary [30,31].

Mostly terminally differentiated clonal $CD38^{++}CD138^{+}CD45^{-}$ PCs are available in MM bone marrow. Relative number of PCs (determined by morphology and/or flow cytometry) corresponds to type of MG, although results could be distorted by dilution of aspirated bone marrow with peripheral blood. Lower amount of PCs is characteristic for MGUS, aMM and/or amyloidosis, on the other hand higher PC infiltration occurs in MM. There is no possibility to determine PC "abnormality" in low-infiltrated cases without detailed phenotype study (Fig 2). There are also circulating pathological PCs in peripheral blood of some myeloma patients, which have usually the same phenotype as bone marrow PCs (mostly $CD56^-$) [32].

Increased absolute (>$2x10^9$/l) and/or relative (>20% of leukocytes) count of peripheral PCs serve as diagnostic criterion of plasma cell leukaemia (PCL). Primary PCL originates *de novo*, but secondary PCL occurs in patients with relapsed/refractory myeloma [33]. Primary PCL is a distinct clinic-pathological entity with different cytogenetic and molecular findings. The clinical course is aggressive with short remissions and survival duration [34].

Mixture of lymphoplasmacytic cell (LPC) subpopulations with different maturity status (from B cells $CD19^+CD20^+CD38^-CD138^-$ to PCs $CD19^+CD20^{+/-}CD38^{+++}CD138^+$) is characteristic for Waldenström macroglobulinemia (WM), where abnormal LPCs multiply out of control and produce large amounts of IgM protein [35]. It is supposed that every MM is precede mostly by non-IgM MGUS, however Waldeström macroglobulinemia and/or B-CLL probably arise from IgM MGUS or monoclonal B cell lymphocytosis (MBL) [36,37].

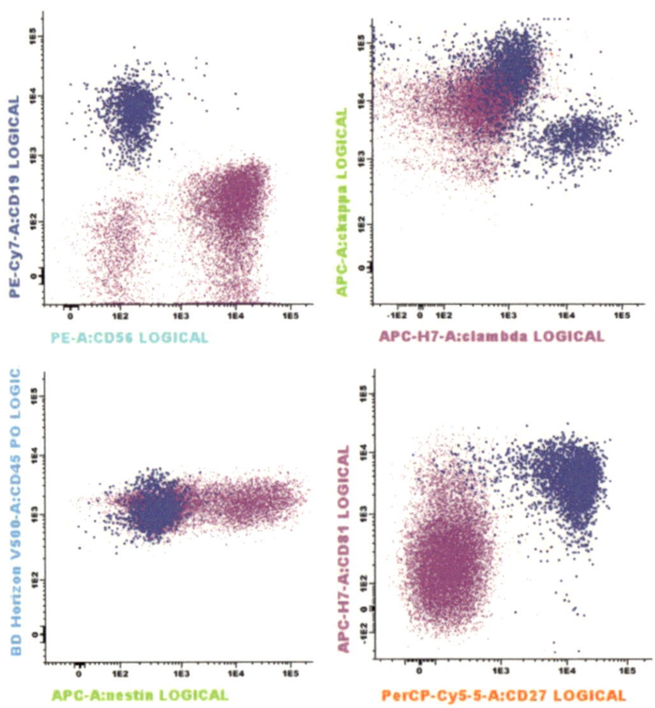

Figure 2. Mixture of polyclonal $CD19^+$ (blue dots) and clonal $CD56^{+/-}$ PCs (violet dots). Heterogeneous expression of CD56 and nestin, positivity for CD45, negativity for CD27 and CD81 was found in clonal $CD38^+CD138^+$ PCs.

Clinically important and necessary antigens allowing discrimination of abnormal from normal PCs are known and listed in Table 1 [4]. Similar antigens were used in Euroflow settings (Table

2) [38]. Detailed information about diagnostic and prognostic value of some interesting markers is mentioned in Table 3. Also other markers should be more and/or less expressed by PCs, mostly without clinical relevance.

Antigen	Normal expression	Abnormal expression	Patients with abnormal expression (%)	Requirement for diagnostics and monitoring
CD19	Positive (>70%)	negative	95%	necessary
CD56	Negative (<15%)	strongly positive	75%	necessary
CD117	Negative (0%)	positive	30%	recommended
CD20	Negative (0%)	positive	30%	recommended
CD28	Weak Positivity (<15%)	strongly positive	15-45%	recommended
CD27	Strong Positivity (100%)	weak/negative	40-50%	recommended

Table 1. List of surface antigens useful for detection of normal and abnormal $CD38^{+}CD138^{+}$ PCs in MGs [4].

Tube/ fluorochrom	Pacific Blue	Pacific Orange	FITC	PE	PerCP-Cy5.5	PE-Cy7	APC	APC-H7
1	CD45	CD138	CD38	CD28	CD27	CD19	CD117	CD81
2	CD45	CD138	CD38	CD28	CD56	β2m	cIgκ	cIgλ

Table 2. EuroFlow PCD classification panel. Tube No.1 is useful for phenotype characterization of PCs and evaluation markers with potential prognostic significance, tube No.2 is used for detection and discrimination of normal PCs from aberrant and clonal PCs [38].

Cluster Designation	Normal distribution and functions	Expression in plasma cells of pre-malignant (MGUS) and malignant stage of myeloma	Diagnostic or prognostic significance	References
CD19	Expressed in all stages of B cells ranging from pro-B cells to PCs	MGUS – normal PCs express CD19 whereas malignant PCs do not MM – only negative or dim CD19 expression on PCs	Facilitate as an identification marker of malignant and physiological PCs in combination with CD56. Patients with "/>5% of normal PCs (CD19+CD56-) had better PFS and OS compared to patients with ≤ 5% of normal PCs. Similarly, presence of "/>5% normal PCs or <95% of malignant PCs in MGUS and asymptomatic MM (AMM/ SMM) predicted better PFS compared to patients with ≤ 5% normal PCs or ≥ 95% of malignant PCS.	[39-41]
CD20	Expressed during maturation process of B cells and mostly absent on PCs	Only few patients express CD20 on their PCs (< one third of patients)	Associated with poor prognosis	[41-43]
CD27	Helps in differentiation of B cells into PCs	MGUS - consistent expression on PCs MM- expression is heterogeneous and intensity of expression is lower compared to MGUS	Lack of CD27 expression associated with shorter PFS and OS	[44,45]
CD28	T cell activation	MGUS– only very few cases express CD28 MM– CD28 expressing PC represents aggressive phenotype and associates always with tumour expansion	Combination of CD28 and CD117 markers identified three groups of patients with different risk. Patients with CD28-CD117+ PCs (good risk group) had better PFS and OS compared to patients with CD28+CD117- PCs (poor risk) and patients with CD28-CD117- or CD28+CD117+ PCs (intermediate risk)	[46]
CD33	Myeloid and monocytic cells	A very few MM cases express CD33 on the surface of PCs	CD33 expression associated with poor OS and higher mortality rate	[47]

Cluster Designation	Normal distribution and functions	Expression in plasma cells of pre-malignant (MGUS) and malignant stage of myeloma	Diagnostic or prognostic significance	References
CD45	CD45 is a leukocyte common antigen and aids in activation and signaling processes of B and T cells	MGUS - heterogeneous distribution of CD45+ normal and CD45- abnormal PCs in bone marrow MM - mostly CD45 negative CD45 expression demonstrates proliferating compartment of normal, reactive and malignant PCs; immature PCs should be CD45+ as well	Patients with CD45 positive expression had better OS than patients with CD45 negative expression	[48-50]
CD56	NK and NKT cells	One of the most valuable markers to define the abnormal phenotype of PCs in PC proliferative disorders including myeloma. Loss of CD56 expression always associated with aggressive phenotype of myeloma cells. Lack of CD56 expression can be frequently found in patients with circulating PCs and extramedullary myeloma.	Possess substantial diagnostic value in PC disorders when combined with CD19 marker. Patients with CD56 negative expression on PCs found to have reduced OS compared to patients with CD56 positive expression. Also, CD56 negative myeloma cases strongly associated with adverse biological parameters.	[30,51-53]
CD81	Expressed on B cells including PCs and regulates CD19 expression	Less than 50% of MM cases express CD81 on PCs and expression is heterogeneous in most of the cases (ranging from 5%-92%)	Patients with CD81 expression on myeloma cells had inferior prognostic outcome (PFS and OS) compared to patients with CD81 negative expression	[54]
CD117	Progenitors of myeloid, erythroid and megakaryocytic lineage; mast cells	MGUS- 50% of cases express CD117 MM- only one third of myeloma cases express CD117	CD117 expression on PCs predicted better outcome in MM patients. Combination of CD117 and CD28 markers delineated MM patients with different risks; CD117 expression is associated with an altered maturation of the myeloid and lymphoid hematopoietic cell compartments and favorable disease features	[46,55-57]

Cluster Designation	Normal distribution and functions	Expression in plasma cells of pre-malignant (MGUS) and malignant stage of myeloma	Diagnostic or prognostic significance	References	
CD138	Plasma cells	Both normal and malignant PCs from MGUS and MM cases express CD138 but the expression of CD38 marker is lower in malignant PCs	Universal marker of PCs and provides basis to quantify or to assess disease burden in PC proliferative disorders	[30]	
CD200	Member of immunoglobulin superfamily and expressed on endothelial cells, neurons, B cells and a subset of T cells	MM - more than 70% of cases do express CD200	MM - more than 70% of cases do express CD200	Absence of CD200 expression on myeloma cells associated with better PFS	[58, 59]
CD221 (insulin like growth factor-1 receptor)	Tyrosine kinase receptor family, expressed widely on all types of cells	MM - more than 70% and 85% of medullary and extramedullary cases express CD221 on the surface of PCs, respectively	Patients with CD221 expression had worse prognosis and CD221+ PCs were associated with adverse cytogenetic abnormalities	[55,60]	
CD229	Signaling lymphocytic activation molecules (SLAM) family member	MM- consistent expression on PCs	Might represent an attractive diagnostic and therapeutic target for MM	[61]	
nestin	Protein of class VI intermediate filaments, marker of multipotent proliferative precursors found in some embryonic and fetal tissues	MGUS - less than 30% express nestin; MM - more than 45% and 80% of medullary and extramedullary myeloma cases express nestin in the cytoplasma of PCs, respectively	Patients with nestin expression should have higher risk to develop extramedullary type of MM	[62]	

Table 3. Myeloma cell specific antigens and their diagnostic and prognostic values. Abbreviations: PFS - progression free survival, OS - overall survival

5. Abnormality vs. clonality of PCs

The most useful antigens allowing basic orientation in context of PC normality are CD19 and CD56 which can allow relatively easy discrimination of immunophenotypically normal ($CD19^+CD56^-$) from immunophenotypically aberrant ($CD19^-CD56^+$) PCs [63-65]. As was verified by cytoplasmic analysis of immunoglobulin light chains kappa and lambda, this discrimination should be used just for orientation and does not have to correspond to a real number of polyclonal and clonal PCs, especially in unusual cases and/or time after treatment.

http://dx.doi.org/10.5772/55938

Thus polychromatic FC (minimum of 6 markers, but usually 8 markers) is required for sufficient PC analysis and combination of surface and intracellular antigens is necessary for identification and clonality assessment of PCs [66-68]. Only a limited number of cases requires more than 8 markers to detect a small clonal subpopulation of PCs on the prevailing background of polyclonal PCs. Use of marker with a known aberrant expression on analysed PCs (CD28, CD117 etc.) could help in precise identification of clonal PCs. Marker CD27 should be useful as loss of this antigen should reveal clonal PCs (Fig 3). Together with analysis of a sufficient number of PCs, the sensitivity of polychromatic FC should reach the sensitivity of the PCR approach [5,67].

6. Clinical application of flow cytometry in MGs

FC should be used not only for assessment of PCs in peripheral blood (PB) and/or bone marrow (BM), but in simultaneous analysis of 8 markers on a single cell could identify the type of PCs that has clinical and predictive value.

6.1. Differential diagnostics

Identification and enumeration of PCs is as important as discrimination between normal polyclonal PCs in reactive plasmocytosis and clonal PCs in plasma cell disorders (MGUS, MM, PCL, extramedullary plasmocytoma) [4]. It was found that BM of MGUS cases contained a mixture of polyclonal PCs with normal phenotype and clonal PCs with aberrant phenotype, on the other hand there is a majority of clonal PCs in MM [63,65]. Presence of more than 5% normal PCs in BM should be used as a cut-off value for differentiation between MGUS and MM [40]. Surprisingly there were found symptomatic MM patients with more than 5% normal PCs in BM, these should be signed as "MGUS-like MM" and have a low incidence of high-risk cytogenetic abnormalities with a longer progression-free survival and longer overall survival as well [39]. There are clonal non-myelomatous PCs present in Waldenström macroglobulinemia (WM) so careful PC analysis should be done in these patients especially when they have low number of PCs [35]. Discrimination of myelomatous from non-myelomatous PCs then should help in determination of other lymphoproliferations [28].

6.2. Determination of the progression risk in MGUS and MM

Conventional parameters related to the higher risk of progression of MGUS into MM are monoclonal Ig level (MIG) > 15 g/l and non-IgG isotype of MIG. Even so, a new parameter is serum free light chain (FLC) ratio. These parameters were used for risk stratification model [69]. Simultaneously evolving and non-evolving theory of MGUS type, based on evolutionary pattern of MIG (increasing vs. stable) was published [70]. Mentioned parameters are important in patient monitoring for decades, but FC approach based on pathological PCs enumeration is quicker with a better predictive value [40]. Finding ≥95 % pathological PCs (from all PCs) is an independent parameter with a predictive value, in term of risk of progression MGUS and/or a MM into symptomatic form. When compared FC results with a parameter describing evolution of monoclonal component, the risk of progression was better described by immunophenotypisation [71]. Multiparametric FC is thus capable to distinguish patients which need more frequent monitoring and which need to start treatment earlier than usual. There is still not any marker allowing discrimination between benign MGUS and its malignant form at this moment.

6.3. Prognostic markers in MGs

Determination of immunophenotype should be used not only for discrimination of normal and pathological PCs, but it has also prognostic value. The loss of CD56 (neural cell adhesion molecule, NCAM) should be joined with extramedullary spread [72]. An association between the phenotype profile and cytogenetic abnormalities was found. Expression of CD19 and CD28 and/or absence of the CD117 on pathological PCs are joined with significantly shorter time without progression and overall survival in transplanted patients [46]. Expression of CD28 correlated with t(14;16) and del(17p), on the other hand no presence of CD117 was joined with t(4;14) and del(13q). The analysis combining both CD28 and CD117 was able to divide patients into 3 risk groups with different time without progression and overall survival. The correlation of CD117 expression with hyperdiploidy was found as well [73]. The expression of CD117 on PCs is associated with changes in production of haematopoietic stem cells from BM, lead to a decreasing number of neutrophils in PB and the presence of normal PCs in BM [57]. Recently, a rare MM case was described with PCs phenotype: $CD19^{+}CD56^{-}CD20^{+}CD22^{+}CD28^{+}CD33^{+}CD117^{+}HLA\text{-}DR^{+}$. Moreover, the cytogenetic analysis of this case revealed a hyperdiploid karyotype and no rearrangement of the IgH gene or deletion of 13q14 [74]. The very important genetic change in MM is loss of the gene for CD27 which is linked with clinically aggressive disease, but in about 50% of MM is expression of CD27 preserved and these patients have better prognosis [44]. Probably the best prognostic information until now serves a combination of two independent parameters: the presence of high-risk cytogenetics by FISH and persistent minimal residual disease evaluated by multiparameter flow cytometry at day +100 after autologous transplantation. These two parameters were able to identify patients in complete remission at risk of early progression [75]. The important thing is that these two methods are available in most hospitals taking care of patients with haematological malignancies.

6.4. Minimal residual disease analysis

It is known that conventional parameters (% PCs, MIG level) are not sensitive enough for analysis of treatment response in MM patients. As FC is applicable up to 80-90% of patients, this method is able to reach the sensitivity of allelic-specific oligonucleotide (ASO)-PCR (sensitivity 10^{-4} for FC vs. 10^{-5} for PCR) and is less time and monetary consuming as well. Hence FC looks as the optimal method for minimal residual disease (MRD) assessment after any treatment [76,77]. The advantage of FC in MRD analysis is the versatility of used markers allowing assessment of normal and abnormal PCs (CD19/CD56), removing the need to know the original phenotype of PCs before treatment. MRD negativity proved by FC (detection $<10^{-4}$ myeloma PC within all nucleated cells) was more informative then

http://dx.doi.org/10.5772/55938

positive immunofixation (IF) after autologous transplantation (regarding to time to progression and overall survival), so FC is sufficiently sensitive method and should be used for routine MRD analysis [78].

6.4.1 Better definition of complete remission

Using new treatment protocols led The International Myeloma Working Group (IMWG) to review treatment response criteria. There was included also FC analysis in the assessment of stringent complete response (sCR), more precisely the absence of phenotypically aberrant PCs in 3000 PC analysed by multiparametric FC (≥ 4 colours) [79]. Criteria of MRD level assessment are changing nowadays as newer more efficient treatment protocols are available and FC has technically developed. When used flow cytometry for confirmation of (s)CR, the new term „immunophenotype remission (iCR)" - a state without presence of any clonal PCs should be used [79, 80]. The evidence suggests that the 4-colour FC is not sufficiently sensitive for confirmation of iCR and standardized polychromatic flow cytometry is the best approach (Fig 3).

7. Conclusion

Flow cytometry analysis was performed only in a limited number of subjects with monoclonal gammopathies in the late 1990's and early 2000's. During the past decade and present, many analyses showed importance of MFC in differential diagnostics and monitoring (management) of plasma cell diseases. The MFC has developed significantly and with better understanding of PC pathophysiology is the mandatory diagnostic tool which should be included as a routine assay in monoclonal gammopathy patients.

Author details

Lucie Rihova[1,2], Karthick Raja Muthu Raja[2,3], Luiz Arthur Calheiros Leite[4], Pavla Vsianska[1,2,3] and Roman Hajek[1,2,5]

1 Department of Clinical Hematology, University Hospital Brno, Brno, Czech Republic

2 Babak Myeloma Group, Department of Pathological Physiology, Faculty of Medicine, Masaryk University, Brno, Czech Republic

3 Department of Experimental Biology, Faculty of Science, Masaryk University, Brno, Czech Republic

4 Department of Biochemistry, Federal University of Pernambuco, Brazil

5 Department of Clinical Hematology, University Hospital Ostrava and Faculty of Medicine, Ostrava, Czech Republic

References

[1] Orfao A., Ruiz-Arguelles A., Lacombe F. Flow cytometry: its applications in hematology. Haematologica 1995;80(1) 69-81.

[2] Davis B.H., Holden J.T., Bene M.C. et al. 2006 Bethesda International Consensus recommendations on the flow cytometric immunophenotypic analysis of hematolymphoid neoplasia: medical indications. Cytometry B Clin Cytom 2007;72 Suppl 1:S5-13.

[3] Craig F.E., Foon K.A. Flow cytometric immunophenotyping for hematologic neoplasms. Blood 2008;111(8) 3941-3967.

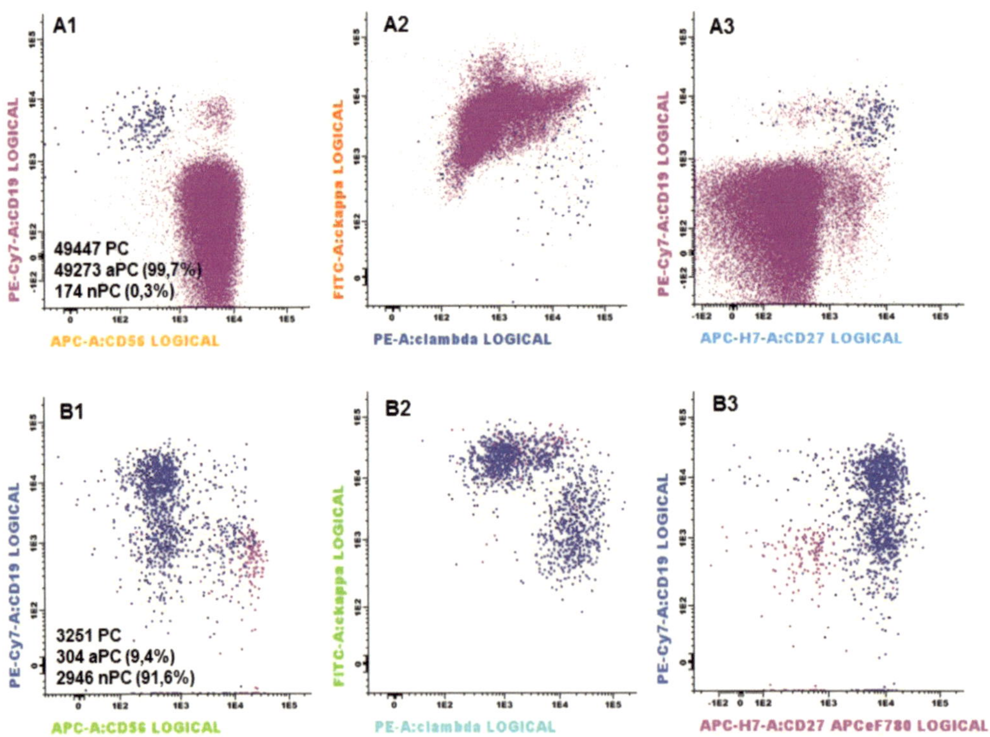

Figure 3. Polychromatic analysis of PC phenotype and clonality. A1-A3:Majority of clonal CD56^{+}ckappa^{+}CD27^{-} PCs (99,7% of aPCs according to clonality assessment) is visible in MM patient at the time of diagnosis (purple dots). B1-B3:Mixture of clonal (aPCs, purple dots) and polyclonal PCs (nPCs, blue dots) is visible at 3rd month after transplantion; assessment of % aPCs is possible only when CD27 is used as some nPCs are CD19^{-} and/or CD56^{+} as well.

[4] Rawstron A.C., Orfao A., Beksac M. et al. Report of the European Myeloma Network on multiparametric flow cytometry in multiple myeloma and related disorders. Haematologica 2008;93(3) 431-438.

[5] Paiva B., Almeida J., Pérez-Andrés M. et al. Utility of flow cytometry immunophenotyping in multiple myeloma and other clonal plasma cell-related disorders. Cytometry B Clin Cytom 2010; 78(4) 239–252.

[6] Kumar S., Kimlinger T., Morice W. Immunophenotyping in multiple myeloma and related plasma cell disorders. Best Pract Res Clin Haematol 2010;23(3) 433-451.

[7] Chattopadhyay P.K., Hogerkorp C.M., Roederer M. A chromatic explosion: the development and future of multiparameter flow cytometry. Immunology 2008;125(4) 441-449.

[8] Latreille J., Barlogie B., Johnston D. et al. Ploidy and proliferative characteristics in monoclonal gammopathies. Blood 1982;59(1) 43-51.

[9] Barlogie B., Alexanian R., Gehan E.A. et al. Marrow cytometry and prognosis in myeloma. J Clin Invest 1983;72(3) 853-861.

[10] Zeile G. Intracytoplasmic immunofluorescence in multiple myeloma. Cytometry 1980;1(1) 37-4.

[11] King M.A., Nelson D.S. Tumor cell heterogeneity in multiple myeloma: antigenic, morphologic, and functional studies of cells from blood and bone marrow. Blood 1989;73(7) 1925-1935.

[12] Terstappen L.W., Johnsen S., Segers-Nolten I.M. et al. Identification and characterization of plasma cells in normal human bone marrow by high-resolution flow cytometry. Blood 1990;76(9) 1739-1747.

[13] Paiva B., Vidriales M.B., Pérez J.J. et al. Multiparameter flow cytometry quantification of bone marrow plasma cells at diagnosis provides more prognostic information than morphological assessment in myeloma patients. Haematologica 2009; 94(11) 1599-1602.

[14] van Dongen J.J., Orfao A. EuroFlow Consortium. EuroFlow: Resetting leukemia and lymphoma immunophenotyping. Basis for companion diagnostics and personalized medicine. Leukemia 2012;26(9) 1899-1907.

[15] Okada T., Miller M.J., Parker I. et al. Antigen-engaged B cells undergo chemotaxis toward the T zone and form motile conjugates with helper T cells. PLoS Biol 2005;3(6) e150.

[16] Perez-Andres M., Paiva B., Nieto W.G. et al. Primary Health Care Group of Salamanca for the Study of MBL. Human peripheral blood B-cell compartments: a crossroad in B-cell traffic. Cytometry B Clin Cytom 2010; 78 (Suppl 1) S47–S60.

[17] Liu Y.J., Zhang J., Lane P.J. et al. Sites of specific B cell activation in primary and secondary responses to T cell-dependent and T cell-independent antigens. Eur J Immunol 1991;21(12) 2951-2962.

[18] Allen C.D., Okada T., Cyster J.G. Germinal-center organization and cellular dynamics. Immunity 2007;27(2) 190-202.

[19] Benson M.J., Erickson L.D., Gleeson M.W. et al. Affinity of antigen encounter and other early B-cell signals determine B-cell fate. Curr Opin Immunol 2007;19(3) 275-280.

[20] Dal Porto J.M., Haberman A.M., Shlomchik M.J. et al. Antigen drives very low affinity B cells to become plasmacytes and enter germinal centers. J Immunol 1998;161(10) 5373-5381.

[21] Agematsu K., Hokibara S., Nagumo H. et al. CD27: a memory B-cell marker. Immunol Today 2000;21(5) 204-206.

[22] Klein U., Rajewsky K., Küppers R. Human immunoglobulin (Ig)M+IgD+ peripheral blood B cells expressing the CD27 cell surface antigen carry somatically mutated variable region genes: CD27 as a general marker for somatically mutated (memory) B cells. J Exp Med 1998;188(9) 1679-1689.

[23] Blink E.J., Light A., Kallies A. et al. Early appearance of germinal center-derived memory B cells and plasma cells in blood after primary immunization. J Exp Med 2005;201(4) 545-554.

[24] Fecteau J.F., Côté G., Néron S. A new memory CD27-IgG+ B cell population in peripheral blood expressing VH genes with low frequency of somatic mutation. J Immunol 2006;177(6) 3728-3736.

[25] Taylor J.J., Jenkins M.K., Pape K.A. Heterogeneity in the differentiation and function of memory B cells. Trends Immunol 2012;33(12) 590-597.

[26] Jaffe E.S. The 2008 WHO classification of lymphomas: implications for clinical practice and translational research. Hematology Am Soc Hematol Educ Program 2009:523-531.

[27] Campo E., Swerdlow S.H., Harris N.L. et al. The 2008 WHO classification of lymphoid neoplasms and beyond: evolving concepts and practical applications. Blood 2011;117(19) 5019-5032.

[28] Meyerson H.J., Bailey J., Miedler J. et al. Marginal zone B cell lymphomas with extensive plasmacytic differentiation are neoplasms of precursor plasma cells. Cytometry B Clin Cytom 2011; 80(2) 71–82.

[29] Sanderson R.D., Lalor P., Bernfield M. B lymphocytes express and lose syndecan at specific stages of differentiation. Cell Regul 1989;1(1) 27-35.

[30] Bataille R., Jégo G., Robillard N. et al. The phenotype of normal, reactive and malignant plasma cells. Identification of "many and multiple myelomas" and of new targets for myeloma therapy. Haematologica 2006; 91(9) 1234–1240.

[31] Raja K.R., Kovarova L., Hajek R. Review of phenotypic markers used in flow cytometric analysis of MGUS and MM, and applicability of flow cytometry in other plasma cell disorders. Br J Haematol 2010;149(3) 334-351.

[32] García-Sanz R., Orfão A., González M. et al. Primary plasma cell leukemia: clinical, immunophenotypic, DNA ploidy, and cytogenetic characteristics. Blood 1999;93(3) 1032-1037.

[33] Kyle R.A., Maldonado J.E., Bayrd E.D. Plasma cell leukemia. Report on 17 cases. Arch Intern Med 1974.133:813.

[34] Fernández de Larrea C., Kyle R.A., Durie B.G. et al. Plasma cell leukemia: consensus statement on diagnostic requirements, response criteria and treatment recommendations by the International Myeloma Working Group. Leukemia. 2012.

[35] Morice W.G., Chen D., Kurtin P.J. et al. Novel immunophenotypic features of marrow lymphoplasmacytic lymphoma and correlation with Waldenström's macroglobulinemia. Mod Pathol 2009; 22(6) 807-816.

[36] Landgren O., Kyle R.A., Pfeiffer R.M. et al. Monoclonal gammopathy of undetermined significance (MGUS) consistently precedes multiple myeloma: a prospective study. Blood 2009;113(22) 5412-5417.

[37] McMaster M.L., Caporaso N. Waldenström macroglobulinaemia and IgM monoclonal gammopathy of undetermined significance: emerging understanding of a potential precursor condition. Br J Haematol 2007;139(5) 663-671.

[38] van Dongen J.J., Lhermitte L., Böttcher S. et al. EuroFlow antibody panels for standardized n-dimensional flow cytometric immunophenotyping of normal, reactive and malignant leukocytes. Leukemia.2012;26(9) 1908-1975.

[39] Paiva B., Vidriales M.B., Mateo G. et al. The persistence of immunophenotypically normal residual bone marrow plasma cells at diagnosis identifies a good prognostic subgroup of symptomatic multiple myeloma patients. Blood 2009;114(20) 4369-4372.

[40] Pérez-Persona E., Vidriales M.B., Mateo G. et al. New criteria to identify risk of progression in monoclonal gammopathy of uncertain significance and smoldering multiple myeloma based on multiparameter flow cytometry analysis of bone marrow plasma cells. Blood 2007; 110(7) 2586-2592.

[41] Uckun F.M. Regulation of human B-cell ontogeny. Blood 1990;76(10) 1908-1023.

[42] Robillard N., Avet-Loiseau H., Garand R. et al. CD20 is associated with a small mature plasma cell morphology and t(11;14) in multiple myeloma. Blood 2003;102(3) 1070-1081.

[43] San Miguel J.F., González M., Gascón A. et al. Immunophenotypic heterogeneity of multiple myeloma: influence on the biology and clinical course of the disease. Castellano-Leones (Spain) Cooperative Group for the Study of Monoclonal Gammopathies. Br J Haematol 1991;77(2) 185-190.

[44] Guikema J.E., Hovenga S., Vellenga E. et al. CD27 is heterogeneously expressed in multiple myeloma: low CD27 expression in patients with high-risk disease. Br J Haematol 2003;121(1) 36-43.

[45] Moreau P., Robillard N., Jégo G. et al. Lack of CD27 in myeloma delineates different presentation and outcome. Br J Haematol 2006;132(2) 168-170.

[46] Mateo G., Montalbán M.A., Vidriales M.B. et al. Prognostic value of immunophenotyping in multiple myeloma: a study by the PETHEMA/GEM cooperative study groups on patients uniformly treated with high-dose therapy. J Clin Oncol 2008; 26(16) 2737-2744.

[47] Sahara N., Ohnishi K., Ono T. et al. Clinicopathological and prognostic characteristics of CD33-positive multiple myeloma. Eur J Haematol 2006;77(1) 14-18.

[48] Kumar S., Rajkumar S.V. et al. Prognostic value of circulating plasma cells in monoclonal gammopathy of undetermined significance. J Clin Oncol 2005;23(24) 5668-5674.

[49] Moreau P., Robillard N., Avet-Loiseau H. et al. Patients with CD45 negative multiple myeloma receiving high-dose therapy have a shorter survival than those with CD45 positive multiple myeloma. Haematologica 2004;89(5) 547-551.

[50] Guikema J.E., Hovenga S., Vellenga E. et al. Heterogeneity in the multiple myeloma tumor clone. Leuk Lymphoma 2004;45(5) 857-871.

[51] Pellat-Deceunynck C., Barillé S., Jego G. et al. The absence of CD56 (NCAM) on malignant plasma cells is a hallmark of plasma cell leukemia and of a special subset of multiple myeloma. Leukemia 1998;12(12) 1977-1982.

[52] Sahara N., Takeshita A. Prognostic significance of surface markers expressed in multiple myeloma: CD56 and other antigens. Leuk Lymphoma 2004;45(1) 61-65.

[53] Van Camp B., Durie B.G., Spier C. et al. Plasma cells in multiple myeloma express a natural killer cell-associated antigen: CD56 (NKH-1, Leu-19). Blood 1990;76(2) 377-382.

[54] Paiva B., Gutiérrez N.C., Chen X. et al. Clinical significance of CD81 expression by clonal plasma cells in high-risk smoldering and symptomatic multiple myeloma patients. Leukemia 2012;26(8) 1862-1869.

[55] Bataille R., Pellat-Deceunynck C., Robillard N. et al. CD117 (c-kit) is aberrantly expressed in a subset of MGUS and multiple myeloma with unexpectedly good prognosis. Leuk Res 2008; 32(3) 379–382.

[56] Kraj M., Pogłód R., Kopeć-Szlezak J. et al. C-kit receptor (CD117) expression on plasma cells in monoclonal gammopathies. Leuk Lymphoma 2004;45(11) 2281-2289.

[57] Schmidt-Hieber M., Pérez-Andrés M., Paiva B. et al. CD117 expression in gammopathies is associated with an altered maturation of the myeloid and lymphoid hematopoietic cell compartments and favorable disease features. Haematologica 2011;96(2) 328-332.

[58] Moreaux J., Hose D., Reme T. et al. CD200 is a new prognostic factor in multiple myeloma. Blood 2006;108(13) 4194-4197.

[59] Alapat D., Coviello-Malle J., Owens R. et al. Diagnostic usefulness and prognostic impact of CD200 expression in lymphoid malignancies and plasma cell myeloma. Am J Clin Pathol 2012;137(1) 93-100.

[60] Bataille R., Robillard N., Avet-Loiseau H. et al. CD221 (IGF-1R) is aberrantly expressed in multiple myeloma, in relation to disease severity. Haematologica 2005;90(5) 706-7.

[61] Atanackovic D., Panse J., Hildebrandt Y. et al. Surface molecule CD229 as a novel target for the diagnosis and treatment of multiple myeloma. Haematologica 2011;96(10) 1512-1520.

[62] Svachova H., Pour L., Sana J. et al. Stem cell marker nestin is expressed in plasma cells of multiple myeloma patients. Leuk Res 2011;35(8) 1008-1013.

[63] Ocqueteau M., Orfao A., Almeida J. et al. Immunophenotypic characterization of plasma cells from monoclonal gammopathy of undetermined significance patients. Implications for the differential diagnosis between MGUS and multiple myeloma. Am J Pathol 1998;152(6)1655-1665.

[64] Sezer O., Heider U., Zavrski I. et al. Differentiation of monoclonal gammopathy of undetermined significance and multiple myeloma using flow cytometric characteristics of plasma cells. Haematologica 2001;86(8) 837-843.

[65] Kovarova.L, Buresova I., Buchler T. et al. Phenotype of plasma cells in multiple myeloma and monoclonal gammopathy of undetermined significance. Neoplasma 2009;56(6) 526-532.

[66] de Tute R.M., Jack A.S., Child J.A. et al. A single-tube six-colour flow cytometry screening assay for the detection of minimal residual disease in myeloma. Leukemia 2007;21(9) 2046-2049.

[67] Kovarova L., Varmuzova T., Zarbochova P. et al. Flow cytometry in monoclonal gammopathies. Klin Onkol 2011;24 Suppl:S24-29.

[68] Peceliunas V., Janiulioniene A., Matuzeviciene R. et al. Six color flow cytometry detects plasma cells expressing aberrant immunophenotype in bone marrow of healthy donors. Cytometry B Clin Cytom 2011;80(5) 318-323.

[69] Rajkumar S.V., Kyle R.A., Therneau T.M. et al. Serum free light chain ratio is an independent risk factor for progression in monoclonal gammopathy of undetermined significance. Blood 2005;106(3) 812-817.

[70] Rosiñol L., Cibeira M.T., Montoto S. et al.Monoclonal gammopathy of undetermined significance: predictors of malignant transformation and recognition of an evolving type characterized by a progressive increase in M protein size. Mayo Clin Proc 2007;82(4) 428-434.

[71] Pérez-Persona E., Mateo G., García-Sanz R. et al. Risk of progression in smouldering myeloma and monoclonal gammopathies of unknown significance: comparative analysis of the evolution of monoclonal component and multiparameter flow cytometry of bone marrow plasma cells. Br J Haematol 2010; 148(1) 110–114.

[72] Bladé J., Fernández de Larrea C., Rosiñol L. et al. Soft-tissue plasmacytomas in multiple myeloma: incidence, mechanisms of extramedullary spread, and treatment approach. J Clin Oncol 2011;29(28) 3805-3812.

[73] Kovarova L., Buresova I., Muthu Raja K.R. et al. Association of plasma cell phenotype with cytogenetic findings in multiple myeloma. In 15th EHA. Barcelona 2010; 95[suppl. 2]:137.

[74] Leite L.A.C., Kerbary D.M.B., Kimura E. et al. Multiples aberrant phenotypes in multiple myeloma patient expressing CD56-, CD28+,CD19+. Rev. Bras. Hematol. Hemoter 2012;34(1) 66-67.

[75] Paiva B., Gutiérrez N.C., Rosiñol L. et al. High-risk cytogenetics and persistent minimal residual disease by multiparameter flow cytometry predict unsustained complete response after autologous stem cell transplantation in multiple myeloma. Blood 2012;119(3) 687-691.

[76] Rawstron A.C., Davies F.E., DasGupta R. et al. Flow cytometric disease monitoring in multiple myeloma: the relationship between normal and neoplastic plasma cells predicts outcome after transplantation. Blood 2002;100(9) 3095–3100.

[77] Sarasquete M.E., García-Sanz R., González D. et al. Minimal residual disease monitoring in multiple myeloma: a comparison between allelic-specific oligonucleotide real-time quantitative polymerase chain reaction and flow cytometry. Haematologica 2005; 90(10)1365–1372.

[78] Paiva B., Vidriales M.B., Cerveró. J et al. Multiparameter flow cytometric remission is the most relevant prognostic factor for multiple myelomapatients who undergo autologous stem cell transplantation. Blood 2008;112(10) 4017-4023.

[79] Rajkumar S.V., Harousseau J.L., Durie B. et al. Consensus recommendations for the uniform reporting of clinical trials: report of the International Myeloma Workshop Consensus Panel 1. Blood 2011; 117(18) 4691–4695.

[80] Hajek et al. Diagnostika a léčba mnohočetného myelomu. Transfuze a hematologie dnes. 2012;Suppl1.

Chapter 6

Monoclonal Gammopathy of Undetermined Significance

Magdalena Patricia Cortés, Rocío Alvarez,
Jessica Maldonado, Raúl Vinet and Katherine Barría

Additional information is available at the end of the chapter

http://dx.doi.org/10.5772/56138

1. Introduction

Monoclonal gammopathy of undetermined significance (MGUS) is an asymptomatic plasma cell dyscrasia, present in 3.2% of white people over 50 years of age [1], which converts to multiple myeloma (MM) or related disorders at a rate of just 1% a year [2], an incurable malignancy of plasma cells. While MM is the prototypical monoclonal gammopathy, the most common is MGUS [3].

Monoclonal gammopathies are a heterogeneous group of disorders characterized by the stable or progressive proliferation of an abnormal clone of plasma cells that continue producing antibodies [4]. But because these immunoglobulin proteins are abnormal and monoclonal (identical copies of each other), these offer no protection against infections and can damage the kidney. This monoclonal immunoglobulin is called M-protein. Each basic unit is a monomeric immunoglobulin consisting of two heavy chains of the same class and subclass and two light chains of the same type. The heavy chain classes are G, A, M, D, E (gamma, alpha, mu, delta, epsilon), while the light chain types are kappa (κ) and lambda (λ).

Monoclonal gammopathies are recognized on serum protein electrophoresis demonstrating a band of migration in the beta or gamma region [5]. When a band is seen on serum protein electrophoresis, immunofixation electrophoresis should be performed. Immunofixation electrophoresis is the gold standard and should be performed to confirm the presence of an M-protein and to distinguish its heavy chain and light chain type [6].

In 1952, Waldeström [7] initially reported finding an M-protein without evidence of malignant disorder, and named the condition "essential hypergammaglobulinemia". For some time, this condition was also referred to as "benign monoclonal gammopathy". However, Kyle recognized that some patients with MGUS could progress to MM, Waldeström macroglobulinemia, light chain amyloidosis, or related disorders. Thus, Kyle coined the term MGUS in 1978 [8]. In 2003, MGUS is defined by serum M-protein concentration less than 3 g/dL, the bone marrow clonal plasma cell less than 10%, with no evidence of other B-cell proliferation disorders [9].

The objective of this chapter is to describe new concepts and advances concerning the diagnosis, classification, management of patient, risk factors for malignant transformation and new preventive strategies of progression of MGUS to malignant conditions.

2. Prevalence

As mentioned above, MGUS is the most common plasma cell disorders and is a potential precursor of MM. At the Mayo Clinic during 2005, 51% of patients with a monoclonal gammopathy (n=1,510) had MGUS, 18% MM, 11% amyloidosis, 3% Waldeström macroglobulinemia and 17% other diseases [3].

In 1972, Kyle et al [10] collected serum from 1,200 residents (≥50 y) of Thief River Falls of Minnesota; M-proteins were detected in 15 people, 1.7% men and 0.9% women of the surveyed population (Table 1). In 2006, Kyle et al [1] reported variability in the prevalence of MGUS from a normal population in community practice [11, 12] or in hospitals; data was obtained from studies carried out between 1963 and 2002. It is suggested that this variability might be due to that some studies lacked a geographically defined population in which testing could be performed during a specified period, and that screening methods used in many previous studies are less sensitive than current techniques. To overcome these limitations, Kyle et al [1] used sensitive laboratory procedures to determine the prevalence of MGUS in a large population (n=21,463) in a well-defined geographic area (Table 1): sample of persons aged ≥50 years residing in Olmsted Country (Minnesota, USA). MGUS was found in 3.2% of people in their 5th decade, 5.3% in their 7th decade and 7.5% in over 85 years old (350/9469 men and 344/11,994 women) [1]. Axelsson et al [13] also reported that MGUS is more prevalent in men (1.9%) than in women (1.3%).

The incidence in the population aged 70 years reaches 3% in Caucasian population [4] and 0.7% in Mexican mestizos [14]. The prevalence of MGUS in African Americans was 3-fold higher than in white male veterans, among 4 million African American and white male veterans admitted to Veterans Affairs, between 1980 and 1996 [15] (Table 1). The age-adjusted prevalence of MGUS was 1.97-fold higher in Ghanaian men compared with white men (50-74 y) [16]. Later, they reported the risk of MGUS between white and black male United States veterans could be associated with prior autoimmune, infectious, inflammatory, and allergic disorders; they concluded that various types of immune-mediated conditions might act as triggers for MM/MGUS development [17]. Recently, a disparity in the prevalence, pathogenesis and progression of MGUS between blacks and whites [18] has been reported.

http://dx.doi.org/10.5772/56138

Site [References]	Type Study (Length)	Test Identify M-protein	Nº of Persons Studied (Age, y)	Prevalence % (Age, y); Incidence or Cases	M-protein		
					IgG % n/MGUS	IgA % n/MGUS	IgM % n/MGUS
Minnesota, USA [10]	PB (<1 mo)	CAE IE	1,200 (≥50)	1.25 % (≥50) 2.8 % (≥70)	73.3 % 11/15	6.7% 1/15	20.0% 3/15
Finistere, France [11]	Health CP (1 y)	CAE IE	30,279 (≥30) 17,968 (≥50)	0.2 % (all) 1.7 % (≥50)	71.7% 43/60	6.6% 4/60	21.7% 13/60
North Carolina, USA [12]	PB (NA)	AGE IFE	1,732 (≥70)	6.1% total 8.4/3.8% blacks/whites	NA/106	NA/106	NA/106
Iceland [20]	RCS (22 y)	CAE AGE	Population Iceland (20-104)	11/100,000 (M) 9/100,000 (F)	55.0%	13.0%	32.0%
Hospital, Japan [21]	HCS-BS (16 y)	CAE IE	6,737 (45-85)	0.93% 2.0% (≥70)	55.8%	41.6%	-
Minnesota, USA [1]	PB (6 y)	AGE IFE	21,463 (≥50)	3.2 % (≥50) 3.7/2.9% (M/F)	68.9% NA/694	10.8% NA/694	17.2% NA/694
142 VA hospitals [15]	RS-IHR (16 y)	NA	3,997,815(≥18)	0.05% total; 0.09% blacks 0.04% whites	NA/2,046	NA/2,046	NA/2,046
LHNC, Japan [22]	RS-BS (15.5 y)	CAE IE	52,781 (≥42)	2.1% (all) 4.4 % (≥80)	73.6% NA/1,088	17.7% NA/1,088	7.5% NA/1,088
1 hospital, Chile [23]	RS	AGE IFE	MGUS: 17 (28-96)	NA 11/6 (M/F)	59.0% 10/17	24.0% 4/17	18.0% 3/17
Bangkok, Thailand [24]	SH (6 mo)	HRGE AGE	3,260 (50-93)	2.3% 38/46% (M/F)	64% 48/75	21.3% 16/75	--
Seongnam, Korean [25]	KL (1 y)	SPEP IFE	1,118 (65-97)	3.1% 3.8/2.5% (M/F)	29% 6/21	43% 9/21	19% 4/21
Germany [26]	PB-HNR	SPEP IFE	4,702 (45-75)	3.5% 4.4/2.7% (M/F)	59% 97/165	17% 28/165	17% 28/165

AGE: Agarose gel electrophoresis; **CAE**: Cellulose acetate electrophoresis; **CP:** Control prevalence; **HCS-PS:** Hospital cohort study- atomic bomb survivors; **HRGE:** High-resolution gel electrophoresis; **IFE:** Immunofixation; **IE**: Immunoelectrophoresis; **KL:** After scheduled tests for the Korean longitudinal study on health and aging; **LHNC:** Local hospital Nagasaki City**; M/F:** Males/females; **NA:** No available; **PB:** Population based; **PB-HNR:** Population-based Heinz Nixdorf Recall study; **RCS:** Retrospective cohort study; **RS:** Retrospective study; **RS-BS:** Retrospective study of date base of atomic bomb survivors; **RS-IHR:** Retrospective study of inpatient hospitalization records; **SH:** Cross-sectional survey of healthy; **SPEP:** Standard serum electrophoresis; **VA:** Veterans Affairs.

Table 1. Studies of epidemiology of MGUS

In 2010, Wadhera and Rajkumar [19] on the basis of a systematic review of prevalence of MGUS selected 14 of 460 articles, which met the inclusion criteria for their review [10, 12, 15, 16, 20-22] (Table 1). They discussed study types, method sensibility and availability to detect M-protein and diagnostic criteria. They conclude that the prevalence increases with age and is affected by race, sex, among other factors. Further studies of prevalence are shown in Table 1 [23-26].

One long-term research studied a population-based of 1,384 patients with MGUS from the 11 counties of southeastern Minnesota who were evaluated from 1960 to 1994 [2]. These patients were observed for a total of 11,009 person-years. Of the identified MGUS, 115 progressed to MM or related disorders. At 10 years, 10% had progressed; 20 years, 21% had progressed; and at 25 years, 26% had progressed. The conclusion of these authors is that the risk of progression is about 1% per year. In 2003, a study reported that relative risk of progression was 16-fold higher in the patients with IgM MGUS than in the white population of the Iowa Surveillance [27]. Furthermore, risk for progression to lymphoma or a related disorder at 10 years after the diagnosis of MGUS was 14% with an initial M-protein concentration of 0.5 g/dL or less, 26% with 1.5 g/dL, 34% for 2.0 g/dL, and 41% for more than 2.5 g/dL [27]. Risk factors associated with the progression will be discussed later in this chapter.

3. Diagnosis and classification of patient with MGUS

The UK Myeloma Forum and the Nordic Myeloma Study Group have proposed guidelines for the effective clinical investigation of patients with M-proteins and management of patients with MGUS [28]. These guidelines are almost entirely based on expert consensus opinion. They were searched by MEDLINE and EMBASE systematically for publications from 1950 to October 2008. They suggest that screening normal populations for M-protein for clinical purposes are not recommended. It was suggested that serum protein electrophoresis should be performed if there is clinical suspicion of an M-protein or when the abnormal test results (erythrocyte sedimentation rate >30 mm/h or plasma viscosity; unexplained anemia, hypercalcemia or renal failure; raised total protein/globulin or immunoglobulins; reduction of one or more immunoglobulin class levels).

The UK Myeloma Forum and the Nordic Myeloma Study Group guidelines specifically state that there is no evidence supporting the use of serum free light chain in monitoring patients [28]. By contrast, the International Myeloma Working Group members suggest that serum free light chain analysis may be a useful adjunctive test in monitoring patients with MGUS [29-33]. The ratio of κ/λ is critical to the interpretation, because an abnormal serum free light chain ratio should only be present in the context of a plasma cell dyscrasia with severe renal failure or other B-cell lymphoproliferative disorders [34]. It is important to note that serum free light chain analysis by immunoassay is much more sensitive than the serum protein electrophoresis methodology [35].

In 2010, International Myeloma Working Group has recommended a new classification of MGUS [36]; each type must meet all the criteria set out: Non-IgM (IgG or IgA) MGUS with serum M-protein <3 g/dL, clonal bone marrow plasma cells <10%, absence of end-organ

http://dx.doi.org/10.5772/56138

damage, such as CRAB (hypercalcemia, renal insufficiency, anemia and bone lesions); IgM MGUS with serum M-protein <3 g/dL, clonal bone marrow lymphoplasmacytic cells <10%, absence of end-organ damage; and light chain-MGUS with abnormal free light chain ratio <0.26 or >1.65, increased level of the appropriate involved light chain, increased κ free light chain in patients with ratio >1.65 and increased λ free light chain in patients with ratio <0.26, no immunoglobulin heavy chain expression on immunofixation, clonal bone marrow plasma cells <10%, and absence of end-organ damage, such as CRAB [19, 36]. Each clinical type is characterized by unique intermediate stages and progression events. The intermediate stages with high risk of progression are [36]: (i) smoldering MM (SMM: IgG or IgA M-protein ≥3 g/dL, and/or clonal bone marrow plasma cells ≥10%, and absence of end-organ damage, CRAB); (ii) smoldering Waldenström macroglobulinemia (IgM M-protein ≥3 g/dL and/or clonal bone marrow lymphoplasmacytic infiltration ≥10%, no evidence of anemia constitutional symptoms); and (iii) idiopathic Bence Jones proteinuria (urinary M-protein on urine protein electrophoresis ≥500 mg/24 h and/or clonal bone marrow plasma cells ≥10%, no immunoglobulin heavy chain expression on immunofixation, absence of end-organ damage, CRAB).

4. Risk factors for malignant transformation of MGUS

Risk factors for transformation of MGUS to malignant condition have been analyzed in several studies. An abnormal serum free light chain ratio (κ/λ), non-IgG MGUS, and a high serum M protein level (≥1.5 g/dL) are three major risk factors for the progression of MGUS to myeloma [36].

Based on the clinical markers still available, two independent studies were able to establish predictive risk models from MGUS to MM for each clinical type of MGUS. The first model, proposed by a group at the Mayo Clinic identifies three main risk factors for progression: serum M-protein >1.5 g/dL, IgG subtype and normal free light chain ratio. The probability of progression of MGUS to malignant monoclonal gammopathy is 1% per year, with an estimated risk of progression of 34% over 20 years [37]. At 20 years of follow-up, absolute risk of progression for MGUS patients with 0, 1, 2, and 3 risk factors are 5%, 21%, 37%, and 58%, respectively [29].

Immunophenotyping is an attractive technique to potentially identify high levels of malignant plasma cells among normal plasma cells [38] and for the differential diagnosis between MGUS and MM [39]. The second model, proposed by a Spanish group, introduces a novel prognostic criterion for MGUS. This group has established a multiparameter flow cytometry as a tool to identify aberrant plasma cell populations: $CD38^+$, $CD19^-$, $CD45^-$, $CD56^+$ [40]. They defined two factors: (1) a plasma cell/normal bone marrow plasma cell ratio >95% associated with higher risk of progression, and (2) DNA aneuploidy. Free progression survival at 5 years for MGUS patients with 0, 1, and 2 risk factors is 2%, 10%, and 46%, respectively.

Both models present advantages and disadvantages with regard to the risk stratification of patients with MGUS [41]. The Mayo Clinical model may be useful in routine clinical practice, but the disadvantages of the model are its poor discrimination of the risk of progression between groups. On the other hand, the Salamanca model is a superior model, in particular, to identify a truly high-risk MGUS population; however, its main disadvantages are invasiveness (it requires a bone marrow aspirate), technical complexity and high cost.

The biological events related to progression from normal plasma cells to MM precursor disease and to MM involve many overlapping oncogenic steps that differently affect each individual [42]. Several authors discuss the very early and partially overlapping molecular pathogenic events that are shared by MGUS, and how they are associated to progression at the MGUS to MM transition [43-45].

5. Cytogenetic studies on MGUS and SMM

MGUS, SMM and MM present common chromosomal abnormalities [46-49] whose prevalence and relative association between these diagnostic groups have been controversial for years. The development of new techniques and methodologies has helped to define new biomarkers and elucidate the pathogenetic mechanisms of progression, characterized as a multistep process from the precursor state to myeloma.

The first step in the pathogenesis is likely an abnormal response to antigenic stimulation, mediated possibly by aberrant expression of toll-like receptors and overexpression of interleukin (IL) 6 receptors and IL-1β. This then results in the development of primary cytogenetic abnormalities, either hyperdiploidy or immunoglobulin heavy chain translocations [36]. Hyperdiploid tumors, which include about 50% of MM tumors, often have multiple trisomies involving chromosomes 3, 5, 7, 9, 11, 15, 19, and 21; also, a substantially lower prevalence of immunoglobulin heavy chain translocations and monosomy of chromosome 13 compared with nonhyperdiploid tumors. Trisomies of these same chromosomes also occur in premalignant MGUS tumors [47].

It has been well established that each translocation subgroup found in MM tumors is associated with deregulation of a D group cyclin either directly, such as occurs with the t(11;14) (cyclin D1) and t(6;14) (cyclin D3) or indirectly, such as occurs with the t(4;14) or in the MAF translocation group [47]. All these translocations have also been reported in MGUS (Table 2).

The first studies that showed structural chromosomal changes in MGUS and performed fluorescence *in situ* hybridization experiments (FISH) found 14q32 and 13q14 abnormalities [51, 52]. Subsequent studies have determined that approximately 50% of SMM show primary translocations involving the immunoglobulin heavy chain locus leading to the dysregulation of oncogenes including the Cyclin D, FGFR3/MMSET and MAF genes [46, 48, 53] (see Table 2). There is evidence of an immunoglobulin light chain-λ translocation in MGUS associated with a prevalence of 10% in MGUS/SMM [53].

Ross et al [55] found that cases characterized by t(4;14), t(14;16), particularly the t(14;20), can be stable as either MGUS or SMM for years before progression occurs. It has been shown that t(4;14), t(14;16) and t(14;20) translocations are associated with a poor prognosis in MM

http://dx.doi.org/10.5772/56138

Translocation (Prevalence %) [References]	Group	Deregulated Gene	Cell Level Consequence
IgH translocated MGUS (50%) [50]			
t(11;14)(q13;q32) (15%-25% of MGUS/SMM patients) [50-53]	D group cyclin Directly	CCND1	Enhance cyclin D1 (normally B-cells express cyclin D2 and cyclin D3 but not cyclin D1)
t(6;14)(p21;q32) (1% of MGUS/SMM patients) [50]	D group cyclin Directly	CCND3	Enhance cyclin D3
t(4;14)(p16;q32) (2%-5% of MGUS patients) (13% of SMM patients) [48, 52-54]	D group cyclin Indirectly	FGFR-3 and MMSET	Enhance cyclin D2
t(14;16)(q32;q23) (3%-5% of MGUS/SMM patients) [53, 55]	MAF translocation group	c-MAF upregulation	Enhance cyclin D2
t(14;20)(q32;q11) (5% of MGUS patients) (0%-1.5% of SMM patients) [50, 55]	MAF translocation group	MAFB upregulation	Enhance cyclin D2

MGUS: Monoclonal gammopathy of undetermined significance; **SMM:** Smoldering multiple myeloma

Table 2. Translocations into the immunoglobulin heavy chain locus in MGUS and SMM patients

(1,860 studied patients). The t(14;20) patients had a short median survival of only 14.4 months [50]. It has been determined that these three translocations produce cyclin D2 enhancement (Table 2).

Using interphase FISH, Chiecchio et al [50] performed a study to evaluate chromosome 13 deletion (delta 13), deletion of TP53 (17p13), ploidy status and immunoglobulin heavy chain translocations. They found that 50% of MGUS patients carried one of the primary immunoglobulin heavy chain translocations and the remaining patients displayed a hyperdiploid karyotype. Thus 72/189 (42%) MGUS, 70/127 (63%) SMM, and 223/338 (57%) of MM cases were hyperdiploid. When the individual incidences of the specific translocations were compared, only t(4;14) was significantly less frequent in MGUS. The authors propose that ploidy status and immunoglobulin heavy chain rearrangements were early events delineating different pathogenic pathways [50]. The study revealed a significantly lower frequency of delta 13 in the pre-malignant conditions than in MM. Delta 13 was rare in MGUS (25%) and SMM (34%) compared to MM (47%).Translocations directly involve cyclin D genes (CCND1 and CCND3) suggesting a possible role of delta 13 in the progression of the disease, specifically in these genetic sub-groups [50]. In MGUS, the greatest variation in the proportion of abnormal plasma cells carrying the abnormality was seen for delta 13 and 16q23 deletion. The presence and time of occurrence of delta 13 depend on the presence of specific concurrent abnormalities: earlier when t(4;14) or t(14;16) was present, later with t(14;20), and even later with t(11;14) or t(6;14).This data suggests a possible role of delta 13 in the transition from MGUS to MM specifically in cases with t(11;14) or t(6;14). Chromosome 13 deletion on its own probably does not affect prognosis [50].

We have treated previously in this chapter, that MGUS progresses to MM at annual frequency of 1% [2], however little is known about the proportion of patients whose MM has evolved from this precursor condition. Zhan F et al [56] developed a gene-expression profiling study in which 52 genes differentially expressed in MGUS and MM identifying and validating a MGUS-like MM with favorable clinical features and longer survival.

Point mutations, such as N-RAS, K-RAS, MYC up-regulation, and gain or loss of chromosome 1q or 1p, also seem to correlate with disease progression from myeloma precursor disease, MGUS and SMM [57]. Rasmussen et al [58] found a high prevalence of activating RAS mutations in MM (31%) compared with MGUS (5%) and suggest that these mutations may facilitate the transition from MGUS to MM in a subset of patients. Only N-RAS mutation was found in MGUS. At present, RAS mutations are the major genetic difference between MGUS and MM [43].

In a case report, Chiecchio et al [59] describe the clinicopathological and genetic findings of a young patient initially diagnosed with SMM: loss of 1p and a rearrangement of MYC were first observed in a small population of plasma cells one year prior to the clinical diagnosis of MM, but these subclones increased rapidly in size to become the major population suggesting that they were directly involved in the transformation [59].

MicroRNA is a novel class of short non-coding RNA molecules regulating a wide range of cellular functions through translational repression of their target genes. Recently, epigenetic dysregulation of tumor-suppressor microRNA genes by promoter DNA methylation has been implicated in human cancers, including MM [60]. It has been reported that MGUS and MM patients seem to upregulate miR-21, miR-106b, miR-181a, and miR-181b; which are microRNA involved in B-cell and T-cell lymphocyte differentiation as well as oncogene regulation [61]. Recently, Jones et al [62] have developed a biomarker signature using microRNAs extracted from serum, which has potential as a diagnostic and prognostic tool for MM. The combination of miR-1246 and miR-1308 can distinguish MGUS from myeloma patients [62].

In the progression process to malignant condition it also seems to be important the proportion of clonal plasma cell with specific genetic abnormalities in every diagnostic group. In fact, López-Corral et al [63] observed a significant difference in MGUS compared with SMM, and in SMM compared with MM, suggesting that the progression from MGUS to SMM and eventually to MM involves a clonal expansion of genetically abnormal plasma cell. This result was found for immunoglobulin heavy chain translocations, 13q and 17p deletions, and 1q gains. In other recent study, López-Corral et al [49] analyzed the genomic characteristics by FISH, Single-nucleotide polymorphism arrays and gene expression profile finding that the overexpression of four SNORD genes (SNORD25, SNORD27, SNORD30 and SNORD31) was correlated with shorter time progression to symptomatic MM. However, they failed to find chromosomal lesions associated to risk of progression, observing an increase in the proportion of clonal plasma cells carrying a given abnormality supporting the hypothesis that the number of genetically abnormal plasma cell increases from high-risk SMM to active MM [49]. In a later study López-Corral et al [64] have performed for the first time a comprehensive high-resolution analysis of genomic imbalances by high-density 6.0 S SNP-array in 20 MGUS, 20 SMM and 34 MM patients to search for the genetic lesions that may be involved in the transformation from MGUS to MM. Their results showed a progressive increase in the incidence of copy number abnormalities from MGUS to SMM and to MM. The study shows for the first time the different copy number and loss of heterozygosity profiles present at three stages of monoclonal gammopathy evolution: MGUS, SMM and MM. There were significantly more copy number alterations in MM than in MGUS patients, values for SMM being intermediate [64].

Taking into account that the majority of MM plasma cell are quiescent, it has been suggested that the growth of the tumor is restricted to a specialized subpopulation of cells [43]. In this sense, the bone marrow microenvironment plays an essential role in the pathogenesis of MM. The bone marrow microenvironment in which MGUS and MM cells live is composed of extracellular matrix and different types of cells, e.g., stromal cells, osteoclasts, osteoblasts, immune cells (T lymphocytes, dendritic cells), other hematopoietic, cells and their precursors, and vascular endothelial cells. Reciprocal positive and negative interactions among these cells are mediated by a variety of adhesion molecules, cytokines, and receptors [65]. MAF translocations dysregulate expression of a MAF transcription factor that causes increased expression of many genes, including CCND2 and adhesion molecules that are thought to enhance the ability of the tumor cell to interact with the bone marrow microenvironment [66].

In summary, it has been proposed that the pathogenesis of MGUS and MM can be considered as occurring in three phases [6]. First, partially overlapping genetic events common to MGUS and MM include at a minimum primary immunoglobulin heavy chain translocations, hyperdiploidy, and del13 that lead directly or indirectly to dysregulation of a CCND gene; second, the transition from MGUS to MM is associated with increased MYC expression and sometimes K-RAS mutations, but can also include del13 in t(11;14) tumors; third, additional progression of the MM tumor seems to be associated with other events. For example, increased proliferation and genomic instability, and decreased dependence on the bone marrow microenvironment, sometimes including extramedullary spread of disease, can be associated with late MYC rearrangements that often involve an immunoglobulin locus, activating mutations of the nuclear factor-κB pathway, deletion or mutation of TP53, and inactivation of p18INK4c or RB [65] (see Fig. 1).

6. Clinical management

As mentioned above, the UK Myeloma Forum and the Nordic Myeloma Study Group have proposed guidelines for the management of MGUS [28]. They suggest that is essential that patients should be monitored not only by laboratory testing but also clinically. Low risk patients (serum IgG <1.5 g/dL; IgA or IgM <1.0 g/dL; normal free light chain ratio in the absence of symptoms such as anemia or renal dysfunction) can be monitored in the primary-care setting

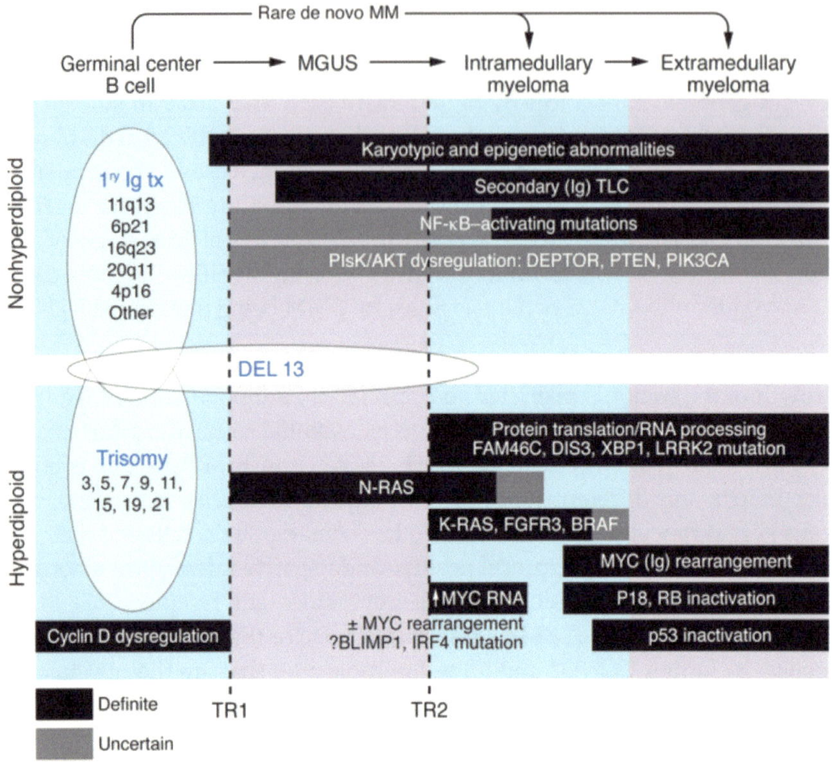

Figure 1. Model for molecular pathogenesis of monoclonal gammopathy of undetermined significance (MGUS) and multiple myeloma (MM). TR1, the initial transition to a recognizable tumor involves two mostly non-overlapping pathways (IgH translocations versus multiple trisomies) that include primary events associated with dysregulated cyclin D expression in MGUS and MM. TR2, the transition from MGUS to MM is associated with increase MYC expression and sometimes with activating mutations of K-RAS or chromosome 13 deletion. Early and late progression events for symptomatic MM tumors are shown. Reproduced with permission from Kuehl WM and Bergsagel PL. Molecular pathogenesis of multiple myeloma and its premalignant precursor. J Clin Invest. 2012;122(10):3456-63. doi:10.1172/JCI61188. Copyright from the American Society for Clinical Investigation.

at intervals of 3-4 months initially for the first year and then lengthened to 6-12 months based on the patient`s clinical history, laboratory results and comorbid conditions. Should be checked for serum protein electrophoresis, complete blood count, calcium, and serum creatinine every 6 months and if they are stable, every 2 to 6 years. There is also an alternative strategy suggesting that screening should be performed only if there is an increase in symptoms associated with MM. International Myeloma Working Group members suggest that the patients with low risk-MGUS should be followed during 6 months after the diagnosis of MGUS [32]. On the other hand, they specified that a bone marrow examination should be required if the patients had any CRAB features.

UK Myeloma Forum and the Nordic Myeloma Study Group recommend that patients with high-risk MGUS (IgG ≥1.5 g/dL; IgA or IgM >1.0 g/dL; IgD or IgE at any level) should be referred to a hematology specialist 3-4 times per year as a minimum [28]. The recommended tests for monitoring include serum protein electrophoresis, serum total immunoglobulin, complete blood count, creatinine, urea, electrolytes and serum calcium. In addition, it should be evaluated using bone marrow cytogenetic and FISH with bone imaging studies. Nevertheless, it is important to highlight that sometimes it will be necessary to perform Magnetic Resonance Imaging or Positron Emission Tomography-Computed Tomography, instead of traditional x-rays. Patients with unexplained anemia or kidney failure should be evaluated with a full bone scan that also include cytogenetic and FISH. Korde et al [57] reported that is critical to recognize that in a disease such as MM, where defining criteria rely on the presence or absence of end-organ damage, diagnosis is only as good as the tools and technology able to detect end-organ damage. For instance, in SMM or high-risk MGUS patients suspicious to harbor bone disease, imaging evaluation may be better served by obtaining magnetic resonance imaging or Positron Emission Tomography-Computed Tomography rather than traditional skeletal surveys. International Myeloma Working Group members recommend for intermediate-risk and high-risk MGUS patients should have a bone marrow aspirate and biopsy with both conventional cytogenetics and FISH [32]. If available, a plasma cell labeling index and a search for circulating plasma cells in the peripheral blood using flow cytometry are useful. Patients with IgM isotype should have a computational tomography scan of the abdomen since asymptomatic retroperitoneal lymph nodes may be present. If there is evidence of MM or Waldeström macroglobulinemia, lactate dehydrogenase, 2-microglobulin, and C-reactive protein levels should be measured. If the results of these tests are satisfactory, International Myeloma Working Group recommend patients should be followed with serum protein electrophoresis and complete blood cell count in 6 months and then annually for life [32].

7. Management

In clinical practice, patients with MGUS are followed clinically without treatment until progression. However, the existence of easily identifiable precursor states represents an opportunity for chemoprevention [67]. However, it must be weighed that benefits achieved by treating a precursor state is greater than a potential for therapeutic toxicity. Recently, Korde et al [57] revised early treatment strategies for MGUS and SMM.

Bhattacharyya et al [68] reported a clinic case of IgM-MGUS associated with cryoglobulinemia and cold agglutinin disease, which was treated with immunotherapy and was successful (Table 3). Immunochemotherapy, consisting of rituximab (375 mg/m2, day 1), fludarabine (25 mg/m2, days 2-4), and cyclophosphamide (250 mg/m2, days 2-4), was administered every 4 weeks up to three times as a first-line treatment followed by three cycles of monthly rituximab treatment. Extensive skin lesions with livedo reticularis entirely disappeared prior to initiation of the second cycle in association with the declined serum level of IgM.

Pepe et al [69] studied 100 patients affected by MGUS, grouped according to the presence (group A, 50 patients) or absence (group B) of vertebral fractures and/or osteoporosis. Group A was treated with alendronate (70 mg/weekly) plus calcium and cholecalciferol for 18

Drug [References]	Treatment scheme	Nº of patients (age or study/control)	Benefit	Observations
Zoledronic acid [70]	4 mg, i.v. at 0, 6, and 12 months	54 MGUS and osteopenia or osteoporosis (50-91 years; median=67 years)	Reducing fractures.	48 patients completed the study. Some patients showed adverse effects. Progression of MGUS does not diminish with time.
Alendronate plus calcium and cholecalciferol *vs.* calcium and cholecalciferol [69]	70 mg/weekly, at 18 months	100 MGUS With presence or absence (control) vertebral fractures and/or osteoporosis (50/50)	Reducing fractures.	8 patients developed MM 12 patients did not want to take the drugs.
Rituximab, fludarabine, and cyclophosphamide [68]	Every 4 weeks up to three times followed by three cycles of monthly rituximab treatment	1 MGUS associated with cryoglobulinemia and cold agglutinin disease	Decreases M-protein and skin lesions disappeared.	NA
Curcumin vs. placebo [73]	4 g/day oral	26 MGUS (17/9)	Decreases bone resorption and M-protein (12-30%) of patients with M-protein >20 g/L	NA
Curcumin vs. placebo [74]	4 g/day and an open-label 8 g curcumin extension study, oral, at 3 months	19 MGUS 17 SMM (12/13)	Decreasing free light chain and marker of bone resorption.	Curcumin may benefit some but not all patients with MGUS and SMM.

MGUS: Monoclonal gammopathy of undetermined significance; **SMM:** Smoldering multiple myeloma; **NA:** Not available.

Table 3. Therapy on patients with MGUS

months, and group B was treated with calcium and cholecalciferol. Treatment with alendronate could lead to a significant reduction in fracture risk in MGUS patients with skeletal fragility. During the whole period of investigation, eight patients in group A developed MM and therefore were not able to continue the study. A further 12 patients included in group A did not want to take the drugs prescribed. Additionally, the author indicated that this study has some limitations, mainly because of the lack of a real control group (longitudinally followed for the entire observation period) and the lack of morphometric evaluation of vertebral fractures at 18 months. Another similar study was administered zoledronic acid to

54 patients with MGUS and osteopenia or osteoporosis [70]. They also demonstrated that increase bone mineral density in patients with bone loss with the theoretical added benefit of reducing fractures although it was not observed that the progression can be delayed or prevented.

There are two ongoing studies, in the first, the aim is to assess whether omega-3 fatty acids reduce activated NF-κB levels in peripheral blood lymphocytes [71]. Omega-3 supplementation will be initiated at three 1250 mg capsules daily for the first month. If dose is well tolerated, it will be increased to six 1250 mg capsules daily for 30 days and finally to nine 1250 mg capsules daily. Treatment period is 12 months (study design nonrandomized). No study results posted on clinicaltrials.gov [71]. In the second study, the aim is to test whether green tea extract reduces the M-protein concentration [72]. Patients receive oral green tea catechin extract (Polyphenon E) daily on days 1-28. Treatment repeats every 28 days for up to 6 courses in the absence of disease progression or unacceptable toxicity. No study results posted on clinicaltrials.gov [72].

Golombick et al [73] investigated the effect of curcumin on plasma cells and osteoclasts in patients with MGUS (see Table 3). Twenty-six patients with MGUS were randomized into two groups (single-blind, randomized, crossover pilot). The pilot study found that curcumin may decrease both serum M-protein (in patients with levels of >20 g/L) and urinary N-telopeptide of type I collagen bone turnover marker in patients with MGUS. Recently, Golombick et al [74] performed a randomized, double-blind placebo-controlled crossover 4 g curcumin study and an open-label extension study using an 8 g curcumin. 19 MGUS and 17 SMM were randomized into two groups: one received 4 g curcumin and the other 4 g placebo, crossing over at 3 months. 25 patients completed the 4 g crossover study and 18 the 8 g extension study. In some patients curcumin therapy decreased the free light-chain ratio and uDPYD (a marker of bone resorption).

Curcumin is the most active component in *Curcuma longa* or turmeric (tropical plant native to southern and southeastern tropical Asia). Curcumin has been shown to downregulate IL-6 and nuclear factor-κB; to inhibit osteoclastogenesis and to reduce bone turnover; suppresses proliferation and induces apoptosis in MM cells [75] and inhibits osteoclastogenesis through the suppression of RANKL signaling [76]. Nevertheless, it is known that curcumin inhibits IL-12 production in dendritic cells, thereby dampening the Th1 response [77]. This suggests that may have an immunosuppressive effect. However, Rajkumar [78] indicated that finding reported by Golombick [74] is a modest decrease in free light chain levels by 25-50% in one quarter of the patients, reason why he disagrees with curcumin as a preventive or therapeutic strategy in MGUS (Table 3). Rajkumar also indicated that using risk stratification model approximately 50% of all MGUS patients are considered low-risk MGUS, and have a lifetime risk of progression of only 2%. Therefore, he recommends that focus should be put on preventive strategies in patients with high-risk SMM.

There is an increased interest in identifying biomarkers that can predict patients who will inevitably progress to symptomatic MM. These include genetic and/or epigenetic targets and microenvironment and/or its interaction with tumor cells, which may change the future of disease progression [65]. Dynamic changes in tumor and microenvironment, cell immunophenotype, mRNA and protein expression, should offer insight into disease progression [57, 78].

8. Conclusion

In conclusion, it is crucial to follow up cases of MGUS carefully, including their systematic recording as a fundamental contribution to understand the evolution of this pathology and its malignant transformation process. This will be critical to develop better biomarkers that contribute to understand the evolution and malignant transformation of MGUS. These efforts should lead to the development of new, more effective management and treatment strategies.

Abbreviations

CRAB	Hypercalcemia, renal insufficiency, anemia and bone lesions
FISH	Fluorescence *in situ* hybridization
IL	interleukin
κ	Kappa
λ	Lambda
MGUS	Monoclonal gammopathy of undetermined significance
MM	Multiple myeloma
M-protein	Monoclonal protein
NF-κB	Nuclear factor-κB
SMM	Smoldering multiple myeloma

Author details

Magdalena Patricia Cortés[1], Rocío Alvarez[2], Jessica Maldonado[4], Raúl Vinet[3] and Katherine Barría[4]

1 Department of Biochemistry, Faculty of Pharmacy, Universidad de Valparaíso, Valparaíso, Chile

2 Department of Pharmaceutical Sciences, Faculty of Pharmacy, Universidad de Valparaíso, Valparaíso, Chile

3 Laboratory of Pharmacology and Biochemistry, Faculty of Pharmacy, Universidad de Valparaíso, Valparaíso, Chile

4 Hospital Almirante Nef, Viña del Mar, Chile

References

[1] Kyle RA, Therneau TM, Rajkumar SV, Larson DR, Plevak MF, Offord JR, Dispenzieri A, Katzmann JA, Melton LJ 3rd. Prevalence of monoclonal gammopathy of undetermined significance. N Engl J Med. 2006;354(13):1362-69.

[2] Kyle RA, Therneau TM, Rajkumar SV, Offord JR, Larson DR, Plevak MF, Melton LJ 3rd. A long-term study of prognosis in monoclonal gammopathy of undetermined significance. N Engl J Med. 2002;21;346(8):564-69.

[3] Kyle RA, Rajkumar SV. Monoclonal gammopathy of undetermined significance. Br J Haematol. 2006;134(6):573-89.

[4] Kyle RA. The monoclonal gammopathies. Clin Chem. 1994;40(11 Pt 2):2154-61.

[5] Kyle RA. Sequence of testing for monoclonal gammopathies. Arch Pathol Lab Med. 1999;123(2):114-18.

[6] Attaelmannan M, Stanley L. Understanding and identifying monoclonal gammopathies. Clin Chem. 2000;46(8):1230-38.

[7] Waldeström J. Studies on conditions associated with disturbed gamma globulin formation (gammopathies). Harvey Lect. 1960-1961;56:211-31.

[8] Kyle, RA. Monoclonal gammopathy of undetermined significance: natural history in 241 cases. Am J Med. 1978; 64(5):814-26.

[9] International Myeloma Working Group. Criteria for the classification of monoclonal gammopathies, multiple myeloma and related disorders: a report of the International Myeloma Working Group. Br J Haematol. 2003;121(5):749-57.

[10] Kyle RA, Finkelstein S, Elveback LR, Kurland LT. Incidence of monoclonal proteins in a Minnesota community with a cluster of multiple myeloma. Blood. 1972;40(5): 719-24.

[11] Saleun JP, Vicariot M, Deroff P, Morin JF. Monoclonal gammopathies in the adult population of Finistere, France. J Clin Pathol. 1982;35(1):63-68.

[12] Cohen, HJ, Crawford, J, Rao, MK, Pieper, CF, Currie, MS. Racial differences in the prevalence of monoclonal gammopathy in a community-based sample of the enderly. Am J Med. 1998;104(5):439-44.

[13] Axelsson U, Bachmann R, Hällén J. Frequency of pathological proteins (M-components) om 6,995 sera from an adult population. Acta Med Scand. 1966;179(2):235-47.

[14] Ruiz-Delgado GJ, Gómez Rangel JD. Monoclonal gammopathy of undetermined significance (MGUS) in Mexican mestizos: one institution's experience. Gac Med Mex. 2004;140(4):375-79.

[15] Landgren O, Gridley G, Turesson I, Caporaso NE, Goldin LR, Baris D, Fears TR, Hoover RN, Linet MS. Risk of monoclonal gammopathy of undetermined signifi-

cance (MGUS) and subsequent multiple myeloma among African American and white veterans in the United States. Blood. 2006;107(3):904-06.

[16] Landgren O, Katzmann JA, Hsing AW, Pfeiffer RM, Kyle RA, Yeboah ED, Biritwum RB, Tettey Y, Adjei AA, Larson DR, Dispenzieri A, Melton LJ 3rd, Goldin LR, McMaster ML, Caporaso NE, Rajkumar SV. Prevalence of monoclonal gammopathy of undetermined significance among men in Ghana. Mayo Clin Proc. 2007;82(12): 1468-73.

[17] Brown LM, Gridley G, Check D, Landgren O. Risk of multiple myeloma and monoclonal gammopathy of undetermined significance among white and black male United States veterans with prior autoimmune, infectious, inflammatory, and allergic disorders. Blood. 2008;111(7):3388-94.

[18] Greenberg AJ, Vachon CM, Rajkumar SV. Disparities in the prevalence, pathogenesis and progression of monoclonal gammopathy of undetermined significance and multiple myeloma between blacks and whites. Leukemia. 2012;26(4):609-14.

[19] Wadhera RK, Rajkumar SV. Prevalence of monoclonal gammopathy of undetermined significance: a systematic review. Mayo Clin Proc. 2010;85(10):933-42.

[20] Ogmundsdóttir HM, Haraldsdóttir V, M Jóhannesson G, Olafsdóttir G, Bjarnadóttir K, Sigvaldason H, Tulinius H. Monoclonal gammopathy in Iceland: a population-based registry and follow-up. Br J Haematol. 2002;118(1):166-73.

[21] Neriishi K, Nakashima E, Suzuki G. Monoclonal gammopathy of undetermined significance in atomic bomb survivors: incidence and transformation to multiple myeloma. Br J Haematol. 2003;121(3):405-10.

[22] Iwanaga M, Tagawa M, Tsukasaki K, Kamihira S, Tomonaga M. Prevalence of monoclonal gammopathy of undetermined significance: study of 52,802 persons in Nagasaki City, Japan. Mayo Clin Proc. 2007;82(12):1474-79.

[23] Barría K, Maldonado J, Álvarez R, Rodríguez M, Cortés M. Case study of monoclonal gammopathy of undetermined significance and multiple myeloma at "Hospital Naval Almirante Nef" Viña del Mar, Chile. Rev Med Chil. 2010;138(6):788-90.

[24] Watanaboonyongcharoen P, Nakorn TN, Rojnuckarin P, Lawasut P, Intragumtornchai T. Prevalence of monoclonal gammopathy of undetermined significance in Thailand. Int J Hematol. 2012;95(2):176-81.

[25] Park HK, Lee KR, Kim YJ, Cho HI, Eun Kim J, Woong Kim K, Jung Kim Y, Lee KW, Hyun Kim J, Bang SM, Lee JS. Prevalence of monoclonal gammopathy of undetermined significance in an elderly urban Korean population. Am J Hematol. 2011;86(9): 752-55.

[26] Eisele L, Dürig J, Hüttmann A, Dührsen U, Assert R, Bokhof B, Erbel R, Mann K, Jöckel KH, Moebus S; Heinz Nixdorf Recall Study Investigative Group. Prevalence

and progression of monoclonal gammopathy of undetermined significance and light-chain MGUS in Germany. Ann Hematol. 2012;91(2):243-48.

[27] Kyle RA, Therneau TM, Rajkumar SV, Remstein ED, Offord JR, Larson DR, Plevak MF, Melton LJ 3rd. Long-term follow-up of IgM monoclonal gammopathy of undetermined significance. Blood. 2003;102(10):3759-64.

[28] Bird J, Behrens J, Westin J, Turesson I, Drayson M, Beetham R, D'Sa S, Soutar R, Waage A, Gulbrandsen N, Gregersen H, Low E; Haemato-oncology Task Force of the British Committee for Standards in Haematology, UK Myeloma Forum and Nordic Myeloma Study Group. UK Myeloma Forum (UKMF) and Nordic Myeloma Study Group (NMSG): guidelines for the investigation of newly detected M-proteins and the management of monoclonal gammopathy of undetermined significance (MGUS). Br J Haematol. 2009;147(1):22-42.

[29] Rajkumar SV, Kyle RA, Therneau TM, Melton LJ 3rd, Bradwell AR, Clark RJ, Larson DR, Plevak MF, Dispenzieri A, Katzmann JA. Serum free light chain ratio is an independent risk factor for progression in monoclonal gammopathy of undetermined significance. Blood. 2005;106(3):812-17.

[30] Rajkumar, S.V. MGUS and smoldering multiple myeloma: update on pathogenesis, natural history, and management. Hematology Am Soc Hematol Educ Program. 2005:340-5.

[31] Dispenzieri A, Kyle R, Merlini G, Miguel JS, Ludwig H, Hajek R, Palumbo A, Jagannath S, Blade J, Lonial S, Dimopoulos M, Comenzo R, Einsele H, Barlogie B, Anderson K, Gertz M, Harousseau JL, Attal M, Tosi P, Sonneveld P, Boccadoro M, Morgan G, Richardson P, Sezer O, Mateos MV, Cavo M, Joshua D, Turesson I, Chen W, Shimizu K, Powles R, Rajkumar SV, Durie BG; International Myeloma Working Group. International Myeloma Working Group guidelines for serum-free light chain analysis in multiple myeloma and related disorders. Leukemia. 2009;23(2):215-24.

[32] Kyle RA, Buadi F, Rajkumar SV. Management of monoclonal gammopathy of undetermined significance (MGUS) and smoldering multiple myeloma (SMM). Oncology. 2011;25(7):578-86.

[33] Dispenzieri A, Katzmann JA, Kyle RA, Larson DR, Melton LJ 3rd, Colby CL, Therneau TM, Clark R, Kumar SK, Bradwell A, Fonseca R, Jelinek DF, Rajkumar SV. Prevalence and risk of progression of light-chain monoclonal gammopathy of undetermined significance: a retrospective population-based cohort study. Lancet. 2010;375(9727):1721-28.

[34] Hutchison CA, Plant T, Drayson M, Cockwell P, Kountouri M, Basnayake K, Harding S, Bradwell AR, Mead G. Serum free light chain measurement aids the diagnosis of myeloma in patients with severe renal failure. BMC Nephrol. 2008;9:11.

[35] Tate J, Bazeley S, Sykes S, Mollee P. Quantitative serum free light chain assay - Analytical issues. Clin Biochem Rev. 2009;30(3):131-40.

[36] Rajkumar SV, Kyle RA, Buadi FB. Advances in the diagnosis, classification, risk stratification, and management of monoclonal gammopathy of undetermined significance: implications for recategorizing disease entities in the presence of evolving scientific evidence. Mayo Clin Proc. 2010;85(10):945-48.

[37] Kyle R.A, Therneau, T.M, Rajkumar, S.V, Larson, D.R, Plevak, M.F, Melton, L.J, III. Long-term follow-up of 241 patients with monoclonal gammopathy of undetermined significance: the original Mayo Clinic series 25 years later. Mayo Clin Proc. 2004;79:59-66.

[38] Rawstron AC, Orfao A, Beksac M, Bezdickova L, Brooimans RA, Bumbea H, Dalva K, Fuhler G, Gratama J, Hose D, Kovarova L, Lioznov M, Mateo G, Morilla R, Mylin AK, Omedé P, Pellat-Deceunynck C, Perez Andres M, Petrucci M, Ruggeri M, Rymkiewicz G, Schmitz A, Schreder M, Seynaeve C, Spacek M, de Tute RM, Van Valckenborgh E, Weston-Bell N, Owen RG, San Miguel JF, Sonneveld P, Johnsen HE. Report of the European Myeloma Network on multiparametric flow cytometry in multiple myeloma and related disorders. Haematologica. 2008;93(3):431-38.

[39] Ocqueteau M, Orfao A, Almeida J, Bladé J, González M, García-Sanz R, López-Berges C, Moro MJ, Hernández J, Escribano L, Caballero D, Rozman M, San Miguel JF. Immunophenotypic characterization of plasma cells from monoclonal gammopathy of undetermined significance patients. Implications for the differential diagnosis between MGUS and multiple myeloma. Am J Pathol. 1998;152(6):1655-65.

[40] Pérez-Persona E, Vidriales MB, Mateo G, García-Sanz R, Mateos MV, de Coca AG, Galende J, Martín-Nuñez G, Alonso JM, de Las Heras N, Hernández JM, Martín A, López-Berges C, Orfao A, San Miguel JF. New criteria to identify risk of progression in monoclonal gammopathy of uncertain significance and smoldering multiple myeloma based on multiparameter flow cytometry analysis of bone marrow plasma cells. Blood. 2007;110(7):2586-92.

[41] Weiss BM, Kuehl WM. Advances in understanding monoclonal gammopathy of undetermined significance as a precursor of multiple myeloma. Expert Rev Hematol. 2010;3(2):165-74.

[42] Landgren O, Waxman AJ. Multiple myeloma precursor disease. JAMA. 2010;304(21): 2397-04.

[43] Anderson KC, Carrasco RD. Pathogenesis of myeloma. Annu Rev Pathol. 2011;6:249-74.

[44] Zingone A, Kuehl WM. Pathogenesis of monoclonal gammopathy of undetermined significance and progression to multiple myeloma. Semin Hematol. 2011;48(1):4-12.

[45] Rajkumar SV. Prevention of progression in monoclonal gammopathy of undetermined significance. Clin Cancer Res. 2009; 15(18):5606-08.

[46] Bergsagel PL, Kuehl WM. Chromosome translocations in multiple myeloma. Oncogene. 2001;20(40):5611-22.

[47] Bergsagel PL, Kuehl WM, Zhan F, Sawyer J, Barlogie B, Shaughnessy J Jr. Cyclin D dysregulation: an early and unifying pathogenic event in multiple myeloma. Blood. 2005;106(1):296-03.

[48] Fonseca R, Barlogie B, Bataille R, Bastard C, Bergsagel PL, Chesi M, Davies FE, Drach J, Greipp PR, Kirsch IR, Kuehl WM, Hernandez JM, Minvielle S, Pilarski LM, Shaughnessy JD Jr, Stewart AK, Avet-Loiseau H. Genetics and cytogenetics of multiple myeloma: a workshop report. Cancer Res. 2004; 64(4):1546-58.

[49] López-Corral L, Mateos MV, Corchete LA, Sarasquete ME, de la Rubia J, de Arriba F, Lahuerta JJ, García-Sanz R, San Miguel JF, Gutiérrez NC. Genomic analysis of high-risk smoldering multiple myeloma. Haematologica. 2012;97(9):1439-43.

[50] Chiecchio L, Dagrada GP, Ibrahim AH, Dachs Cabanas E, Protheroe RK, Stockley DM, Orchard KH, Cross NC, Harrison CJ, Ross FM; UK Myeloma Forum. Timing of acquisition of deletion 13 in plasma cell dyscrasias is dependent on genetic context. Haematologica. 2009;94(12):1708-13.

[51] Nishida K, Tamura A, Nakazawa N, Ueda Y, Abe T, Matsuda F, Kashima K, Taniwaki M. The Ig heavy chain gene is frequently involved in chromosomal translocations in multiple myeloma and plasma cell leukemia as detected by in situ hybridization. Blood. 1997;90(2):526-34.

[52] Avet-Loiseau H, Facon T, Daviet A, Godon C, Rapp MJ, Harousseau JL, Grosbois B, Bataille R. 14q32 translocations and monosomy 13 observed in monoclonal gammopathy of undetermined significance delineate a multistep process for the oncogenesis of multiple myeloma. Intergroupe Francophone du Myélome. Cancer Res. 1999;59(18):4546-50.

[53] Fonseca R, Bailey RJ, Ahmann GJ, Rajkumar SV, Hoyer JD, Lust JA, Kyle RA, Gertz MA, Greipp PR, Dewald GW. Genomic abnormalities in monoclonal gammopathy of undetermined significance. Blood. 2002;100(4):1417-24.

[54] Malgeri U, Baldini L, Perfetti V, Fabris S, Vignarelli MC, Colombo G, Lotti V, Compasso S, Bogni S, Lombardi L, Maiolo AT, Neri A. Detection of t(4;14)(p16.3;q32) chromosomal translocation in multiple myeloma by reverse transcription-polymerase chain reaction analysis of IGH-MMSET fusion transcripts. Cancer Res. 2000;60:4058-61.

[55] Ross FM, Chiecchio L, Dagrada G, Protheroe RK, Stockley DM, Harrison CJ, Cross NC, Szubert AJ, Drayson MT, Morgan GJ; UK Myeloma Forum. The t(14;20) is a poor prognostic factor in myeloma but is associated with long-term stable disease in monoclonal gammopathies of undetermined significance. Haematologica. 2010;95(7): 1221-25.

[56] Zhan F, Barlogie B, Arzoumanian V, Huang Y, Williams DR, Hollmig K, Pineda-Roman M, Tricot G, van Rhee F, Zangari M, Dhodapkar M, Shaughnessy JD Jr. Gene-expression signature of benign monoclonal gammopathy evident in multiple myeloma is linked to good prognosis. Blood. 2007;109(4):1692-00.

[57] Korde N, Kristinsson SY, Landgren O. Monoclonal gammopathy of undetermined significance (MGUS) and smoldering multiple myeloma (SMM): novel biological insights and development of early treatment strategies. Blood. 2011;117(21):5573-81

[58] Rasmussen T, Kuehl M, Lodahl M, Johnsen HE, Dahl IM. Possible roles for activating RAS mutations in the MGUS to MM transition and in the intramedullary to extramedullary transition in some plasma cell tumors. Blood. 2005;105(1):317-23.

[59] Chiecchio L, Dagrada GP, Protheroe RK, Stockley DM, Smith AG, Orchard KH, Cross NC, Harrison CJ, Ross FM; UK Myeloma Forum. Loss of 1p and rearrangement of MYC are associated with progression of smouldering myeloma to myeloma: sequential analysis of a single case. Haematologica. 2009;94(7):1024-28.

[60] Wong KY, Huang X, Chim CS. DNA methylation of microRNA genes in multiple myeloma. Carcinogenesis. 2012;33(9):1629-38.

[61] Pichiorri F, Suh SS, Ladetto M, Kuehl M, Palumbo T, Drandi D, Taccioli C, Zanesi N, Alder H, Hagan JP, Munker R, Volinia S, Boccadoro M, Garzon R, Palumbo A, Aqeilan RI, Croce CM. MicroRNAs regulate critical genes associated with multiple myeloma pathogenesis. Proc Natl Acad Sci U S A. 2008;105(35):12885-90.

[62] Jones CI, Zabolotskaya MV, King AJ, Stewart HJ, Horne GA, Chevassut TJ, Newbury SF. Identification of circulating microRNAs as diagnostic biomarkers for use in multiple myeloma. Br J Cancer. 2012;107(12):1987-96.

[63] López-Corral L, Gutiérrez NC, Vidriales MB, Mateos MV, Rasillo A, García-Sanz R, Paiva B, San Miguel JF. The progression from MGUS to smoldering myeloma and eventually to multiple myeloma involves a clonal expansion of genetically abnormal plasma cells. Clin Cancer Res. 2011;17(7):1692-00.

[64] López-Corral L, Sarasquete ME, Beà S, García-Sanz R, Mateos MV, Corchete LA, Sayagués JM, García EM, Bladé J, Oriol A, Hernández-García MT, Giraldo P, Hernández J, González M, Hernández-Rivas JM, San Miguel JF, Gutiérrez NC. SNP-based mapping arrays reveal high genomic complexity in monoclonal gammopathies, from MGUS to myeloma status. Leukemia. 2012;26(12):2521-29.

[65] Kuehl WM, Bergsagel PL. Molecular pathogenesis of multiple myeloma and its premalignant precursor. J Clin Invest. 2012;122(10):3456-63.

[66] Chesi M, Bergsagel PL. Many multiple myelomas: making more of the molecular mayhem. Hematology Am Soc Hematol Educ Program. 2011;2011:344-53.

[67] Bianchi G, Kyle RA, Colby CL, Larson DR, Kumar S, Katzmann JA, Dispenzieri A, Therneau TM, Cerhan JR, Melton LJ 3rd, Rajkumar SV. Impact of optimal follow-up

of monoclonal gammopathy of undetermined significance on early diagnosis and prevention of myeloma-related complications. Blood. 2010;116(12):2019-25.

[68] Bhattacharyya J, Mihara K, Takihara Y, Kimura A. Successful treatment of IgM-monoclonal gammopathy of undetermined significance associated with cryoglobulinemia and cold agglutinin disease with immunochemotherapy with rituximab, fludarabine, and cyclophosphamide. Ann Hematol. 2012;91(5):797-99.

[69] Pepe J, Petrucci MT, Mascia ML, Piemonte S, Fassino V, Romagnoli E, Minisola S. The effects of alendronate treatment in osteoporotic patients affected by monoclonal gammopathy of undetermined significance. Calcif Tissue Int. 2008;82(6):418-26.

[70] Berenson JR, Yellin O, Boccia RV, Flam M, Wong SF, Batuman O, Moezi MM, Woytowitz D, Duvivier H, Nassir Y, Swift RA. Zoledronic acid markedly improves bone mineral density for patients with monoclonal gammopathy of undetermined significance and bone loss. Clin Cancer Res. 2008;14(19):6289-95.

[71] Ballester OF. Omega 3 Supplementation for the Prevention of Disease Progression in Early Stage Chronic Lymphocytic Leukemia (ES-CLL), Monoclonal Gammopathy of Undetermined Significance (MGUS) and Smoldering Multiple Myeloma (SMM). US National Institutes of Health; 2009. http://clinicaltrials.gov (accessed December 5, 2012).

[72] Zonder JA, Karmanos BA. Green tea extract in treating patients with monoclonal gammopathy of undetermined significance and/or smoldering multiple myeloma. US National Institutes of Health; 2009. http://clinicaltrials.gov (accessed December 5, 2012).

[73] Golombick T, Diamond TH, Badmaev V, Manoharan A, Ramakrishna R. The potential role of curcumin in patients with monoclonal gammopathy of undefined significance - Its effect on paraproteinemia and the urinary N-telopeptide of type I collagen bone turnover marker. Clin Cancer Res. 2009;15(18):5917-22.

[74] Golombick T, Diamond TH, Manoharan A, Ramakrishna R. Monoclonal gammopathy of undetermined significance, smoldering multiple myeloma, and curcumin: a randomized, double-blind placebo-controlled cross-over 4g study and an open-label 8g extension study. Am J Hematol. 2012;87(5):455-60.

[75] Bharti AC, Donato N, Singh S, Aggarwal BB. Curcumin (diferuloylmethane) down-regulates the constitutive activation of nuclear factor-kappa B and IkappaBalpha kinase in human multiple myeloma cells, leading to suppression of proliferation and induction of apoptosis. Blood. 2003;101(3):1053-62.

[76] Bharti AC, Takada Y, Aggarwal BB. Curcumin (diferuloylmethane) inhibits receptor activator of NF-kappa B ligand-induced NF-kappa B activation in osteoclast precursors and suppresses osteoclastogenesis. J Immunol. 2004;172(10):5940-7.

[77] Vermorken AJ, Zhu J, Van de Ven WJ. Is curcumin for monoclonal gammopathy of undetermined significance without risk?-letter. Clin Cancer Res. 2010;16(7):2225.

[78] Rajkumar SV. Preventive strategies in monoclonal gammopathy of undetermined significance and smoldering multiple myeloma. Am J Hematol. 2012;87(5):453-54.

Chapter 7

Induction Therapy in Multiple Myeloma

Sule Mine Bakanay and Meral Beksac

Additional information is available at the end of the chapter

http://dx.doi.org/10.5772/55151

1. Introduction

Today, multiple myeloma (MM) can be defined as a heterogenous disease composed of different clinical conditions. The differences are a result of patient related factors (age, sex, comorbidity), disease related complications (renal failure, bone disease, neuropathy, thrombosis) and biological characteristics (cytogenetics, lactate dehydrogenase level, plasma cell labelling index, beta2-microglobulin, gene expression profiles). The widely used international scoring system is a powerful tool for determining survival. However, it cannot be used for treatment planning. The biological determinants of disease determined by flourescein in situ hybridization (FISH) and/or conventional cytogenetics are better tools to stratify myeloma subgroups with different survival profiles. Thus these are better tools for designing therapeutic approaches. A risk stratification of newly diagnosed MM according to FISH/Karyotyping has been recently reviewed by Rajkumar (Rajkumar, 2012).

High dose melphalan supported by autologous stem cell transplantation (ASCT) can increase response rates and prolong progression free and overal survival compared to conventional chemotherapies (Attal et al., 1996; Child et al., 2003; Fermand et al., 2005; Koreth et al., 2007). The initial induction regimen is chosen according to whether the patient is eligible or ineligible for a subsequent HDT-ASCT as well as the risk stratification of the patient. Advanced age or significant comorbidity are important limitations for ASCT. High dose therapy has been generally considered for patients ≤ 65 years. However, in medically fit patients, this can be extended up to age 70-75 years. Achievement of high quality responses (VGPR, CR/nCR) at the time of transplantation has been demostrated to be an early predictor of improved outcomes after ASCT (Harousseau et al., 2009; Chanan-Khan&Giralt, 2010). Elderly patients or patients ineligible for transplantation may also benefit from chemotherapy by achieving high quality responses preferably CR in terms of progression free survival (PFS) and overall survival (OS). As such, the choice of induction therapy is crucial for survival for most patients with MM. The emergence of novel agents (thalidomide, lenalidomide and bortezomib) and incorporation of these agents in to the current induction protocols has increased the rate of CR and at least VGPR before ASCT and significantly improved the OS in MM (Kumar et al., 2008; Kastritis et al., 2009). This opened a new area of debate 'upfront' versus 'delayed' transplantation. However, current recommendations from experts is that high dose therapy supported by autologous stem cell transplantation (HDT-ASCT) should be the standard of care for eligible patients (Ludwig et al., 2011).

2. Induction therapy for patients eligible for HDT–ASCT

In patients for whom HDT-ASCT is planned, the goal of induction treatment before HDT-ASCT should be to achieve the deepest response preferably up to the level of ≥ VGPR as quickly as possible, to reverse disease related complications and ameliorate patient's symptoms. The protocol should not induce stem cell toxicity and impair stem cell collection. Hence, it is important to avoid melphalan prior to stem cell collection (Cavo et al., 2011; Ludwig et al., 2011).

Prior to novel agents, the standard of care for patients eligible for ASCT was based on high dose dexamethasone alone or VAD (Vincristine, adriamycin, high dose dexamethasone). Over the last few years, the emergence of novel agents (thalidomide, bortezomib and lenalidomide) has shifted the choice of induction regimen from conventional VAD or VAD-like regimens to novel-agent containing protocols. In the earlier studies, the combinations of novel agents with high dose dexamethasone were shown to be superior to VAD regimen before ASCT. The more recent trials have concentrated on upfront use of initially 2-drug and more recently 3-drug or even 4-drug combinations applied before ASCT.

2.1. Thalidomide–based regimens

Thalidomide is the first immunomodulatory drug used in the treatment of MM. Apart from the anti-angiogenic activity, this group of drugs also induce apoptosis in myeloma cells. Thalidomide induces responses in MM patients refractory to conventional and even high dose therapy suggesting that it can overcome drug resistance. It may alter the secretion and bioactivity of cytokines (e.g. TNF-α) secreted into bone marrow microenvironment by myeloma and bone marrow stromal cells that induce myeloma cell growth and survival. Thalidomide mediates its immunomodulatory action by induction of Th-1 T cell response with secretion of IFN-Y and IL-2 and regulation of adhesion molecule expression (Hideshima et al., 2000).

After the initial studies showing that single agent thalidomide could produce significant reponses and that combination of thalidomide with dexamethasone (TD) results in synergism in refractory/relapsed MM, thalidomide was introduced to the induction therapy for newly diagnosed MM (Singhal et al., 1999; Palumbo et al., 2001). The phase II studies demonstrated the efficacy of TD as front line therapy with 64%-66% response rates (Rajkumar et al., 2002; Cavo et al., 2004). In 2005, a retrospective matched case-control analysis provided the first demonstration of superior rate and depth of response by TD compared with VAD as induction

(≥PR; 76% vs 52%, respectively, p<0.001) (Cavo et al., 2005). Based on the subsequent phase III studies which confirmed the superior response rates achieved with thalidomide containing regimens compared with the conventional induction therapies, TD regimen received an accelerated approval in patients with newly diagnosed MM (Rajkumar et al.,2006; Rajkumar et al., 2008). The summary of the phase II-III studies involving thalidomide-based induction regimens is shown in table-1.

Rajkumar et al. in a randomized double blind placebo-controlled study, provided the first data on significant prolongation of time to progression (TTP) and progression free survival (PFS) with TD compared with dexamethasone alone in patients with newly diagnosed MM (14.9 vs. 6.5 months; p<0.001). However, this study was not powered enough to compare the differences in OS (Rajkumar et al., 2008). Barlogie et al. randomized their patients to receive two cycles of high dose melphalan based chemotherapy each supported with ASCT (Total therapy-2) with or without thalidomide added from outset until disease progression and reported that addition of thalidomide improved the rate of CR and EFS but failed to prolong OS (Barlogie et al., 2006). In a retrospective pair-matched analysis, thalidomide incorporated to induction regimen and continued until the second ASCT revealed significantly improved clinical outcomes and a trend towards extended OS at 5 years (69% vs. 53%; p=0.07) (Cavo et al., 2009). The HOVON-50 trial incorporated doxorubicin to TD (TAD) and compared this regimen with conventional VAD as frontline therapy showing a better response before and after HDT-ASCT (Lokhorst et al., 2008). After long term follow-up, the TAD arm folowed by thalidomide maintenance after ASCT was able to induce longer event free survival compared to the VAD arm folloowed by interferon (34 vs. 22 months; p<0.001) but this did not translate into an improved OS (73 vs. 60 months; p=0.77). Which can be explained by a decreased survival from relapse while on thalidomide maintenance (Lokhorst et al., 2010). A recent MRC Myeloma IX randomized trial compared oral combination therapy CTD (cyclophosphamide, thalidomide, dexamethasone) with oral cyclophosphamide incorporated into conventional VAD (CVAD). Significantly superior response rates were attained with CTD compared with CVAD both after induction and after ASCT. CTD could not significantly prolong PFS or OS but longer followup suggests a trend towards a late OS advantage(Morgan et al., 2012).

Thalidomide does not compromise successful harvest of stem cells. However, it is associated with an increased risk of venous thromboembolism (VTE) and sensory peripheral neuropathy (PNP). Without thromboprophylaxis, the thrombosis risk is 15-17%, which is more frequent during the first 3 months of treatment and warrants prophylactic anticoagulation. Peripheral neuropathy improves within 3-4 months after dose reduction or cessation of the drug in most patients. However, thalidomide induced PNP may be irreversible if appropriate action is not taken when an emerging neuropathy is encountered. Thalidomide at low dose may be effective in the management of patients with renal failure, but close monitorization for complications is required in patients with serious renal and hepatic failure. Major thalidomide toxicities and the summary of the supportive care guidelines regarding the approach to PNP is given in tables 7 and 8, respectively (Beksac et al., 2008, Bird et al., 2011).

It is clearly understood that thalidomide-based regimens have produced better post-induction response rates (≥PR; 63-82.5%) and PFS than conventional high dose dexamethasone based regimens. However, OS was not prolonged. Poorer response to salvage therapy and decreased survival have been observed in patients who relapsed while on thalidomide. This may be the result of emergence of resistant clones after thalidomide (Rajkumar et al., 2006; Barlogie et al., 2006;, Cavo et al., 2009; Lokhorst et al., 2010; Morgan et al., 2012). Thalidomide-dexamethasone is less active and more toxic than lenalidomide-based regimens and not recommended as first line therapy anymore. However, in countries where lenalidomide is not available as initial first line therapy and in patients with renal failure, thalidomide combinations may be preferred. On the other hand, thalidomide is still being investigated in combination with other drugs as induction and maintenance regimens for both transplant eligible and ineligible MM patients.

Regimen	N	After induction			After ASCT			PFS	OS	Reference
		≥PR %	≥VGPR %	CR %	≥PR %	≥VGPR %	CR %			
TD vs. D	103 104	63 41	nr nr	4 0	nr nr	nr nr	nr nr	nr nr	nr nr	Rajkumar 2006
TT2 with T vs. TT2 without T	323 345	nr nr	nr nr	nr nr	nr nr	nr nr	62 43	5-year 56% 44% P=0.01	5-year 65% 65% P=0.90	Barlogie 2006
TD vs. D	235 235	63 46	43.8 15.8	7.7 2.6	nr nr	nr nr	nr nr	14.9 mos 6.5 mos P<0.001	nr nr	Rajkumar 2008
Double ASCT + T vs. Double ASCT	135 135		30 15			68 49		4-year 51% 31% P=0.001	5-year 69% 53% P=0.07	Cavo 2009
TAD vs. VAD	268 268	71 57	37 18	3 2	84 76	54 44	14 12	Median 34 mos 22 mos P<0.001	Median 73 mos 60 mos P=0.77	Lokhorst 2010
CTD vs.CVAD	555 556	82.5 71	43 27.5	13 8	92 90	62[a] 74[a]	50[a] 37[a]	Median 27[a] mos 25[a] mos P=0.56	Median Not reach. 63[a] mos P=0.29	Morgan 2012

ASCT: autologous stem cell transplantation ; CTD: cyclophosphamide, thalidomide, dexamethasone; CVAD: cyclophosphamide added to VAD (vincristine, doxorubicin, dexamethasone); nr: not reported; TAD: thalidomide, doxorobicin, dexametahsone; TD: thalidomide, dexamethasone; T: thalidomide; TT2: Total therapy-2. [a] per-protocol analysis

Table 1. Phase II- III studies of thalidomide-based regimens as induction therapy before HDT-ASCT

2.2. Bortezomib–based regimens

Bortezomib is an effective inhibitor of proteosome. The ubiquinitin-proteosome pathway plays an important role in intracellular protein homeostasis by regulating degradation of proteins, including mediators of cell cycle progression and apoptosis. Bortezomib also blocks TNF-α mediated upregulation of NF-KB resulting in decreased binding of myeloma cells to bone marrow stromal cells and results in myeloma cell apoptosis. This activity is observed even in cell lines resistant to conventional anti-myeloma therapies. Bortezomib also cleaves DNA repair enzymes increasing the susceptibility of myeloma cells to DNA damaging agents such as alkylating agents and anthracyclines (Hideshima et al., 2001; Cherry et al., 2012).

Bortezomib received FDA approval in 2003 after showing significant activity in relapsed-refractory MM (Jagannath et al., 2004; Richardson et al., 2005). The initial phase II study of single agent bortezomib in previously untreated MM revealed a response rate of 41% (Richardson et al., 2009). Other phase 2 studies incorporating bortezomib ± dexamethasone to induction regimens were consistent with superior responses ranging from 66% to 95% with 6% to 24% CR rates (Jagannath et al., 2005; Harousseau et al., 2006; Rosinol et al., 2007).

The IFM2005-01 Phase III trial compared VD with VAD as induction before ASCT and lenalidomide was given as post-ASCT maintenance in both arms in a randomized fashion. Post-induction at least VGPR (38% vs 15%) and CR/nCR (15% vs 6%) were superior with VD. This response difference was also maintained after ASCT. However, there was only slight improvement in PFS without an OS benefit. Responses with bortezomib were higher regardless of the disease stage or high-risk cytogenetics (Harousseau et al., 2010).

Popat et al. added doxorubicin at escalating doses (0, 4.5 and 9 mg/m^2) to standard dose bortezomib-dexamethasone (PAD) and demonstrated 95% post-induction response rate with 62% high quality responses (≥ VGPR) (Popat et al., 2008). Addition of pegylated-liposomal doxorubicin to bortezomib-dexamethasone revealed similar responses (≥ PR 85% and ≥ VGPR 57.5%) which was further enhanced in patients who underwent ASCT (≥ VGPR 76.6%) (Jakubowiak et al., 2009). A very recent HOVON-65/GMMG-HD4 trial compared pre-transplant PAD (Bortezomib, Adriamycin, Dexamethasone) induction and bortezomib maintenance after ASCT with pre-transplant VAD induction and thalidomide maintenance after ASCT and demonstrated that bortezomib during induction and maintenance significantly improved response rates, quality of response. Similar to other bortezomib containing 3-drug combinations, PFS was significantly improved. Additionally, unlike the other studies, OS was also prolonged in this study (61% vs 55%). Subgroup analysis also indicated that superior outcome with bortezomib was predominantly accomplished in high risk patients presenting with renal failure and del17p (≥ VGPR; 72% vs 43%) (Sonneveld et al., 2012).

Reeder et al. incorporated cyclophosphamide to bortezomib-dexamethasone (CyBorD/VCD) and reported 71% ≥VGPR after 4 cycles and 74% ≥VGPR after ASCT (Reeder et al., 2009). The German Myeloma Study Group reported 84% response rate (≥PR) with 10% CR after 3 cycles of VCD. Over 60% of their patients had high-risk cyctogenetics. The response rate in cytogenetically high-risk patients were 83.7% (del13q) and 90% t(4;14). However, del17p group had lower response rate at 69.2% (Einsele et al., 2009).

These studies demonstrate that bortezomib-based induction studies produce high response rates (≥ PR; 78%-93% and CR 7%-35%) without any adverse effect on stem cell mobilization (Harousseau et al., 2010; Cavo et al.,2010; Rosinol et al., 2012; Sonneveld et al.,2012; Moreau et al., 2010). However, neurotoxicity is a major concern especially when bortezomib is combined with thalidomide. Neurotoxicity can be reduced by reducing bortezomib dose once weekly without affecting the efficacy or by using subcutenous bortezomib (Mateos et al., 2010). Moreover, Moreau et al. used reduced doses of bortezomib (1 mg/m2) and thalidomide (100 mg/d) in vtD regimen and found that this regimen provided higher VGPR rates compared with VD and the dose reduction of both drugs could resulted in reduced incidence of poly-neuropathy (Moreau et al., 2011). Major bortezomib toxicities and the summary of the supportive care guidelines regarding the approach to emerging PNP is given in tables 7 and 8, respectively (Bird et al.,2011).

Regimen	N	After induction			After ASCT			PFS	OS	Reference
		≥PR %	≥VGPR %	CR %	≥PR %	≥VGPR %	CR %			
VD vs. VAD	223 218	78.5 63	38 15	15 6	80 77	54 37	35 18	Median 36 mos 30 mos P=0.06	3-year 81% 77% P=0.5	Harousseau 2010 IFM 2005-02
VTD vs. TD	236 238	93 79	62 28	31 11	93 84	82 64	55 41	3-year 68% 56% P=0.005	3-year 86% 84% P=0.03	Cavo 2010 GIMEMA-MMY 3006
VBMCP/VBAD+V vs. VTD vs. TD	129 130 127	75 85 62	36 60 29	21 35 14	73 77 58	51 65 40	38 46 24	Median 38 mos 27 mos Not reach. P=0.006	Nr Nr Nr	Rosinol 2012 PETHEMA/ GEM
PAD vs. VAD	413 414	78 54	42 14	7 2	88 75	62 36	21 9	Median 35 mos 28 mos P=0.002	5-year 61% 55%	Sonneveld 2012 HOVON65/ GMMG HD4
VD vs. vtD	99 100	81 88	36 49	31 29	86 89	58 74	22 31	Median 30 mos 26 mos P=0.22	Nr nr	Moreau 2011 IFM2007-02

VD: Bortezomib, dexamethasone; VAD: Vincristine, doxorubicin, dexamethasone; VTD: Bortezomib, thalidomide, dexamethasone; TD: Thalidomide,dexamethasone; VBMCP/VBAD+V: Vincristine, carmustine, melphalan,cyclophosphamide, prednisone/ vincristine, carmustine, doxorubicin, dexamethasone + bortezomib; PAD: Bortezomib, doxorubicin, dexamethasone; vtD: Reduced dose bortezomib, reduced dose thalidomide, dexamethasone; mos: months

Table 2. Phase III studies of bortezomib-based regimens in preparation for HDT-ASCT

Bortezomib has become an important component of therapy for patients with high risk MM associated with del13q and t(4;14) (Richardson et al., 2005; Jagannath et al., 2007). Bortezomib has also proven effective in management of MM patients with renal dysfunction. It has been suggested that in patients with acute renal failure secondary to light chain cast nephropathy VTD can be first choice due to lack of nephrotoxicity. The Mayo Clinic recommends plasma exchange until serum free light chain (FLC)<50 mg/dl and repeated as needed until VTD is fully effective (Rajkumar et al., 2011). Bortezomib is also beneficial for individuals with significant disease related bone-disease due to its inhibitory effect on osteoclastogenesis and stimulatory effect on osteoblast differentiation and proliferation (Zavrski et al., 2005).

Regimen	Progression free survival				Reference
	Overall		**del13q**	**t(4;14)**	**del(17p)**
VD + R ± R vs.	36 mos (median)	nr	28mos (median)	14mos (median)	Avet-Loiseau 2010
VAD + R ± R	30 mos (median)	nr	16mos (median)	nr	
PAD + Bort vs.	48% (at 3-yr)	40% (at 3-yr)	28% (at 3-yr)	22% (at 3-yr)	Sonneveld 2010
VAD + T	40% (at 3-yr)	29% (at 3-yr)	20% (at 3-yr)	16% (at 3-yr)	
VTD + VTD vs.	68% (at 3-yr)	62% (at 3-yr)	69% (at 3-yr)	nr	Cavo 2010
TD + TD	56% (at 3-yr)	46% (at 3-yr)	37% (at 3-yr)	nr	

Table 3. Impact of bortezomib incorporated into ASCT on PFS according to cytogenetic abnormalities (Cavo 2012)

2.3. Lenalidomide–based regimens

Lenalidomide is another IMID and has more potent in vitro activity; inhibition of angiogenesis, cytokine modulation and T-cell costimulation than thalidomide (Hideshima et al., 2000 ; Haslett et al., 2003). Lenalidomide primarily triggers the caspase-8 mediated apoptotic pathway and also down-regulates NF-KB activity via a mechanism distinct from bortezomib (Mitsiades et al., 2002). Lenalidomide alone (R) or with dexamethasone (RD) has shown significant activity in relapsed/refractory MM. Responses were observed even in patients in whom thalidomide therapy has previously failed (Richardson et al., 2002). Several phase II studies of lenalidomide and dexamethasone +/- chemotherapy have demonstrated response rates ranging 76-91% (Table-4). In a randomized controlled trial lenalidomide plus high dose dexamethasone (RD) (480 mg/28d cycle) was compared with lenalidomide plus low dose dexamethasone (Rd) (160 mg/28d cycle). Patient enrollment to study was not restricted with age or eligibility for ASCT. In each group lenalidomide was administered as 25 mg/d on 1-21 days. In accordance with others, this study demonstrated that lenalidomide in combination with dexamethasone is an efficient initial therapy for MM. Although RD produced higher response rates, this did not result in superior TTP, PFS or OS compared with Rd. The cause of inferior OS with high dose dexamethasone seems to be related to increased deaths due to toxicity, particularly in first 4 months and in eldely patients. The major grade 3 or higher toxicities including thromboembolic events and infections were significantly higher in the high dose dexamethasone group (Rajkumar et al., 2010). The multicenter, placebo controlled SWOG trial has confirmed the superiority of lenalidomide in combination with dexamethasone over dexamethasone alone as initial therapy of MM in terms of response rate and PFS but not in OS. This study received early closure and open-label lenalidomide and dexamethasone was made available to all patients (Zonder et al., 2010). In a retrospective case-control study, RD produced better responses than TD including superior PFS and OS. However, this study was not a randomized trial and the choice of post-induction therapy was not standardized (Gay et al., 2010a). Claritromycin is an antibiotic that has shown efficacy in association with steroids and both thalidomide and lenalidomide. The same investigators added clarithromycin (Bioxin) to Rd(BiRd) and compared with Rd in a case-match study. The have reported significantly better responses with BiRd and the PFS was significantly longer. However, 3- year OS was not statistically different between the two study arms (Gay et al., 2010).

Lenalidomide can cause myelosuppression and concerns have been raised that its use may negatively impact the ability to mobilize stem cells in patients who received lenalidomide as part of their induction therapies (Kumar et al., 2007; Mazumder et al., 2008; Paripati et al., 2008; Popat et al., 2009). It is suggested that stem cells should be collected within 6 months of initiation of lenalidomide therapy and the IMWG recommends that patients >65 years or patients who have received ≥ 4 cycles Rd must undergo stem cell mobilization with cyclophosphamide + G-CSF or G-CSF + plerixafor (Kumar 2007; Kumar 2009). Dose reduction is required in presence of renal impairment. Patients may require thromboprophylaxis due to higher incidence of thromboembolic events. Major lenalidomide toxicities are summarized in table-10 (Bird et al., 2011).

2.4. Novel agent triplet combinations

To enhance response rates and prolong PFS combination of Bortezomib with an IMID has been attempted. Bortezomib-thalidomide-dexamethasone (VTD) resulted better response rates and PFS compared to TD or VD in initial randomized trials (Wang et al., 2005; Cavo et al., 2009). In a Phase III study of VTD compared with TD as induction before and consolidation after double ASCT, VTD was superior to TD in all response categories (CR/n CR; 31% vs 11% ; ≥VGPR; 62% vs 28%) as well as the 3 year estimated PFS (68% vs 56%). Progression free survival was also superior with VTD compared to TD in poor prognostic groups including del13q, increased LDH, age>60 years, t(4;14) ± del17p, increased bone marrow plasma cell ratio and ISS-II and III (Cavo et al., 2010). The results of the PETHEMA/GEM study also provided a strong support to VTD as a highly effective induction regimen compared with a combination chemotherapy containing bortezomib and with TD. Additionally, VTD resulted in a higher post-transplantation CR rate and a significantly longer PFS. However, this did not result in a significant prolongation of OS and could not overcome poor prognosis of high-risk cytogenetics (Rosinol et al., 2012).

Synergy has been demonstrated between bortezomib and lenalidomide. Moreover, both bortezomib and immunomodulatory drugs enhance the activity of dexamethasone. In a phase I study combining these three agents (RVD) in patients with newly diagnosed MM, the maximum tolerated dose was set as lenalidomide 25mg/day, bortezomib 1.3mg/m^2, dexamethasone 20mg/day and in phase II portion of the same study, 100% response rate (≥PR) could be obtained with ≥VGPR and CR rates 74% and 37%, respectively. This was the first study to result in 100% response rate. The 18-month PFS and OS were 75% and 97%, respectively (Richardson et al., 2010).

In phase II trials the most promising combinations were either lenalidomide or cyclophosphamide with bortezomib and dexamethasone. A phase II study of four-drug combination VDCR, VDR, VDC and VDC-mod (modification of the cyclophosphamide dose) was performed to evaluate the feasibility and activity of these combinations. The response seen with VDCR appear to be similar to those seen with VDR or VDC-mod arms (Table-5). However, the toxicities with VDCR appear to be more than the other arms, especially hematological toxicity. This study does not support an advantage of four drug combination (Kumar et al.,2012).

In another phase I/II study RVD was combined with pegylated-doxorubicin (RVDD) and this regimen was highly active and well-tolerated with response rates ≥PR 96% and 95%, ≥VGPR 57% and 65% after 4 and 8 cycles, respectively (Table-6). After a median 15.5 months follow-up, PFS and OS were not reached. The estimated 18-month PFS and OS were 80.8% and 98.6%, respectively. Among patients who proceeded to ASCT and were evaluable for posttransplant response, response rate further improved reaching 85% of patients ≥VGPR and 61% of those with CR/n CR at 3 months after ASCT. In patients who continued RVDD beyond 4 cycles, depth of response further improved reaching 65% ≥VGPR and 35% CR/n CR at the completion of 8 cycles (Jakuboviak et al., 2011).

Regimen	N	After induction			PFS	OS	Reference
		≥PR %	≥VGPR %	CR %			
RD	34	91	38	6			Rajkumar 2005
					Median		
RD vs.					19 mos	2-yr	Rajkumar 2010
Rd	223	79	42		25 mos	75%	
	222	68	24		P=0.026	87%	
						3-yr	
RD vs.					3-yr	79%	Zonder 2010
D	97	78			52%	73%	
	95	48			32%	P=0.28	
					Median	Median	
RD vs.					26.7mos	Notreach	Gay 2010
TD	228	80	37.8	13.6	17.1 mos	57.2 mos	
	183	61	15	3.3	P=0.036	P=0.018	
					Median	Median	
BiRd vs.					48.3 mos	89.7%	Gay 2010
Rd	72		73.6	45.8	27.5 mos	73%	
	72		33	13.9	P=0.044	P=0.170	

Table 4. Results of phase II-III Studies of induction with lenalidomide and dexamethasone

	VDCR N=39	VDR N=36	VDC N=31	VDC-mod N=16
After 4 cycles				
CR	5%	7%	3%	12%
≥VGPR	33%	32%	13%	41%
≥PR	80%	73%	63%	82%
Best response across all cycles (median=6 cycles)				
CR	25%	24%	22%	47%
≥VGPR	58%	51%	41%	53%
≥PR	88%	85%	75%	100%
1-yr PFS	86%	83%	93%	100%
After censoring patients going to ASCT				
1-yr PFS	83%	68%	97%	100%
1-yr OS	92%	100%	100%	100%
Patients who undergo ASCT				
1-yr PFS	100%	100%	88%	100%
1-yr OS	100%	100%	100%	100%

Table 5. Results of EVOLUTION Study comparing bortezomib-based multi-drug combinations

	N	Best response after induction (%)			Reference
		≥PR	≥ VGPR	CR	
RVD	66	100	67	39	Richardson 2010
VDCR vs.	39	88	58	25	Kumar 2012
VDR vs.	36	85	51	24	
VDC vs.	31	75	41	22	
VDC-mod	16	100	53	47	
RVDD					
After 4 cycles		96	57	29	Jakubowiak 2011
After 8 cycles	74	95	65	35	

Table 6. Phase II Trials of triplet or quadruplet lenalidomide-based induction

Thalidomide	Lenalidomide	Bortezomib
Venous thromboembolism	Cytopenias	Peripheral neuropathy
Sensory peripheral neuropathy	Venous thromboembolism	Gastrointestinal toxicity
Constipation	Constipation	Postural hypotension and pre-syncope secondary to autonomic neuropathy

Thalidomide	Lenalidomide	Bortezomib
Hematological toxicity	Fatigue	Thrombocytopenia
Somnolence	Neuropathy	Fatigue
Rashes	Skin rash	Increased incidence of varicella zoster infections
Arrhythmias	Muscle cramps	
Thyroid dysfunction	Thyroid dysfunction	
Congenital malformations due to fetal exposure	Diarrhea	

Table 7. Major toxicities of novel agents

Grade of neuropathy	Bortezomib	Thalidomide
Grade 1 Paresthesia, weakness and/or loss of reflexes without painor loss of function	No action	No action
Grade 1 with pain or grade 2 interfering with function but not with daily activities	Reduce bortezomib dose to 1mg/m^2	Reduce thalidomide dose to 50% or suspend thalidomide until disappearence of toxicity, then reinitiate at 50% dose
Grade 2 with pain or grade 3	Suspend bortezomib until disappearence of toxicity then re-initiate at 0.7 mg/m^2 and administer once weekly	Suspend thalidomide until disappearence of toxicity, then reinitiate at low dose if PNP grade 1
Grade 4	Discontinue	Discontinue

Table 8. Guidelines for the management of bortezomib and thalidomide induced PNP

2.5. Conclusions

High dose melphalan supported by autologous stem cell transplantation after novel agent-based induction regimen is the standard of care for patients younger than 65. The quality of response achieved with induction regimens before ASCT affect PFS and potentially the OS. In this regard, the availability of novel anti-myeloma drugs, thalidomide, bortezomib and lenalidomide has improved the pre-transplantation responses. Recent data suggest that 3-drug induction regimens, containing at least one novel agent result in better responses than 2-drug combinations. The results of studies with combinations of VD with either doxorubicin (PAD), cyclophosphamide (CyBorRd), thalidomide (VTD) or lenalidomide (VRD) have demonstrated that the responses can be further enhanced and PFS ± OS can be improved. Within the 3-drug combinations, bortezomib-dexamethasone combined with thalidomide or cyclophosphamide(VTD or VCD) appear to be the most active regimens. So, 3-6 cycles of a triplet bortezomib based regimen should be considered the standard induction for patients eligible for ASCT. The objective of treatment should be the achievement of a sustained CR with a good quality of life. Current studies concentrate on best approach to combine available drugs to affect long-term disease control as well as consolidation and maintenance after ASCT and minimize the long-term toxicities, especially neurotoxicity. Bortezomib is effective not only in patients with standard risk disease but also in the presence of high risk cytogenetic abnormalities especially in presence of t(4;14). Current question under evaluation is whether to apply or delay ASCT when a CR is achieved with a novel agent induction treatment.

3. Induction therapy for patients ineligible for HDT–ASCT

Melphalan was the first alkylating agent used for treatment of MM and melphalan –prednisone (MP) has been the standard therapy for over 30 years although it yielded only PR in 40-60% of patients with CR <5% and PFS about 18 months and OS 2-3 years. Trials comparing MP with high dose dexamethasone-based combinations revealed no survival advantage (Mateos et al., 2012). During the last decade, with the emergence of novel agents and the studies revealing the importance of achieving VGPR/CR on survival of myeloma patients, the historical goals of induction have changed to achieving a high quality response in elderly patients as well.

3.1. Bendamustine

Bendamustine is a novel bifunctional drug which has similarities to both alkylating agents and purine analogs. It has promising activity in low grade lymphoid malignancies. The East German Study Group conducted a phase III trial comparing bendamustine and prednisone (BP) with standard MP in previously untreated patients with MM who are ineligible for transplantation. Bendamustine –prednisone was superior to MP with respect to CR rate (32% vs 13%, p=0.007) and TTF (14 mos vs 10 mos, p=0.02). There was no significant difference with regard to OS between the two treatment groups and the toxicity profile was comparable (Pönisch et al., 2006). Mainly based on the results of this study, bendamustine is currently approved for treatment of newly diagnosed MM patients who are not candidates for HDT-ASCT and who can not receive thalidomide or bortezomib due to peripheral neuropathy. The same investigators in a recent study demonstrated that bendamustine in combination with bortezomib and prednisone (BPV) is also effective in patients with newly diagnosed MM and renal failure. Eighty-three percent of the patients treated with this protocol responded to therapy and 72% had their renal function improved after treatment (Pönisch et al., 2012).

3.2. Thalidomide–based regimens

Thalidomide incorporated in to the MP regimen (MPT) has been compared with the standard MP regimen in six randomized phase III studies. Each protocol had some minor differences in their schedules which is shown in table-9. The overall response rate (57%-76%) with MPT was significantly higher than MP (31%-48%).The CR rates with MPT ranged between 7%-13%, one study reported ≥ VGPR rate as 27%. In the IFM-I/II studies and in HOVON study, the prolongation in the PFS with MPT was also translated in to OS advantage (Facon et al., 2007; Hulin et al., 2009; Wijermans et al., 2010). Despite in the other three studies the PFS advantage was not translated into OS advantage (Palumbo et al., 2008; Waage et al., 2010; Beksac et al., 2011), a metaanalysis of the pooled data of 1682 patients from these six trials showed that the addition of thalidomide to MP improves OS and PFS in previously untreated elderly patients with multiple myeloma, extending the median survival time by on average 20%. In this metaanalysis, median PFS was prolonged by 5.4 months (HR 0.67 (0.55-0.80) p<0.0001) and the median OS was prolonged 6.6 months (HR 0.82 (0.66-1.02) p=0.004) (Fayers et al., 2011). This improvement was less pronounced in patients aged ≥ 75 years and no favorable effect of thalidomide on OS in this population could be demonstrated. The most frequent grade 3-4 adverse events with MPT protocol were polyneuropathy (6-23%) and VTE (3-12%), infections (10-13%), cardiac complications (2-7%), gastrointestinal events (5%). The discontinuation rate ranged 16-45% (Hulin et al., 2009; Wijermans et al., 2010; Fayers et al., 2011). Based on these results, MPT became one of the new standard therapies for elderly patients with newly diagnosed MM.

Thalidomide-dexamethasone (TD) combination was also compared with MP in 289 elderly patients with MM. Patients achieving stable disease or better were randomly assigned to maintenance therapy with either thalidomide 100 mg daily or interferon alpha-2b. Thalidomide-dexamethasone resulted in a higher proportion of ≥VGPR (26% vs 13%; P=.006) and ORR (68% vs 50%; P=.002) compared with MP. However, PFS was similar (16.7 vs 20.7 months; P=. 1) and OS was significantly shorter in the TD group (41.5 vs 49.4 months; P=.024). Decreased survival was more evident in patients older than 75 years due to increased non-disease related deaths during the first year (Ludwig et al., 2009). Combinations with high dose dexamethasone is not recommended for elderly patients especially those ≥ 75 years due to increased toxicity. In a randomized MRC Myeloma IX trial, cyclophosphamide, thalidomide and dexamethasone (CTDa) in which dexamethasone dose was reduced, produced higher response rates than MP but was not associated with improved PFS and OS. Additionally, CTDa was associated with higher rates of adverse events compared to MP (Morgan et al., 2011).

3.3. Bortezomib–based regimens

After showing significant efficacy in relapsed-refractory myeloma, bortezomib was also incorporated into trials for initial therapy of MM in transplant ineligible patients. The clinical value of adding bortezomib to the standard MP regimen (VMP) was explored in Velcade as Initial Standard Therapy (VISTA) Study (San Miguel et al., 2008). In this phase III study, 682 newly diagnosed myeloma patients were randomly assigned to receive nine 6-week cycles of melphalan (9 mg/m2) and prednisone (60 mg/m2) on days 1 to 4, either alone or with bortezomib (1.3 mg/m2) on days 1, 4, 8, 11, 22, 25, 29 and 32 during cycles 1 to 4 and on days 1, 8, 22, and 29 during cycles 5 to 9. Addition of bortezomib to MP significantly improved all responses, PFS as well as the OS (Table-10). The main adverse events associated with VMP were neutropenia (40%), thrombocytopenia (37%), peripheral neuropathy (14%), infection (10%) and gastrointestinal events (7%). A recent update of the VISTA study and a subsequent study showed that grade 3-4 hematological and non-hematological adverse events in partic-

Regimen	N	Schedule	ORR%	CR%	TTP (months)	OS (median)	Reference
MPT+T(until PD) MP	129 126	M: 4mg/m2, d1-7 P: 40mg/m2, d1-7 T: 100mg/d 6 cycles every 4 wks until relapse	76 48	16 2.4	22 15 p=0.004	45 47.6 p=0.79	GIMEMA Palumbo 2008
MPT MP No maintenance	125 196	M:0.25mg/kg, d1-4 P: 2mg/kg, d1-4 T:100-400mg/d 12 cycles every 6 wks	76 35	13 2	28 18	52 33 P=0.0006	IFM-I Facon 2007
MPT MP No maintenance	113 116	M:0.20mg/kg, d1-4 P: 2mg/kg, d1-4 T:100mg/d 12 cycles every 6 wks	62 31	7 1	24 19 P=0.001	44 29 P=0.028	IFM-II Hulin 2009
MPT+T(until PD) MP	148 179	M:0.25mg/kg, d1-4 P: 100mg/d, d1-4 T:200-400mg/d Until plateau every 6 wks Maintenance T 200mg	57 40	13 4	15 14 ns	29 32 ns	NMSG Waage 2010
MPT+T(until PD) MP	165 168	M:0.25mg/kg, d1-5 P: 1mg/kg, d1-5 T:200mg/d 8 cycles every 4 wks Maintenance T 50mg	66 45	27 10 ≥VGPR	13 9 P<0.001 PFS	40 31 P=0.05	HOVON Wijermans 2010
MPT MP No maintenance	62 60	M: 9mg/m2, d1-4 P: 60mg/m2, d1-4 T: 100mg/d 8 cycles every 6 wks	58 38	9 9	21 14 P=0.34 DFS	26 28 P=0.65	TMSG Beksac 2011

M:Melphalan; P:Prednisone; T:Thalidomide; PD:Progressive disease; PFS:Progression free survival; DFS: Disease free survival; GIMEMA: Italian Myeloma Network IFM: Intergroupe Francophone du Mye´lome; NMSG: Nordic Myeloma Study Group; HOVON: Dutch-Belgium Hemato-Oncology Cooperative Group; TMSG:Turkish Myeloma Study Group

Table 9. Phase III Studies comparing MPT versus MP for newly diagnosed MM ineligible for HDT-ASCT

ular PNP as well as discontinuation of the drug was significantly reduced without affecting the efficacy when once weekly bortezomib schedule was used (Mateos et al., 2010a; Brignhen et al., 2010). In the VISTA trial, patients with high risk cytogenetic profile had similar response rate and OS with the patients with standard risk profile suggesting that addition of bortezomib may overcome the poor prognosis confered to high risk cytogenetics. Another important point of this study was that first-line bortezomib use did not induce more resistant relapse unlike that is seen in thalidomide relapses. The survival data of the VISTA trial was updated at 3 years and 5 years and the survival benefit of VMP protocol remained significant (Mateos et al., 2010a; San Miguel et al., 2011). A part of the VISTA trial investigated the efficacy of VMP protocol in renal impairment excluding patients with Cr >2mg/dl. Response rates with VMP and TTP in both arms did not appear significantly different between patients with GFR ≤ 50 or > 50 mL/min. Moreover, VMP resulted in 44% renal impairment reversal suggesting that this protocol is also an active and well-tolerated treatment option for patients with moderate renal impairment (Dimopoulos et al., 2009).

	VMP N=344	**MP N=338**	p	**References**
ORR (≥PR)	71%	35%	<0.001	San Miguel 2008
CR	30%	4%	<0.001	
TTP	24 mos	16.6 mos	<0.001	
OS Median follow-up 16.3 mos			0.008 HR[a]=0.61	
OS Median follow-up 36.7 mos	Not reached	43 mos	<0.001 HR[a]=0.653	Mateos 2010
OS Median follow-up 60 mos	56.4 mos	43.1 mos	0.0004 HR[a]=0.695	San Miguel 2011
3-yr OS	68.5%	54%		

a Hazard Ratio

Table 10. Results of the VISTA trial and the long-tem follow-up

In the PETHEMA trial Mateos et al. have demonstrated that reduced intensity induction with a bortezomib based regimen followed by maintenance is a safe and effective treatment. The investigators compared VMP with VTP (bortezomib, thalidomide, prednisone) as initial therapy in newly diagnosed patients with MM ineligible for transplantation. In both protocols, a reduced intensity bortezomib schedule consisting of one cycle of bortezomib twice per week for 6 weeks followed by five cycles of bortezomib once per week for 5 weeks was used. Patients who completed the six induction cycles were randomly assigned to maintenance therapy with bortezomib plus prednisone (VP) or bortezomib plus thalidomide (VT). The response rates were higher with VTP compared to VMP (CR 28% vs 20% ; ORR 81% vs 80%). Maintenance with VT significantly improved time to progression compared with that for patients who received VP. The support to better response rates with VTP also came from the initial results of UPFRONT study which compared VD, VTD and VMP and revealed better response rates with VTD (Table-11). On the other hand, in both studies patients treated with VTP had more frequent serious adverse events especially PNP and thrombosis (Mateos et al., 2010b; Nievizsky et al., 2011). Combining four drugs (bortezomib, melphalan, prednisone, thalidomide) followed by maintenance with bortezomib-thalidomide (VMPT-VT) was superior to VMP alone in patients with MM who are ineligible for autologous stem-cell transplantation. The 3-years PFS was also improved with VMPT-VT. However, no significant difference in 3-year OS was observed. Additionally, grade 3 to 4 neutropenia, cardiologic events and thromboembolic events were more frequent among patients assigned to the VMPT-VT group than among those assigned to the VMP group (Palumbo et al., 2010). Due to significantly increased adverse events with 4-drug regimen, VMP or MPT are better alternatives for induction of elderly myeloma patients.

	N	ORR % CR % After induction		PFS	OS	Reference
VMP	130	80	20	37 mos	60mos median	Mateos 2010
VTP	130	81	28	32 mos	5-yr 53%	
maintenance VP or VT						
VMPT + VT	254	89	38	3-year	3-year 89%	Palumbo 2010
VMP + no maintenance	257	81	24 P<0.001	56% 41% p=0.008	87% p=0.77	
VD	168	73	24			
VTD	167	80	36	NA	NA	Nievizsky 2011
VMP	167	69	31			

VD:Bortezomib dexamethasone; VTD: Bortezimib, thalidomide, dexamethasone; VMP: Bortezomib, melphalan, prednisone; VT: Bortezomib, thalidomide; mos: months; NA: Not available

Table 11. Phase III Studies comparing bortezomib containing regimens

3.4. Lenalidomide–based regimens

In a randomized controlled trial lenalidomide (25 mg/d on d 1-21) plus high dose dexamethasone (480 mg/28d cycle) (RD) produced higher response rates compared with lenalidomide (25 mg/d on d 1-21) plus low dose dexamethasone (Rd) (160 mg/28d cycle). However, this did not translate into superior PFS (Median 19.1 months vs 25.3 months). Moreover, Rd was associated with significantly improved 1-year OS than with RD (96% vs 87%, p=0.0002) and treatment related toxicity was significantly reduced. The cause of inferior OS with high dose dexamethasone seems to be related to increased deaths due to toxicity particularly in first 4 months and in elderly patients. Hence, the advantages of Rd over RD were more pronounced in patients aged > 70 years (Rajkumar et al.,2010; Zonder et al., 2010). A recent double-blind, multicenter, randomized study compared melphalan-prednisone-lenalidomide induction followed by lenalidomide maintenance (MPR-R) with melphalan-prednisone-lenalidomide

(MPR) or melphalan-prednisone (MP) followed by placebo. Response rates were superior with MPR-R compared with MPR or MP (ORR, 77% vs 68% vs 50%; CR, 18% vs 13% vs 5%; respectively). MPR-R significantly prolonged PFS in patients with newly diagnosed multiple myeloma who were ineligible for transplantation, with the greatest benefit observed in patients 65 to 75 years of age. This study also underlines the importance of lenalidomide maintenance after MPR induction as another treatment option for elderly myeloma patients The toxicity profile was excessive for frail patients, which negatively affected the efficacy. Main grade 3-4 adverse events of MPR were neutropenia (52-71%), thrombocytopenia (23-38%), infections (10%) and thromboembolism (5%)(Palumbo et al., 2012).

Various circumstances	Suggestions
Rapid reversal of spinal cord compression or renal impairment	Bortezomib
Pre-existing neuropathy	Lenalidomide (MPR, Rd) or bendamustin (BP)
History of venous thromboembolism	Bortezomib
In cases with renal failure	Thalidomide, bortezomib, bendamustin can be administered at full dose, Lenalidomide requires dose reduction according to creatinin clearence
Contraindications to use of alkyllating agents such as presence myelodysplasia or increased risk of myelosuppression	TD or VD can be used instead of MP
Frail patients	Prednisone is beter tolerated than dexamethasone

Table 12. Individualized treatment strategies for non-transplant candidate patients

It is clear that the novel agents have prolonged the survival of patients with MM. However, this benefit is more pronounced in younger patients. Age has been reported to be a negative prognostic factor. It is not because the elderly patients have biologically different disease but because they can not tolerate high intensity therapy protocols, have lower bone marrow reserves, increased tendency for infections and also difficulty in recovering from infections and have more frequent drug toxicities. A patient's overall physical condition, fraility, comorbidity and disability should be asessed before starting therapy in order to choose the appropriate treatment protocol and dosing. These terms are fully explained in a review by Palumbo et al (Palumbo A et al. 2011). Although the novel agents offer important survival for patients with MM, the incidence of grade 3-4 adverse events and drug discontinuations are significantly higher with combination regimens that are based on novel agents than with traditional chemotherapy regimens. It has been suggested that modifying drug doses at the start of therapy and management of adverse events during the therapy improves tolerability so that the patients can receive the drugs for a longer time to get survival benefit. Secondly, the tolerability of treatment can be further improved with full supportive therapy with bisphosphanates, antivirals, anticoagulants, growth factors and appropriate pain control.

3.5. Conclusions

At present, the induction regimen for patients ineligible for HDT/ASCT is either MP or high/lower dose of Dexamethasone combined with one of the three novel agents (thalidomide or bortezomib or lenalidomide). Selection between these combinations depends on the patients' presenting symptoms such as presence of neuropathy, renal impairment or the rapidity required to reverse the symptoms. In countries where lenalidomide is not yet allowed as first line therapy, induction can be started with thalidomide or bortezomib containing triple regimens and in case of unresponsiveness or intolerability, lenalidomide can be used as second line therapy. Fraility, comorbidity and disability of the elderly patients should be taken into account before choosing the induction protocol and appropriate dose reductions should be done. Thus, the treatment should be individualized. Melphalan-based regimens are used for a fixed duration (9-18 months) and then observed. However, the duration of treatment with revlimid (Rd) is unclear either continue until relapse or a fixed duration of 18 months has been tested in ongoing phase III trials. Evidence is now emerging that maintenance or continuous therapy with novel agents is improving PFS with a potential to improve OS. However, in elderly patients, it is particularly important to start treatment at a dose that can be tolerated over the long term. Specific recommendations yet can not be made regarding the impact of novel treatment regimens on prognosis of elderly patients with high-risk cytogenetics. Although the Italian study (Palumbo et al., 2010) suggested some PFS benefit in response to VMPT+VT over VMP regarding the high-risk cytogenetics, other studies did not confirm this.

Regimen	Usual dosing schedule	Reference
Melphalan-Prednisone (MP-7 day Schedule)	Melphalan 8-10 mg oral days 1-7 Prednisone 60mg/d oral days 1-7 Repeated every 6 weeks	Kyle et al., 2004
Thalidomide-Dexamethasone (Td)	Thalidomide 200 mg oral days 1-28 Dexamethasone 40 mg oral days 1,8,15,22 Repeated every 4 weeks	Rajkumar et al., 2006
Lenalidomide-Dexamethasone (Rd)	Lenalidomide 25 mg oral days 1-21 Dexamethasone 40 mg oral days 1,8,15,22 Repeated every 4 weeks	Rajkumar et al., 2010
Bortezomib –dexamethasone (Vd)	Bortezomib 1.3 mg/m^2 iv days 1,8,15,22 Dexamethasone 20 mg on day of and day after bortezomib (or 40 mg days 1,8,15,22) Repeated every 4 weeks	Harousseau et al., 2006
Melphalan-Prednisone-Thalidomide (MPT)	Different MPT protocols are described in table...	

Regimen	Usual dosing schedule	Reference
Bortezomib-Melphalan-Prednisone (VMP)	Bortezomib 1.3 mg/m^2 iv days 1,8,15,22 Melphalan 9 mg/ m^2 oral days 1-4 Prednisone 60 mg/ m^2 oral days 1-4 Repeated every 35 days	San Miguel et al., 2008
Bortezomib-Thalidomide-Dexamethasone (VTD)	Bortezomib 1.3 mg/m^2 iv days 1,8,15,22 Thalidomide 100-200 mg oral days 1-21 Dexamethasone 20 mg on day of and day after bortezomib (or 40 mg days 1,8,15,22) Repeated every 4 weeks	Cavo et al., 2009
Cyclophosphamide-Bortezomib-Dexamethasone (CyBorD)	Cyclophosphamide 300mg/ m^2 oral days 1,8,15,22 Bortezomib 1.3 mg/m^2 iv days 1,8,15,22 Dexamethasone 40 mg oral days 1,8,15,22 Repeated every 4 weeks	Reeder et al., 2009
Bortezomib-Cyclophosphamide-Dexamethasone (VCD)	Bortezomib 1.3 mg/m^2 iv days 1,4,8,11 Cyclophosphamide 900mg/ m^2 on day 1 every 3 weeks Dexamethasone 40 mg on day of and day after bortezomib	Einsele et al., 2009
Bortezomib-Lenalidomide-Dexamethasone (VRD)	Bortezomib 1.3 mg/m^2 iv days 1,8 and 15 Lenalidomide 25 mg oral days 1-14 Dexamethasone 20 mg on day of and day after bortezomib (or 40 mg days 1,8,15,22) Repeated every 3 weeks	Richardson et al., 2010
Bortezomib-Melphalan-Prednisone-Thalidomide (VMPT)	Bortezomib 1.3 mg/m^2 iv days 1,8,15,22 every 35 days Melphalan 9 mg/ m^2 oral days 1-4 every 35 days Prednisone 60 mg/ m^2 oral days 1-4 every 35 days Thalidomide 50 mg/day	Palumbo et al., 2010
Melphalan-Prednisone-Lenalidomide (MPR-R)	Melphalan 0.18 mg/kg on days 1-4 every 4 weeks x 9 cycles Prednisone 2mg/kg on days 1-4 every 4 weeks x 9 cycles Lenalidomide 10 mg on days 1-21 then 10mg/d until relapse	Palumbo et al., 2012
Cyclophosphamide-Thalidomide-Dexamethasone (atenuated dose) (CTD a)	Cyclophosphamide 500mg/week Thalidomide 50 mg/day for 4 weeks, 50 mg increments every 4 weeks to a maximum 200mg/day Dexamethasone 20 mg/day on days 1- 4 and 15-18 every 4 weeks	Morgan et al., 2011
Bortezomib-Lenalidomide-Dexamethasone-Cyclophosphamide (VRDC)	Bortezomib 1.3 mg/m^2 iv days 1,4,8,11 Lenalidomide 15 mg oral days 1-14 Dexamethasone 40 mg days 1,8,15 Cyclophosphamide 500mg/ m^2 days 1,8	Kumar et al., 2010

Table 13. Main treatment protocols in Multiple Myeloma

Author details

Sule Mine Bakanay[1] and Meral Beksac[2]

1 Ataturk Hospital, Hematology Unit, Ankara, Turkey

2 Ankara University School of Medicine,Department of Hematology, Ankara, Turkey

References

[1] Anderson, K. C, Jagannath, S, Jakubowiak, A, Lonial, S, Raje, N, Alsina, M, Ghobrial, I, & Knight, R. Esseltine D & Richardson J Clin Oncol, abstr 8536., 2009.

[2] Attal, M, Harousseau, J. L, Stoppa, A. M, Sotto, J. J, Fuzibet, J. G, Rossi, J. F, Casassus, P, Maisonneuve, H, Facon, T, & Ifrah, N. Payen C & Bataille R. ((1996). A prospective, randomized trial of autologous bone marrow transplantation and chemotherapy in multiple myeloma. Intergroupe Français du Myélome. N Engl J Med., 11;, 335(2), 91-7.

[3] Avet-loiseau, H, Leleu, X, Roussel, M, Moreau, P, Guerin-charbonnel, C, Caillot, D, Marit, G, Benboubker, L, Voillat, L, Mathiot, C, Kolb, B, Macro, M, Campion, L, Wetterwald, M, Stoppa, A. M, Hulin, C, Facon, T, & Attal, M. Minvielle S & Harousseau JL. ((2010). Bortezomib plus dexamethasone induction improves outcome of patients with t(4;14)myeloma but not outcome of patients with del(17p). J Clin Oncol.,, 28(30), 4630-4.

[4] Barlogie, B, Tricot, G, Anaissie, E, Shaughnessy, J, Rasmussen, E, Van Rhee, F, Fassas, A, Zangari, M, Hollmig, K, Pineda-roman, M, Lee, C, Talamo, G, Thertulien, R, Kiwan, E, Krishna, S, Fox, M, & Crowley, J. Thalidomide and hematopoietic-cell transplantation for multiple myeloma. N Engl J Med. (2006). Mar 9;, 354(10), 1021-30.

[5] Beksac, M. Delforge M & Richardson The evolving treatment paradigm of multiple myeloma: From past to present and future. Turk J Hematol., 25(2): 60-70., 2008.

[6] Beksac, M, Haznedar, R, Firatli-tuglular, T, Ozdogu, H, Aydogdu, I, Konuk, N, Sucak, G, Kaygusuz, I, Karakus, S, Kaya, E, Ali, R, Gulbas, Z, & Ozet, G. Goker H & Undar L. ((2011). Addition of thalidomide to oral melphalan/prednisone in patients with multiple myeloma not eligible for transplantation: results of a randomized trial from the Turkish Myeloma Study Group. Eur J Haematol., , 86(1), 16-22.

[7] Bird, J. M, Owen, R. G, Sa, D, Snowden, S, Pratt, J. A, Ashcroft, G, Yong, J, Cook, K, Feyler, G, Davies, S, Morgan, F, Cavenagh, G, Low, J, Behrens, E, & Haemato-oncology, J. Task Force of British Committee for Standards in Haematology (BCSH) and UK Myeloma Forum. ((2011). Guidelines for the diagnosis and management of multiple myeloma 2011. Br J Haematol,, 154(1), 32-75.

[8] Bringhen, S, Larocca, A, Rossi, D, Cavalli, M, Genuardi, M, Ria, R, Gentili, S, Patriarca, F, Nozzoli, C, Levi, A, Guglielmelli, T, Benevolo, G, Callea, V, Rizzo, V, Cangialosi, C, Musto, P, De Rosa, L, Liberati, A. M, Grasso, M, Falcone, A. P, Vangelista, A, Cavo, M, & Gaidano, G. Boccadoro M & Palumbo A. ((2010). Efficacy and safety of once-weekly bortezomib in multiple myeloma patients. Blood,, 116(23), 4745-53.

[9] Cavo, M. Di Raimondo F, Zamagni E, Patriarca F, Tacchetti P, Casulli AF, Volpe S, Perrone G, Ledda A, Ceccolini M, Califano C, Bigazzi C, Offidani M, Stefani P,Ballerini F, Fiacchini M, de Vivo A, Brioli A, Tosi P & Baccarani M. ((2009). Short-term thalidomide incorporated into double autologous stem-cell transplantation improves outcomes in comparison with double autotransplantation for multiple myeloma. J Clin Oncol.,, 27(30), 5001-7.

[10] Cavo, M, Rajkumar, S. V, Palumbo, A, Moreau, P, Orlowski, R, Bladé, J, Sezer, O, Ludwig, H, Dimopoulos, M. A, Attal, M, Sonneveld, P, Boccadoro, M, Anderson, K. C, Richardson, P. G, Bensinger, W, Johnsen, H. E, Kroeger, N, Gahrton, G, Bergsagel, P. L, Vesole, D. H, Einsele, H, Jagannath, S, Niesvizky, R, & Durie, B. G. San Miguel J & Lonial S; International Myeloma Working Group. ((2011). International Myeloma Working Group consensus approach to the treatment of multiple myeloma patients who are candidates for autologous stem cell transplantation. Blood,, 117(23), 6063-73.

[11] Cavo, M, Tacchetti, P, Patriarca, F, Petrucci, M. T, Pantani, L, & Galli, M. Di Raimondo F,Crippa C, Zamagni E, Palumbo A, Offidani M, Corradini P, Narni F, Spadano A,Pescosta N, Deliliers GL, Ledda A, Cellini C, Caravita T, Tosi P & Baccarani M;GIMEMA Italian Myeloma Network. ((2010). Bortezomib with thalidomide plus dexamethasone compared with thalidomide plus dexamethasone as induction therapy before, and consolidation therapy after,double autologous stem-cell transplantation in newly diagnosed multiple myeloma: a randomised phase 3 study. Lancet,, 376(9758), 2075-85.

[12] Cavo, M, Zamagni, E, Tosi, P, Cellini, C, Cangini, D, Tacchetti, P, Testoni, N, Tonelli, M, De Vivo, A, & Palareti, G. Tura S & Baccarani M. ((2004). First-line therapy with thalidomide and dexamethasone in preparation for autologous stem cell transplantation for multiple myeloma. Haematologica, , 89(7), 826-31.

[13] Cavo, M, Zamagni, E, Tosi, P, Tacchetti, P, Cellini, C, Cangini, D, De Vivo, A, Testoni, N, Nicci, C, Terragna, C, Grafone, T, Perrone, G, & Ceccolini, M. Tura S & Baccarani M; Bologna 2002 study. ((2005). Superiority of thalidomide and dexamethasone over vincristine-doxorubicindexamethasone (VAD) as primary therapy in preparation for autologous transplantation for multiple myeloma. Blood ;, 106(1), 35-9.

[14] Chanan-Khan AA & Giralt S(2010). Importance of achieving a complete response in multiple myeloma, and the impact of novel agents. J Clin Oncol.,, 28(15), 2612-24.

[15] Cherry, B. M, Korde, N, & Kwok, M. Roschewski M & Landgren O. ((2012). Evolving therapeutic paradigms for multiple myeloma: back to the future. Leuk Lymphoma. [Epub ahead of print].

[16] Child, J. A, Morgan, G. J, Davies, F. E, Owen, R. G, Bell, S. E, Hawkins, K, & Brown, J. Drayson MT & Selby PJ; Medical Research Council Adult Leukaemia Working Party. ((2003). Highdose chemotherapy with hematopoietic stem-cell rescue for multiple myeloma. NEngl J Med, 8;, 348(19), 1875-83.

[17] Dimopoulos, M. A, Richardson, P. G, Schlag, R, Khuageva, N. K, Shpilberg, O, Kastritis, E, Kropff, M, Petrucci, M. T, Delforge, M, Alexeeva, J, Schots, R, Masszi, T, Mateos, M. V, Deraedt, W, Liu, K, & Cakana, A. van de Velde H & San Miguel JF. ((2009). VMP (Bortezomib, Melphalan, and Prednisone) is active and well tolerated in newly diagnosed patients with multiple myeloma with moderately impaired renal function,and results in reversal of renal impairment: cohort analysis of the phase III VISTA study. J Clin Oncol.,, 27(36), 6086-93.

[18] Einsele, H, Liebisch, P, Langer, C, et al. Velcade, intravenous cyclophosphamide and dexamethasone (VCD) induction for previously untreated multiple myeloma (German DSMM XIa Trial). ((2009). ASH Annual Meeting Abstracts. Abstract 131.

[19] Facon, T, Mary, J. Y, Hulin, C, Benboubker, L, Attal, M, Pegourie, B, Renaud, M, Harousseau, J. L, Guillerm, G, Chaleteix, C, Dib, M, Voillat, L, Maisonneuve, H, Troncy, J, Dorvaux, V, Monconduit, M, Martin, C, Casassus, P, Jaubert, J, Jardel, H, Doyen, C, Kolb, B, Anglaret, B, Grosbois, B, & Yakoub-agha, I. Mathiot C & Avet-Loiseau H;Intergroupe Francophone du Myélome. ((2007). Melphalan and prednisone plus thalidomide versus melphalan and prednisone alone or reduced-intensity autologous stem cell transplantation in elderly patients with multiple myeloma (IFM 99-06): a randomised trial. Lancet, , 370(9594), 1209-18.

[20] Fayers, P. M, Palumbo, A, Hulin, C, Waage, A, Wijermans, P, Beksaç, M, Bringhen, S, Mary, J. Y, Gimsing, P, Termorshuizen, F, Haznedar, R, Caravita, T, Moreau, P, Turesson, I, Musto, P, Benboubker, L, & Schaafsma, M. Sonneveld P & Facon T; Nordic Myeloma Study Group; Italian Multiple Myeloma Network; Turkish Myeloma Study Group; Hemato-Oncologie voor Volwassenen Nederland; Intergroupe Francophone du Myélome; European Myeloma Network. ((2011). Thalidomide for previously untreated elderly patients with multiple myeloma: meta-analysis of 1685 individual patient data from 6 randomized clinical trials. Blood, , 118(5), 1239-47.

[21] Fermand, J. P, Katsahian, S, Divine, M, Leblond, V, Dreyfus, F, Macro, M, Arnulf, B, Royer, B, Mariette, X, Pertuiset, E, Belanger, C, Janvier, M, & Chevret, S. Brouet JC & Ravaud P; Group Myelome-Autogreffe. ((2005). High-dose therapy and autologous blood stemcell transplantation compared with conventional treatment in myeloma patients aged 55 to 65 years: long-term results of a randomized control trial from the Group Myelome-Autogreffe. J Clin Oncol, 20;, 23(36), 9227-33.

[22] Gay, F, Hayman, S. R, Lacy, M. Q, Buadi, F, Gertz, M. A, Kumar, S, Dispenzieri, A, Mikhael, J. R, Bergsagel, P. L, Dingli, D, Reeder, C. B, Lust, J. A, Russell, S. J, Roy, V, Zeldenrust, S. R, Witzig, T. E, Fonseca, R, Kyle, R. A, & Greipp, P. R. Stewart AK & Rajkumar SV. ((2010). Lenalidomide plus dexamethasone versus thalidomide plus

dexamethasone in newly diagnosed multiple myeloma: a comparative analysis of 411 patients. Blood,, 115(7), 1343-50.

[23] Gay, F, Rajkumar, S. V, Coleman, M, Kumar, S, Mark, T, Dispenzieri, A, Pearse, R, Gertz, M. A, Leonard, J, Lacy, M. Q, Chen-kiang, S, Roy, V, Jayabalan, D. S, Lust, J. A, Witzig, T. E, Fonseca, R, Kyle, R. A, & Greipp, P. R. Stewart AK & Niesvizky R. ((2010). Clarithromycin (Biaxin)-lenalidomide-low-dose dexamethasone (BiRd) versus lenalidomide-low-dose dexamethasone (Rd) for newly diagnosed myeloma. Am J Hematol.,, 85(9), 664-9.

[24] Harousseau, J. L. Attal M & Avet-Loiseau H. ((2009). The role of complete response in multiple myeloma. Blood, , 114(15), 3139-46.

[25] Harousseau, J. L, Attal, M, Avet-loiseau, H, Marit, G, Caillot, D, Mohty, M, Lenain, P, Hulin, C, Facon, T, Casassus, P, Michallet, M, Maisonneuve, H, Benboubker, L, Maloisel, F, Petillon, M. O, & Webb, I. Mathiot C & Moreau Bortezomib plus dexamethasone is superior to vincristine plus doxorubicin plus dexamethasone as induction treatment prior to autologous stem-cell transplantation in newly diagnosed multiple myeloma: results of the IFM 2005-01 phase III trial. J Clin Oncol.,28(30):4621-9., 2010.

[26] Harousseau, J. L, Attal, M, Avet-loiseau, H, Marit, G, Caillot, D, Mohty, M, Lenain, P, Hulin, C, Facon, T, Casassus, P, Michallet, M, Maisonneuve, H, Benboubker, L, Maloisel, F, Petillon, M. O, & Webb, I. Mathiot C & Moreau Bortezomib plus dexamethasone is superior to vincristine plus doxorubicin plus dexamethasone as induction treatment prior to autologous stem-cell transplantation in newly diagnosed multiple myeloma: results of the IFM 2005-01 phase III trial. J Clin Oncol.,28(30):4621-9., 2010.

[27] Harousseau, J. L, Attal, M, Leleu, X, Troncy, J, Pegourie, B, Stoppa, A. M, Hulin, C, Benboubker, L, Fuzibet, J. G, & Renaud, M. Moreau P & Avet-Loiseau H. ((2006). Bortezomib plus dexamethasone as induction treatment prior to autologous stem cell transplantation in patients with newly diagnosed multiple myeloma: results of an IFM phase II study. Haematologica,, 91(11), 1498-505.

[28] Haslett, P. A, & Hanekom, W. A. Muller G & Kaplan G. ((2003). Thalidomide and a thalidomide analogue drug costimulate virus-specific CD8+ T cells in vitro. J Infect Dis.,, 187(6), 946-55.

[29] Hideshima, T, Chauhan, D, Shima, Y, Raje, N, Davies, F. E, Tai, Y. T, Treon, S. P, Lin, B, Schlossman, R. L, Richardson, P, & Muller, G. Stirling DI & Anderson KC. ((2000). Thalidomide and its analogs overcome drug resistance of human multiple myeloma cells to conventional therapy. Blood,, 96(9), 2943-50.

[30] Hideshima, T, Chauhan, D, Shima, Y, Raje, N, Davies, F. E, Tai, Y. T, Treon, S. P, Lin, B, Schlossman, R. L, Richardson, P, & Muller, G. Stirling DI & Anderson KC. ((2000). Thalidomide and its analogs overcome drug resistance of human multiple myeloma cells to conventional therapy. Blood,, 96(9), 2943-50.

[31] Hideshima, T, Richardson, P, Chauhan, D, Palombella, V. J, & Elliott, P. J. Adams J &Anderson KC. ((2001). The proteasome inhibitor PS-341 inhibits growth, induces

apoptosis, and overcomes drug resistance in human multiple myeloma cells. Cancer Res.,, 61(7), 3071-6.

[32] Hulin, C, Facon, T, Rodon, P, Pegourie, B, Benboubker, L, Doyen, C, Dib, M, Guillerm, G, Salles, B, Eschard, J. P, Lenain, P, Casassus, P, Azaïs, I, Decaux, O, Garderet, L, Mathiot, C, Fontan, J, & Lafon, I. Virion JM & Moreau Efficacy of melphalan and prednisone plus thalidomide in patients older than 75 years with newly diagnosed multiple myeloma: IFM 01/01 trial. J Clin Oncol., 27(22):3664-70., 2009.

[33] Jagannath, S, Barlogie, B, Berenson, J, Siegel, D, Irwin, D, Richardson, P. G, Niesvizky, R, Alexanian, R, Limentani, S. A, Alsina, M, Adams, J, Kauffman, M, & Esseltine, D. L. Schenkein DP & Anderson KC. ((2004). A phase 2 study of two doses of bortezomib in relapsed or refractory myeloma. Br J Haematol.,, 127(2), 165-72.

[34] Jagannath, S, Durie, B. G, Wolf, J, Camacho, E, Irwin, D, Lutzky, J, Mckinley, M, Gabayan, E, & Mazumder, A. Schenkein D&Crowley J. ((2005). Bortezomib therapy alone and in combination with dexamethasone for previously untreated symptomatic multiple myeloma. Br J Haematol.,, 129(6), 776-83.

[35] Jagannath, S, Richardson, P. G, Sonneveld, P, Schuster, M. W, Irwin, D, Stadtmauer, E. A, Facon, T, & Harousseau, J. L. Cowan JM & Anderson KC. ((2007). Bortezomib appears to overcome the poor prognosis conferred by chromosome 13 deletion in phase 2 and 3 trials. Leukemia,, 21(1), 151-7.

[36] Jakubowiak, A. J, Griffith, K. A, Reece, D. E, Hofmeister, C. C, Lonial, S, Zimmerman, T. M, Campagnaro, E. L, Schlossman, R. L, Laubach, J. P, Raje, N. S, Anderson, T, Mietzel, M. A, Harvey, C. K, Wear, S. M, Barrickman, J. C, Tendler, C. L, Esseltine, D. L, Kelley, S. L, & Kaminski, M. S. Anderson KC & Richardson PG. ((2011). Lenalidomide, bortezomib, pegylated liposomal doxorubicin, and dexamethasone in newly diagnosed multiple myeloma: a phase 1/2 Multiple Myeloma Research Consortium trial. Blood,, 118(3), 535-43.

[37] Jakubowiak, A. J, Kendall, T, Al-zoubi, A, Khaled, Y, Mineishi, S, Ahmed, A, Campagnaro, E, Brozo, C, & Braun, T. Talpaz M & Kaminski MS. ((2009). Phase II trial of combination therapy with bortezomib, pegylated liposomal doxorubicin, and dexamethasone in patients with newly diagnosed myeloma. J Clin Oncol,, 27(30), 5015-22.

[38] Kastritis, E, Zervas, K, Symeonidis, A, Terpos, E, Delimbassi, S, Anagnostopoulos, N, Michali, E, Zomas, A, Katodritou, E, Gika, D, Pouli, A, Christoulas, D, Roussou, M, & Kartasis, Z. Economopoulos T & Dimopoulos MA. ((2009). Improved survival of patients with multiple myeloma after the introduction of novel agents and the applicability of the International Staging System (ISS): an analysis of the Greek Myeloma Study Group (GMSG). Leukemia, , 23(6), 1152-7.

[39] Koreth, J, Cutler, C. S, Djulbegovic, B, Behl, R, Schlossman, R. L, Munshi, N. C, Richardson, P. G, & Anderson, K. C. Soiffer RJ & Alyea EP 3rd. ((2007). High-dose therapy with single autologous transplantation versus chemotherapy for newly

diagnosed multiple myeloma: A systematic review and meta-analysis of randomized controlled trials. Biol Blood Marrow Transplant, , 13(2), 183-96.

[40] Kumar, S, Dispenzieri, A, Lacy, M. Q, Hayman, S. R, Buadi, F. K, Gastineau, D. A, Litzow, M. R, Fonseca, R, & Roy, V. Rajkumar SV& Gertz MA. ((2007). Impact of lenalidomide therapy on stem cell mobilization and engraftment post-peripheral blood stem cell transplantation in patients with newly diagnosed myeloma. Leukemia, , 21, 2035-42.

[41] Kumar, S, Flinn, I, Richardson, P. G, Hari, P, Callander, N, Noga, S. J, Stewart, A. K, Turturro, F, Rifkin, R, Wolf, J, Estevam, J, Mulligan, G, & Shi, H. Webb IJ & Rajkumar SV. ((2012). Randomized, multicenter, phase 2 study (EVOLUTION) of combinations of bortezomib,dexamethasone, cyclophosphamide, and lenalidomide in previously untreated multiple myeloma. Blood,, 119(19), 4375-82.

[42] Kumar, S, Giralt, S, Stadtmauer, E. A, Harousseau, J. L, Palumbo, A, Bensinger, W, Comenzo, R. L, Lentzsch, S, Munshi, N, & Niesvizky, R. San Miguel J, Ludwig H, Bergsagel L, Blade J,Lonial S, Anderson KC, Tosi P, Sonneveld P, Sezer O, Vesole D, Cavo M, Einsele H,Richardson PG, Durie BG & Rajkumar SV; International Myeloma Working Group. ((2009). Mobilization in myeloma revisited: IMWG consensus perspectives on stem cell collection following initial therapy with thalidomide-, lenalidomide-, or bortezomib-containing regimens. Blood, 27;, 114(9), 1729-35.

[43] Kumar, S. K, Rajkumar, S. V, Dispenzieri, A, Lacy, M. Q, Hayman, S. R, Buadi, F. K, Zeldenrust, S. R, Dingli, D, Russell, S. J, Lust, J. A, & Greipp, P. R. Kyle RA & Gertz MA. ((2008). Improved survival in multiple myeloma and the impact of novel therapies. Blood,, 111(5), 2516-20.

[44] Kyle RA & Rajkumar SV(2004). Multiple myeloma. N Engl J Med.,, 351(18), 1860-73.

[45] Lokhorst, H. M, Schmidt-wolf, I, Sonneveld, P, Van Der Holt, B, Martin, H, Barge, R, Bertsch, U, Schlenzka, J, Bos, G. M, Croockewit, S, Zweegman, S, Breitkreutz, I, Joosten, P, Scheid, C, Van Marwijk-kooy, M, Salwender, H. J, Van Oers, M. H, Schaafsma, R, Naumann, R, Sinnige, H, Blau, I, Delforge, M, De Weerdt, O, Wijermans, P, Wittebol, S, & Duersen, U. Vellenga E & Goldschmidt H; Dutch-Belgian HOVON; German GMMG. ((2008). Thalidomide in induction treatment increases the very good partial response rate before and after high-dose therapy in previously untreated multiple myeloma. Haematologica,, 93(1), 124-7.

[46] Lokhorst, H. M, Van Der Holt, B, Zweegman, S, Vellenga, E, Croockewit, S, & Van Oers, M. H. von dem Borne P, Wijermans P, Schaafsma R, de Weerdt O, Wittebol S, Delforge M, Berenschot H, Bos GM, Jie KS, Sinnige H, van Marwijk-Kooy M, Joosten P, Minnema MC, van Ammerlaan R & Sonneveld P; Dutch-Belgian Hemato-Oncology Group (HOVON). ((2010). A randomized phase 3 study on the effect of thalidomide combined with adriamycin,dexamethasone, and high-dose melphalan, followed by thalidomide maintenance in patients with multiple myeloma. Blood, , 115(6), 1113-20.

[47] Ludwig, H, Beksac, M, Bladé, J, Cavenagh, J, Cavo, M, Delforge, M, Dimopoulos, M, Drach, J, Einsele, H, Facon, T, Goldschmidt, H, Harousseau, J. L, Hess, U, & Kropff, M. Leal da Costa F, Louw V, Magen-Nativ H, Mendeleeva L, Nahi H, Plesner T, San-Miguel J,Sonneveld P, Udvardy M, Sondergeld P & Palumbo A. ((2011). Multiple myeloma treatment strategies with novel agents in 2011: a European perspective. Oncologist,, 16(4), 388-403.

[48] Ludwig, H, Hajek, R, Tóthová, E, Drach, J, Adam, Z, Labar, B, Egyed, M, Spicka, I, Gisslinger, H, Greil, R, & Kuhn, I. Zojer N & Hinke A. ((2009). Thalidomide-dexamethasone compared with melphalan-prednisolone in elderly patients with multiple myeloma. Blood, , 113(15), 3435-42.

[49] Mateos MV & San Miguel JFOld and new treatments in non-transplant candidate newly diagnosed MM patients. Hematology education programme fort he annual congress of the European Hematology Association. ((2012). Haematologica,, 6(1), 221-227.

[50] Mateos, M. V, Oriol, A, Martínez-lópez, J, Gutiérrez, N, Teruel, A. I, De Paz, R, García-laraña, J, Bengoechea, E, Martín, A, Mediavilla, J. D, Palomera, L, De Arriba, F, González, Y, Hernández, J. M, Sureda, A, Bello, J. L, Bargay, J, Peñalver, F. J, Ribera, J. M, Martín-mateos, M. L, García-sanz, R, Cibeira, M. T, Ramos, M. L, Vidriales, M. B, Paiva, B, Montalbán, M. A, & Lahuerta, J. J. Bladé J & Miguel JF.Bortezomib, melphalan, and prednisone versus bortezomib, thalidomide, and prednisone as induction therapy followed by maintenance treatment with bortezomib and thalidomide versus bortezomib and prednisone in elderly patients with untreated multiple myeloma: a randomised trial. Lancet Oncol.,, 11(10), 934-41.

[51] Mateos, M. V, Oriol, A, Martínez-lópez, J, Gutiérrez, N, Teruel, A. I, De Paz, R, García-laraña, J, Bengoechea, E, Martín, A, Mediavilla, J. D, Palomera, L, De Arriba, F, González, Y, Hernández, J. M, Sureda, A, Bello, J. L, Bargay, J, Peñalver, F. J, Ribera, J. M, Martín-mateos, M. L, García-sanz, R, Cibeira, M. T, Ramos, M. L, Vidriales, M. B, Paiva, B, Montalbán, M. A, & Lahuerta, J. J. Bladé J & Miguel JF. ((2010). Bortezomib, melphalan, and prednisone versus bortezomib, thalidomide, and prednisone as induction therapy followed by maintenance treatment with bortezomib and thalidomide versus bortezomib and prednisone in elderly patients with untreated multiple myeloma: a randomised trial. Lancet Oncol.,, 11(10), 934-41.

[52] Mateos, M. V, Richardson, P. G, Schlag, R, Khuageva, N. K, Dimopoulos, M. A, Shpilberg, O, Kropff, M, Spicka, I, Petrucci, M. T, Palumbo, A, Samoilova, O. S, Dmoszynska, A, Abdulkadyrov, K. M, Schots, R, Jiang, B, Esseltine, D. L, Liu, K, & Cakana, A. van de Velde H & San Miguel JF. ((2010). Bortezomib plus melphalan and prednisone compared with melphalan and prednisone in previously untreated multiple myeloma: updated follow-up and impact of subsequent therapy in the phase III VISTA trial. J Clin Oncol.,, 28(13), 2259-66.

http://dx.doi.org/10.5772/55151

[53] Mazumder, A, Kaufman, J, Niesvizky, R, & Lonial, S. Vesole D & Jagannath S. ((2008). Effect of lenalidomide therapy on mobilization of peripheral blood stem cells in previously untreated multiple myeloma patients. Leukemia, , 22(6), 1280-1.

[54] Mitsiades, N, Mitsiades, C. S, Poulaki, V, Chauhan, D, Richardson, P. G, Hideshima, T, & Munshi, N. C. Treon SP & Anderson KC. ((2002). Apoptotic signaling induced by immunomodulatory thalidomide analogs in human multiple myeloma cells: therapeutic implications. Blood,, 99(12), 4525-30.

[55] Moreau, P, Avet-loiseau, H, Facon, T, Attal, M, Tiab, M, Hulin, C, Doyen, C, Garderet, L, Randriamalala, E, Araujo, C, Lepeu, G, Marit, G, Caillot, D, Escoffre, M, Lioure, B, Benboubker, L, Pégourié, B, Kolb, B, Stoppa, A. M, Fuzibet, J. G, Decaux, O, Dib, M, Berthou, C, Chaleteix, C, Sebban, C, Traullé, C, Fontan, J, Wetterwald, M, & Lenain, P. Mathiot C & Harousseau JL. ((2011). Bortezomib plus dexamethasone versus reduced-dose bortezomib, thalidomide plus dexamethasone as induction treatment before autologous stem cell transplantation in newly diagnosed multiple myeloma. Blood,, 118(22), 5752-8.

[56] Moreau, P, Hulin, C, Marit, G, Caillot, D, Facon, T, Lenain, P, Berthou, C, Pégourié, B, Stoppa, A. M, Casassus, P, Michallet, M, Benboubker, L, Maisonneuve, H, Doyen, C, Leyvraz, S, Mathiot, C, & Avet-loiseau, H. Attal M & Harousseau JL; IFM group. ((2010). Stem cell collection in patients with de novo multiple myeloma treated with thecombination of bortezomib and dexamethasone before autologous stem cell transplantation according to IFM 2005-01 trial. Leukemia,, 24(6), 1233-5.

[57] Morgan, G. J, Davies, F. E, Gregory, W. M, Bell, S. E, & Szubert, A. J. Navarro Coy N, Cook G, Feyler S, Johnson PR, Rudin C, Drayson MT, Owen RG, Ross FM, Russell NH, Jackson GH & Child JA; National Cancer Research Institute Haematological Oncology Clinical Studies Group. ((2012). Cyclophosphamide, thalidomide, and dexamethasone as induction therapy for newly diagnosed multiple myeloma patients destined for autologous stem-cell transplantation: MRC Myeloma IX randomized trial results. Haematologica,, 97(3), 442-50.

[58] Morgan, G. J, Davies, F. E, Gregory, W. M, Russell, N. H, Bell, S. E, & Szubert, A. J. Navarro Coy N, Cook G, Feyler S, Byrne JL, Roddie H, Rudin C, Drayson MT, Owen RG, Ross FM, Jackson GH & Child JA; NCRI Haematological Oncology Study Group. Cyclophosphamide, thalidomide, and dexamethasone (CTD) as initial therapy for patients with multiple myeloma unsuitable for autologous transplantation. Blood, , 118(5), 1231-8.

[59] Niesvizky, R, Flinn, I. W, Rifkin, R. M, Gabrail, N. Y, Charu, V, Clowney, B, Essell, J, Gaffar, Y. A, Warr, T. A, & Neuwirth, R. Corzo D & Reeves JA. ((2010). Phase 3b UPFRONT Study: Safety and Efficacy of Weekly Bortezomib Maintenance Therapy After Bortezomib-Based Induction Regimens In Elderly, Newly Diagnosed Multiple Myeloma Patients. Blood (ASH Annual Meeting Abstracts) 116: Abstract 619.

[60] Palumbo A & Anderson K(2011). Multiple myeloma. N Engl J Med.,, 364(11), 1046-60.

[61] Palumbo, A, Bringhen, S, Caravita, T, Merla, E, Capparella, V, Callea, V, Cangialosi, C, Grasso, M, Rossini, F, Galli, M, Catalano, L, Zamagni, E, Petrucci, M. T, De Stefano, V, Ceccarelli, M, Ambrosini, M. T, Avonto, I, Falco, P, Ciccone, G, & Liberati, A. M. Musto P & Boccadoro M; Italian Multiple Myeloma Network, GIMEMA. ((2006). Oral melphalan and prednisone chemotherapy plus thalidomide compared with melphalan and prednisone alone in elderly patients with multiple myeloma: randomised controlled trial. Lancet, , 367(9513), 825-31.

[62] Palumbo, A, Bringhen, S, Liberati, A. M, Caravita, T, Falcone, A, Callea, V, Montanaro, M, Ria, R, Capaldi, A, Zambello, R, Benevolo, G, Derudas, D, Dore, F, Cavallo, F, Gay, F, Falco, P, Ciccone, G, & Musto, P. Cavo M & Boccadoro M. ((2008). Oral melphalan, prednisone, and thalidomide in elderly patients with multiple myeloma: updated results of a randomized controlled trial. Blood,, 112(8), 3107-14.

[63] Palumbo, A, Bringhen, S, Ludwig, H, Dimopoulos, M. A, Bladé, J, Mateos, M. V, Rosiñol, L, Boccadoro, M, Cavo, M, Lokhorst, H, Zweegman, S, Terpos, E, Davies, F, Driessen, C, Gimsing, P, Gramatzki, M, Hàjek, R, & Johnsen, H. E. Leal Da Costa F, Sezer O, Spencer A,Beksac M, Morgan G, Einsele H, San Miguel JF & Sonneveld Personalized therapy in multiple myeloma according to patient age and vulnerability: a report of the European Myeloma Network (EMN). Blood,118(17):4519-29., 2011.

[64] Palumbo, A, Bringhen, S, Rossi, D, Cavalli, M, Larocca, A, Ria, R, Offidani, M, Patriarca, F, Nozzoli, C, Guglielmelli, T, Benevolo, G, Callea, V, Baldini, L, Morabito, F, Grasso, M, Leonardi, G, Rizzo, M, Falcone, A. P, Gottardi, D, Montefusco, V, Musto, P, & Petrucci, M. T. Ciccone G & Boccadoro M. ((2010). Bortezomib-melphalan-prednisone-thalidomide followed by maintenance with bortezomib-thalidomide compared with bortezomib-melphalan-prednisone for initial treatment of multiple myeloma: a randomized controlled trial. J Clin Oncol.,, 28(34), 5101-9.

[65] Palumbo, A, Giaccone, L, Bertola, A, Pregno, P, Bringhen, S, Rus, C, Triolo, S, & Gallo, E. Pileri A & Boccadoro M. ((2001). Low-dose thalidomide plus dexamethasone is an effective salvage therapy for advanced myeloma. Haematologica.,, 86(4), 399-403.

[66] Palumbo, A, Hajek, R, Delforge, M, Kropff, M, Petrucci, M. T, Catalano, J, Gisslinger, H, Wiktor-jedrzejczak, W, Zodelava, M, Weisel, K, Cascavilla, N, Iosava, G, Cavo, M, Kloczko, J, Bladé, J, Beksac, M, Spicka, I, Plesner, T, Radke, J, & Langer, C. Ben Yehuda D, Corso A, Herbein L, Yu Z, Mei J, Jacques C & Dimopoulos MA; MM-015 Investigators. ((2012). Continuous lenalidomide treatment for newly diagnosed multiple myeloma. N Engl J Med., , 366(19), 1759-69.

[67] Paripati, H, Stewart, A. K, Cabou, S, Dueck, A, Zepeda, V. J, Pirooz, N, Ehlenbeck, C, Reeder, C, Slack, J, Leis, J. F, Boesiger, J, & Torloni, A. S. Fonseca R & Bergsagel PL. ((2008). Compromised stem cell mobilization following induction therapy with lenalidomide in myeloma. Leukemia, , 22(6), 1282-4.

[68] Pönisch, W, Andrea, M, Wagner, I, Hammerschmidt, D, Kreibich, U, Schwarzer, A, Zehrfeld, T, Schwarz, M, Winkelmann, C, Petros, S, & Bachmann, A. Lindner T & Niederwieser D. ((2012). Successful treatment of patients with newly diagnosed/ untreated multiple myeloma and advanced renal failure using bortezomib in combination with bendamustine and prednisone. J Cancer Res Clin Oncol.,, 138(8), 1405-12.

[69] Pönisch, W, Mitrou, P. S, Merkle, K, Herold, M, Assmann, M, Wilhelm, G, Dachselt, K, Richter, P, Schirmer, V, Schulze, A, Subert, R, Harksel, B, Grobe, N, Stelzer, E, Schulze, M, Bittrich, A, Freund, M, Pasold, R, & Friedrich, T. Helbig W & Niederwieser D; East German Study Group of Hematology and Oncology (OSHO). ((2006). Treatment of bendamustine and prednisone in patients with newly diagnosed multiple myeloma results in superior complete response rate, prolonged time totreatment failure and improved quality of life compared to treatment with melphalan and prednisone--a randomized phase III study of the East German Study Group of Hematology and Oncology (OSHO). J Cancer Res Clin Oncol.,, 132(4), 205-12.

[70] Popat, R, Oakervee, H. E, Hallam, S, Curry, N, Odeh, L, Foot, N, Esseltine, D. L, & Drake, M. Morris C & Cavenagh JD. ((2008). Bortezomib, doxorubicin and dexamethasone (PAD) front-line treatment of multiple myeloma: updated results after long-term follow-up. Br J Haematol,, 141(4), 512-6.

[71] Popat, U, Saliba, R, Thandi, R, Hosing, C, Qazilbash, M, Anderlini, P, Shpall, E, Mcmannis, J, Körbling, M, Alousi, A, Andersson, B, Nieto, Y, Kebriaei, P, Khouri, I, De Lima, M, Weber, D, Thomas, S, Wang, M, & Jones, R. Champlin R & Giralt S. ((2009). Impairment of filgrastim-induced stem cell mobilization after prior lenalidomide in patients with multiple myeloma. Biol Blood Marrow Transplant, , 15, 718-23.

[72] Rajkumar, S. V, Blood, E, & Vesole, D. Fonseca R & Greipp PR; Eastern Cooperative Oncology Group. ((2006). Phase III clinical trial of thalidomide plus dexamethasone compared with dexamethasone alone in newly diagnosed multiple myeloma: a clinical trial coordinated by the Eastern Cooperative Oncology Group. J Clin Oncol.,, 24(3), 431-6.

[73] Rajkumar, S. V, Hayman, S, Gertz, M. A, Dispenzieri, A, Lacy, M. Q, Greipp, P. R, Geyer, S, Iturria, N, Fonseca, R, & Lust, J. A. Kyle RA & Witzig TE. ((2002). Combination therapy with thalidomide plus dexamethasone for newly diagnosed myeloma. J Clin Oncol.,, 20(21), 4319-23.

[74] Rajkumar, S. V, Hayman, S. R, Lacy, M. Q, Dispenzieri, A, Geyer, S. M, Kabat, B, Zeldenrust, S. R, Kumar, S, Greipp, P. R, Fonseca, R, Lust, J. A, Russell, S. J, & Kyle, R. A. Witzig TE & Gertz MA. ((2005). Combination therapy with lenalidomide plus dexamethasone (Rev/Dex) for newly diagnosed myeloma. Blood,, 106(13), 4050-3.

[75] Rajkumar, S. V, Jacobus, S, Callander, N. S, Fonseca, R, Vesole, D. H, Williams, M. E, Abonour, R, & Siegel, D. S. Katz M & Greipp PR; Eastern Cooperative Oncology Group. ((2010). Lenalidomide plus high-dose dexamethasone versus lenalidomide

plus low-dose dexamethasone as initial therapy for newly diagnosed multiple myeloma: an open-label randomised controlled trial. Lancet Oncol.,, 11(1), 29-37.

[76] Rajkumar, S. V, Rosiñol, L, Hussein, M, Catalano, J, Jedrzejczak, W, Lucy, L, Olesnyckyj, M, Yu, Z, & Knight, R. Zeldis JB & Bladé J. ((2008). Multicenter, randomized, double-blind, placebo-controlled study of thalidomide plus dexamethasone compared with dexamethasone as initial therapy for newly diagnosed multiple myeloma. J Clin Oncol.,, 26(13), 2171-7.

[77] Rajkumar, S. V. (2012). Multiple myeloma: 2012 update on diagnosis, risk-stratification, and management. Am J Hematol., , 87(1), 78-88.

[78] Reeder, C. B, Reece, D. E, Kukreti, V, Chen, C, Trudel, S, Hentz, J, Noble, B, Pirooz, N. A, Spong, J. E, Piza, J. G, Zepeda, V. H, Mikhael, J. R, Leis, J. F, & Bergsagel, P. L. Fonseca R & Stewart AK. ((2009). Cyclophosphamide, bortezomib and dexamethasone induction for newly diagnosed multiple myeloma: high response rates in a phase II clinical trial. Leukemia,, 23(7), 1337-41.

[79] Richardson, P. G, Barlogie, B, Berenson, J, Singhal, S, Jagannath, S, Irwin, D, Rajkumar, S. V, Hideshima, T, Xiao, H, & Esseltine, D. Schenkein D & Anderson KC; SUMMIT Investigators. ((2005). Clinical factors predictive of outcome with bortezomib in patients with relapsed,refractory multiple myeloma. Blood,, 106(9), 2977-81.

[80] Richardson, P. G, Schlossman, R. L, Weller, E, Hideshima, T, Mitsiades, C, & Davies, F. LeBlanc R, Catley LP, Doss D, Kelly K, McKenney M, Mechlowicz J, Freeman A,Deocampo R, Rich R, Ryoo JJ, Chauhan D, Balinski K, Zeldis J & Anderson KC. ((2002). Immunomodulatory drug CC-5013 overcomes drug resistance and is well tolerated in patients with relapsed multiple myeloma. Blood,, 100(9), 3063-7.

[81] Richardson, P. G, Sonneveld, P, Schuster, M. W, Irwin, D, Stadtmauer, E. A, Facon, T, Harousseau, J. L, Ben-yehuda, D, Lonial, S, Goldschmidt, H, Reece, D, San-miguel, J. F, Bladé, J, Boccadoro, M, Cavenagh, J, Dalton, W. S, Boral, A. L, Esseltine, D. L, & Porter, J. B. Schenkein D & Anderson KC; Assessment of Proteasome Inhibition for Extending Remissions (APEX) Investigators. Bortezomib or high-dose dexamethasone for relapsed multiple myeloma. N Engl J Med.,(2487). , 352(24), 2487-98.

[82] Richardson, P. G, Weller, E, Lonial, S, Jakubowiak, A. J, Jagannath, S, Raje, N. S, Avigan, D. E, Xie, W, Ghobrial, I. M, Schlossman, R. L, Mazumder, A, Munshi, N. C, Vesole, D. H, Joyce, R, Kaufman, J. L, Doss, D, Warren, D. L, Lunde, L. E, Kaster, S, Delaney, C, Hideshima, T, Mitsiades, C. S, & Knight, R. Esseltine DL & Anderson KC. ((2010). Lenalidomide, bortezomib, and dexamethasone combination therapy in patients with newly diagnosed multiple myeloma. Blood,, 116(5), 679-86.

[83] Richardson, P. G, Xie, W, Mitsiades, C, Chanan-khan, A. A, Lonial, S, Hassoun, H, Avigan, D. E, Oaklander, A. L, Kuter, D. J, Wen, P. Y, Kesari, S, Briemberg, H. R, Schlossman, R. L, Munshi, N. C, Heffner, L. T, Doss, D, Esseltine, D. L, & Weller, E. Anderson KC & Amato AA. ((2009). Single-agent bortezomib in previously untreated

multiple myeloma: efficacy,characterization of peripheral neuropathy, and molecular correlations with response and neuropathy.J Clin Oncol.,, 27(21), 3518-25.

[84] Rosiñol, L, Oriol, A, Mateos, M. V, Sureda, A, García-sánchez, P, Gutiérrez, N, Alegre, A, Lahuerta, J. J, De La Rubia, J, Herrero, C, & Liu, X. Van de Velde H, San Miguel J & Bladé J. ((2007). Phase II PETHEMA trial of alternating bortezomib and dexamethasone as induction regimen before autologous stem-cell transplantation in younger patients with multiple myeloma: efficacy and clinical implications of tumor response kinetics. J Clin Oncol.,, 25(28), 4452-8.

[85] Rosiñol, L, Oriol, A, Teruel, A. I, Hernández, D, López-jiménez, J, De La Rubia, J, Granell, M, Besalduch, J, Palomera, L, González, Y, Etxebeste, M. A, Díaz-mediavilla, J, Hernández, M. T, De Arriba, F, Gutiérrez, N. C, Martín-ramos, M. L, Cibeira, M. T, Mateos, M. V, Martínez, J, Alegre, A, & Lahuerta, J. J. San Miguel J & Bladé J; on behalf of the Programa para el Estudio y la Terapéutica de las Hemopatías Malignas/ Grupo Español de Mieloma (PETHEMA/GEM) group. ((2012). Superiority of bortezomib, thalidomide, and dexamethasone (VTD) as induction pretransplantation therapy in multiple myeloma: a randomized phase 3 PETHEMA/GEM study. Blood,, 120(8), 1589-1596.

[86] San Miguel JFSchlag R, Khuageva NK, Dimopoulos MA, Shpilberg O, Kropff M,Spicka I, Petrucci MT, Palumbo A, Samoilova OS, Dmoszynska A, Abdulkadyrov KM, Schots R, Jiang B, Mateos MV, Anderson KC, Esseltine DL, Liu K, Cakana A, van de Velde H & Richardson PG; VISTA Trial Investigators. ((2008). Bortezomib plus melphalan and prednisone for initial treatment of multiple myeloma. N Engl J Med, , 359(9), 906-17.

[87] Singhal, S, Mehta, J, Desikan, R, Ayers, D, Roberson, P, Eddlemon, P, Munshi, N, Anaissie, E, Wilson, C, & Dhodapkar, M. Zeddis J& Barlogie B. ((1999). Antitumor activity of thalidomide in refractory multiple myeloma.N Engl J Med., , 341(21), 1565-71.

[88] Sonneveld, P, Schmidt-wolf, I. G, Van Der Holt, B, El Jarari, L, Bertsch, U, Salwender, H, Zweegman, S, Vellenga, E, Broyl, A, Blau, I. W, Weisel, K. C, Wittebol, S, Bos, G. M, Stevens-kroef, M, Scheid, C, Pfreundschuh, M, Hose, D, Jauch, A, Van Der Velde, H, Raymakers, R, Schaafsma, M. R, Kersten, M. J, Van Marwijk-kooy, M, Duehrsen, U, Lindemann, W, & Wijermans, P. W. Lokhorst HM & Goldschmidt HM. ((2012). Bortezomib Induction and Maintenance Treatment in Patients With Newly Diagnosed Multiple Myeloma: Results of the Randomized Phase III HOVON-65/ GMMG-HD4 Trial. J Clin Oncol.,, 30(24), 2946-55.

[89] Sonneveld, P, Schmidt-wolf, I. G, Van Der Holt, B, El Jarari, L, Bertsch, U, Salwender, H, Zweegman, S, Vellenga, E, Broyl, A, Blau, I. W, Weisel, K. C, Wittebol, S, Bos, G. M, Stevens-kroef, M, Scheid, C, Pfreundschuh, M, Hose, D, Jauch, A, Van Der Velde, H, Raymakers, R, Schaafsma, M. R, Kersten, M. J, Van Marwijk-kooy, M, Duehrsen, U, Lindemann, W, & Wijermans, P. W. Lokhorst HM& Goldschmidt HM. ((2012). Bortezomib Induction and Maintenance Treatment in Patients With Newly Diag-

nosed Multiple Myeloma: Results of the Randomized Phase III HOVON-65/ GMMG-HD4 Trial. J Clin Oncol. 2012 Aug 20;, 30(24), 2946-55.

[90] Waage, A, Gimsing, P, Fayers, P, Abildgaard, N, Ahlberg, L, Björkstrand, B, Carlson, K, Dahl, I. M, Forsberg, K, Gulbrandsen, N, Haukås, E, Hjertner, O, Hjorth, M, Karlsson, T, Knudsen, L. M, Nielsen, J. L, Linder, O, Mellqvist, U. H, Nesthus, I, Rolke, J, Strandberg, M, Sørbø, J. H, & Wisløff, F. Juliusson G & Turesson I; Nordic Myeloma Study Group. ((2010). Melphalan and prednisone plus thalidomide or placebo in elderly patients with multiple myeloma. Blood, , 116(9), 1405-12.

[91] Wang, M, Giralt, S, & Delasalle, K. Handy B & Alexanian R. ((2007). Bortezomib in combination with thalidomide-dexamethasone for previously untreated multiple myeloma. Hematology, , 12(3), 235-9.

[92] Wijermans, P, Schaafsma, M, Termorshuizen, F, Ammerlaan, R, Wittebol, S, Sinnige, H, & Zweegman, S. van Marwijk Kooy M, van der Griend R, Lokhorst H & Sonneveld P; Dutch-Belgium Cooperative Group HOVON. ((2010). Phase III study of the value of thalidomide added to melphalan plus prednisone in elderly patients with newly diagnosed multiple myeloma: the HOVON 49 Study. J Clin Oncol.,, 28(19), 3160-6.

[93] Zavrski, I, Krebbel, H, Wildemann, B, Heider, U, & Kaiser, M. Possinger K & Sezer O. ((2005). Proteasome inhibitors abrogate osteoclast differentiation and osteoclast function. Biochem Biophys Res Commun.,, 333(1), 200-5.

[94] Zonder, J. A, Crowley, J, Hussein, M. A, & Bolejack, V. Moore DF Sr, Whittenberger BF,Abidi MH, Durie BG & Barlogie B. ((2010). Lenalidomide and high-dose dexamethasone compared with dexamethasone as initial therapy for multiple myeloma: a randomized Southwest Oncology Group trial (S0232). Blood,, 116(26), 5838-41.

Chapter 8

Allogeneic Hematopoetic Cell Transplantation in Multiple Myeloma

Pervin Topcuoglu, Sinem Civriz Bozdag and Taner Demirer

Additional information is available at the end of the chapter

http://dx.doi.org/10.5772/54762

1. Introduction

The improvement in the survival of multiple myeloma patients has been attributed to autologous stem cell transplantation (ASCT) after induction with novel agents [1,2]. Nevertheless, ASCT has not been considered to have a curative potential, maintenance treatment seems to be one of the solutions to decrease the high relapse rates after ASCT [3]. Therefore, allogeneic stem cell transplantation (Allo-SCT) is a potentially curative approach; the role of allo-SCT is still an ongoing debate due to high transplant-related mortality and lack of large prospective randomized studies in the newly diagnosed patients. A retrospective case-matched analysis was performed comparing myeloma patients treated with Allo-SCT with an equal number of patients who received ASCT by European Group for Blood and Bone Marrow Transplant (EBMT) [4]. Overall survival (OS) for the whole patient group was significantly better for the ASCT group compared with those for allo-SCT (Median survival: 34 months vs 18 months, p=.001). Therefore, we should answer the question of which patients with multiple myeloma have to be directed to allo-SCT modality.

Prognosis of myeloma patients have been found strongly associated with their cytogenetic features and gene expression profiling [5,6]. Increasing data on the poor prognosis of the 'high risk myeloma patients' changed the trends towards to the allo-transplantation in the earlier period. The Société Française de Greffe de Moelle et de Thérapie Cellulaire evaluated the role of allo-SCT for cytogenetically high-risk myeloma patients in a retrospective multicenter analysis [7]. They showed that allo-SCT could potentially be of benefit to the patients carrying cytogenetic abnormalities such as deletion (del) of (13q), t(4;14), t(14;16) and del(17p) compared to those without the same abnormalities.

In this chapter, we discussed the role of allo-HCT in MM patients, and also we tried to clarify the issues as the intensity of conditioning regimen, the timing of the transplantation, and post-transplantation approaches in relapse or refractory patients.

2. The intensity of conditioning regimen

The early data on myeloablative conditioning (MAC) regimen can be obtained from the transplant registries [8-12]. Cyclophosphamide (Cy) with total body irradiation (Cy-TBI) and busulfan with Cy were the mostly used conditioning regimens. Transplant-related mortality (TRM) rates ranged from 30% to 50%. Actuarial survival for the EBMT-registered patients was 28% at 7 years [9], 15 % for the Hutchinson Center–registered patients [10]. IBMTR data showed that the probabilities of survival at 4 years was 35% for patients with Karnofsky performance scores higher than 70 at pretransplantation and approximately 15% for patients with scores lower than 70 [11]. Thus, due to the exceedingly high TRM, myeloablative Allo-SCT was largely abandoned worldwide in the 1990s.

The use of reduced intensity conditioning (RIC) regimens in allo-SCT was introduced in an attempt to reduce the regimen-related toxicities while preserving an effect of graft versus tumor effect. First study was performed in a canine model conditioned with low-dose (2 Gy) total body irradiation (TBI) in combination of postgrafting mycofenolatemofetil (MMF) and cyclosporine (CSP). This approach permitted to stable engraftment with minimal toxicity [13, 14]. Seattle group introduced the strategy of autologous SCT followed by a RIC allo-SCT in 2-4 months with low-dose TBI as conditioning regimen [15]. Forty eight percent of 52 multiple myeloma patients had relapsed or refractory disease prior to SCT and the overall response rate was 81 % (51% CR + 29% PR). In this tandem modality, the 100-day TRM after the allo-RIC was 2%, progression free survival (PFS) and overall survival (OS) at 2 years were 48% and 69%, respectively. Preliminary clinical studies [15-25] were also encouraging with low TRM rates (Table1). Kröger, et al performed tandem auto/Allo-RIC in 17 myeloma patients using unrelated or mismatched related donors and fludarabine, melphalan, anti-thymocyte globulin (ATG) as conditioning regimen [16]. Early TRM (day 100) was reported as 11% and estimated 1-year disease free survival (DFS) and OS were 56% and 74%.

One of the largest data related to a RIC-allograft in myeloma was published by the EBMT in which the outcome of 229 patients with MM from 33 centers was reported [18]. One-year TRM was 22%, the 3-year estimated PFS and OS were 41% and 21%, respectively. The adverse outcomes were seen in chemo-resistant disease prior to allo-SCT, transplantation to the pair of male recipient- female donor, no-chronic GvHD and the use of alemtuzumab.

The EBMT has also retrospectively compared 320 patients allografted a RIC regimen with 196 received a MAC regimen in multiple myeloma. They have reported markedly lower non relapse mortality in RIC than MAC setting (24% vs 32%, p<.002) [19]. However PFS and OS were not affected by the intensity of conditioning regimen. This was attributed to higher relapse rates in RIC group than the MAC group. Progressive disease at transplantation was associated with an adverse effect on non-relapse mortality, PFS and OS. T cell depletion with alemtuzumab or other(s) led to high relapse rates as well.

Long-term follow-up data was reported in a RIC allo-graft for salvage setting of relapse and/or refractory myeloma patients (Table 1). These data showed that long term remission can be feasible for a subset of myeloma patients with allo-RIC performed in the salvage setting [21]. Seattle group reported the long term comparison data of RIC and MAC regimens [23]. Although the intensity of regimens changed time dependently, RIC regimens resulted in significantly lower overall mortality, improved PFS and much lower TRM.

Reference	Patients (n)	Median age (y)	Prior ASCT (n)	URD (n)	Regimens	GvHD prophylaxis	Acute GvHDGrade II-IV	Chronic GvHD	TRM/ NRM	CR	PFS	OS
Maloney [15]	52	52	52	0	TBI (2 Gy)	CSP-MMF	38%	46%	2% (100 d)	57 %	48 % (2 y)	69% (2 y)
Kröger [16]	17	51	17	8	Fludarabine, Melphalan, ATG	CSP-MTX	38%	40%	11% (100 d)	73%	56% (2y)	74% (2y)
Giralt [17]	22	51	9	9	Fludarabine, Melphalan	TAC-MTX	73%	33%	19% (100 d) 40% (1y)	32%	19% (2 y)	30% (2y)
Crawley [18]	229	52	169	37	Fludarabine, Melphalan or Busulfan or cyclophosphamide or TBI ± ATG or Alemtuzumab	CSP ± MTX	31 %	50%	11% 22% (1y)	25%	21% (3y)	41% (3y)
Rotta [20]	102	50	102	0	TBI (2Gy) ± Fludarabine	CSP-MMF; TAC-MMF	42%	74%	1% (100 d) 11 (1y) 18 (5y)	65%	36% (5y)	64% (5y)
Shimoni [21]	50	53	47	23	Fludarabine, Melphalan ±ATG	CSP-MTX	51%	63%	26 (5y)	58%	26% (7y)	34% (7y)
Cheikh [22]	40	56	11	17	Fludarabine, Busulfan, ATG; Fludarabine,TBI	CSP±MMF	47%	24%	0% (100 d)	44% (URD) 35% (MRD)	42% (URD) 44% (MRD)	59% (URD) 66% (MRD)
Bruno [24]	96	54	54	0	TBI (2 Gy)	CSP-MMF	38%	50%	11%	51%	53% (5 y)	65% (5y)
Vesole [25]	23		23	0	Fludarabine-Cyclop-hos-phamide	CSP-MP	17%	57%	8.7% (100 d)	30%	62% (2 y)	78% (2y)

Abbreviations: ASCT: Autologous Stem Cell Transplantation; GvHD: Graft versus Host Disease; TRM: Transplant-Related Mortality; NRM: Non-Relapse Mortality; CR: Complete Remission; PFS. Progression-Free Survival; OS: Overall Survival; TBI: Total Body Irradiation; ATG: Anti-Thymocyte Globulin; CSP: Cyclosporine; MMF: Mycofenolate Mofetif; TAC: Tacrolimus; MTX: Methotrexate; MP: Methyl-Prednisolone; URD: Unrelated Donor; MRD: Matched Related Donor

Table 1. Reduced intensity allogeneic transplantation alone or following autogous-SCT

A prospective multicenter study by the Gruppo ItalianoTrapianti di Midollo Osseo (GITMO) enrolled 100 newly diagnosed multiple myeloma patients who were < 65 years of age and who had a sibling donor [24]. Allo-RIC transplantation was performed 2 to 4 months after ASCT in 96 patients. Disease sensitivity at the transplantation was significantly associated with longer OS and event-free survival (EFS). Overall survival were not significantly affected by the presence of del(13q) whereas EFS was better in patients without del(13q). Similarly, the Eastern Cooperative Oncology Group (ECOG) performed a trial of ASCT followed by RIC-allo from matched sibling donor to provide maximal tumor cytoreduction to allow for a subsequent graft versus myeloma (GvM) effect [25]. With a median follow up of 4.6 years from registration, 23 patients who completed both transplantations had a median PFS of 3.6 years and a 2-year survival rate of 78%. Cumulative non-relapse mortality on day 100 was 8.7%. In contrast to Italian study, plateau in PFS or OS was not observed with this treatment approach even in patients achieving CR.

Another prospective study for myeloma as part of first-line therapy, a donor versus no-donor analysis was performed of the patients treated in the HOVON-50 study [26]. This study allowed the patients with an HLA-identical sibling donor to proceed to the HOVON-54 study of allo-RIC between 2 and 6 months after ACST. Their results did not support allo-SCT as a frontline therapy.

3. Tandem autologous vs Allo-RIC transplantation

Recent trials have compared tandem auto-allo HSCT with a tandem autologous modality (Table 2). The IFM initiated two trials in high-risk (β-2 microglobulin level greater than 3 mg/L and chromosome 13 deletion at diagnosis) de novo multiple myeloma [27]. Patients with an HLA-identical sibling donor were randomized with allo-RIC arm following 1st ASCT (IFM99-03) (n=65), and patients without an HLA identical sibling donor were randomly assigned to undergo 2nd ASCT with or without anti-IL-6 monoclonal antibody (IFM99-04) (n=219). In IFM99-03 trial, 46 patients completed the entire program. When compared the OS and EFS between two trials, IFM99-03 and 04 did not significantly differ (OS: 35 months versus 41 months, p=.27; 25 months vs 30 months, p=.56). IFM group submitted the updated results in 2008 [28]. When the results of patients in IFM99-04 were compared with those of the 46 patients completed the tandem ASCT/Allo-RIC program, there was a trend of better OS for ASCT followed by allo-RIC transplantation (47.2 months vs 35 months, p=.07). As they compared of the results of the 166 patients out of 219 who completed the whole tandem ASCT protocol with those of the 46 patients out of 65 who underwent the entire auto/allo-RIC program, no difference was observed regarding EFS (median 25 vs 21 months, p=.88), but there was a trend for a superior OS in favor of double ASCT (57 vs 41 months, P =.08), due to a longer survival after relapse in the tandem ASCT arm.

These findings suggest that patients with high-risk myeloma did not benefit from a mini-allo transplantation following ASCT in comparison of tandem ASCT.

	Auto/auto vs Auto/allo RIC (n)	Conditioning for allo- RIC	CR (%) (auto/auto vs auto/allo RIC)	PFS/EFS (months) (auto/auto vs auto/allo RIC)	OS (months) (auto/auto vs auto/allo RIC)	TRM % P(auto/auto vs auto/allo RIC)
Moreau [28]	166 vs 46	Fludarabine, busulfan, ATG	-	25 vs 21 p=.88	57 vs 41 p=.08	Not evaluated
Bruno [29]	80 vs 82	Low-dose TBI	26 vs 55 p=.004	35 vs 29 p=.02	80 vs 54 p=.01	46 pts. vs 58pts. P=.09
Rosinol [30]	85 vs 25	Fludarabine, Melphalan	40 vs 11 p=.001	31 vs not reached p=.08 26 vs 19.6 p=.4	60% vs 61.8% (5y) p=.9	5 vs 16 p=.09
Krishnan [31]	366 vs156	Low-dose TBI	13 vs 9 p=.0004	46% vs 43% (3 y) p=.7	3 years 80% vs 77% P:0.19	Not evaluated
Giaccone [32]	46 vs58	Low-dose TBI	26 vs 55 p=.003	33 vs39 p=0.02	5.3 years vs not reached P=.02	16 vs 2

Abbreviations: CR: Complete Remission; PFS: Progression-Free Survival; EFS: Event-Free Survival; OS: Overall Survival; TRM: Transplant-Related Mortalitiy; TBI: Total Body Irradiation; ATG: Anti-Thymocyte Globulin

Table 2. Double transplantation comparing tandem ASCT with auto/allo RIC

The Italian group enrolled 162 consecutive younger patients ≤ 65 years of age with newly diagnosed myeloma who had at least one sibling [29]. Patients with an HLA-identical sibling donor received NMA TBI (2Gy) and stem cells median 94 days after ASCT (n=58). Patients without an HLA-identical sibling received tandem ASCT with high-dose melphalan (n=46). The rate of complete remission was significantly higher in the auto-allograft group (55% vs 26%, p=.004). Treatment-related mortality was similar (p=.009) but disease-related mortality was significantly higher in the double ASCT group (43% vs 7%, p<.001). There was a trend of higher EFS in auto-allograft arm (p=.07) while survival in the auto-allo setting was superior to the patients received double ASCT (p=.002).

Another prospective study has been performed by the Spanish PETHEMA group [30]. They enrolled 110 patients with newly diagnosed failing to achieve at least near-CR after a 1st ASCT were scheduled to receive either 2nd ASCT (n=85) or allo-RIC (n=25), depending on the availability of HLA-identical donor. There was a higher increase in CR rate (40% vs 11%, p=. 001) and a trend toward a longer PFS (p=.08) in favor of tandem auto-allo transplantation. In contrast, TRM was higher in the tandem auto-allo transplantation (16% vs 5%, p=.07), EFS and OS was not significantly different between 2nd ASCT and allo-RIC.

The Blood and Marrow Transplant Clinical Trials Network reported a multicenter phase III trial (BMT CTN 0102) in which patients were biologically assigned based on the availability of a matched related donor to either tandem ASCT using melphalan 200sqm or tandem auto-alloHCT using melphalan 200 sqm followed by alloHCT with 2 Gy TBI [31]. Among the 710 patients enrolled between 2003 and 2007 from 37 US centers, 625 patients had standard risk. Patients assigned to receive an ASCT followed by an allo-SCT or tandem ASCT on the basis of the availability of an HLA-matched sibling donor. The study showed no difference of median estimated PFS and OS in comparison of double auto with tandem auto-allo.

Recently, the long-term results of a trial in which treatment of newly diagnosed myeloma patients (n=245) was based on the presence or absence of HLA-identical donor was reported from Italy [32]. Patients with HLA-identical siblings were offered by a standard autograft with high-dose melphalan (200sqm) followed by an allograft with NMA TBI (2 Gy) (n=82), while patients without HLA-identical siblings were assigned to double ASCT after intermediate-dose (100 sqm) or high-dose (140-200 sqm) melphalan (n=80). At a median follow-up of 7.1 year, both OS and EFS were significantly longer in patients with HLA-identical siblings than those without, and median OS and EFS remained significantly longer in the patients transplanted with tandem auto-allo than those patients treated double ASCT. This comparative study showed that allograft conferred a long-term survival and disease-free survival advantage over standard autografting.

4. Post-transplant approaches

High rate of CR after allo-SCT was reported in above studies. But relapse still seems to be a remaining problem. The importance of molecular remission on long-term disease control has been mentioned in the studies of allogeneic transplantation with MAC or RIC regimes. Therefore, post-transplant strategies for preventing and treatment of relapse/refractory disease are of clinical importance. The role of adaptive immunotherapy, donor lymphocyte infusion (DLI), and novel agents has been assessed in several studies.

Donor lymphocyte infusion can enhance GvM and also induce graft versus host disease (GvHD) rates [33,34] Van de Donk, et al evaluated DLIs given in eight European transplantation centers for relapsed (n=48) or persistent (n=15) myeloma following NMA allo-SCT [35]. Overall response was 38%, acute GvHD was 38% and chronic GvHD was 42%. The development of GvHD and response to DLI seems to be associated with GvM effect, and durable remissions are restricted to a minority of patients who achieve CR in this retrospective evaluation. Escalating doses of DLI were found to have lower GvHD risk and better survival rates [36-38].

http://dx.doi.org/10.5772/54762

Immunomodulatory agents, thalidomide or lenalidomide have both have T cell and NK cell activity [39]. Effect of low dose thalidomide after allo-SCT was evaluated in the French study and found that 13 of 31 patients responded [40]. Nineteen percent of patients stopped treatment due to toxicity. Although thalidomide is used for treatment of GvHD, authors observed GvHD in the follow up of 5 patients. Kröger et al, showed improved responses with low dose thalidomide followed by DLI in patients who were refractory to sole DLI [41]. Lenalidomide increased the frequency of human leukocyte antigen-DR (+) T cells and regulatory T cells. Improved response rates were reported with lenalidomide with / without dexamethasone for relapsed/refractory patients [42,43]. Recently, HOVON group investigated maintenance of lenalidomide after allo-SCT; it is not found a feasible treatment due to induction of GvHD [44].

The use of proteasome inhibitor, bortezomib for in vitro depletion of alloreactive T cells after allo-SCT can control GvHD [45]. In retrospective analyses bortezomib administration in relapse or progression of MM after allo-HSCT was shown to be effective treatment without worsening of GVHD symptoms (46).

5. Conclusion

The role and timing of allo SCT still cannot be defined clearly. Due to high TRM rates, myeloablative conditioning in allo-SCT has shifted to reduced intensity conditioning. The studies can be summarized as: (1) -early-day 100 TRM as low as 0 -20%, (2) Acute grade II-IV GvHD and chronic GvHD rates as 30 to 70%, (3) chemosensitivity prior to the transplantation as main factors of survival after transplantation (4) negative PFS effects of in vitro T cell depletion with Alemtuzumab or other(s).

Most of the studies were performed in the relapsed/refractory setting and currently there is no strong data to support allo-RIC as part of a frontline therapy. Reduction of tumor burden by high dose therapy with autologous stem cell rescue has found to have impacts on the transplant outcome and these results brought the comparative studies of auto/auto vs auto/ allo transplantation. There are contradictory results in this era and lack of strong evidence to support one to the other procedure.

Relapse after allo RIC transplantation is still a remaining problem to be solved. Introduction of novel agents such as bortezomib, thalidomide, and lenalidomide with/without DLI(s) can provide solutions to this problem.

In conclusion, allo-SCT has been recognized as a potential therapeutic modality in MM, especially since the introduction of RIC regimens and the use of a tandem auto-allo transplants has shown promise by reducing the TRM and inducing high CR rates. Nevertheless, long-term control of the disease remains a key issue, even in patients treated first by RIC allo-SCT. The role of allo-SCT should be re-evaluated when taking into consideration of promising effects of novel agents in myeloma treatment in randomized clinical trials.

Author details

Pervin Topcuoglu[1], Sinem Civriz Bozdag[2] and Taner Demirer[3]

*Address all correspondence to: topcuogl@medicine.ankara.edu.tr

*Address all correspondence to: scivriz@hotmail.com

*Address all correspondence to: demirer@medicine.ankara.edu.tr

1 Ankara University, School of Medicine, Dept of Hematology, Stem Cell Transplantation Unit, Ankara, Turkey

2 Ankara Oncology Research and Education Hospital, Hematology and Stem Cell Transplantation Unit, Ankara, Turkey

3 Ankara University, School of Medicine, Dept of Hematology, Stem Cell Transplantation Unit, Ankara, Turkey

References

[1] Brenner H, Gondos A, Pulte D. Recent major improvement in long-term survival of younger patients with multiple myeloma. Blood 2008;111(5): 2521-2526.

[2] Kumar SK, Rajkumar SV, Dispenzieri A, Lacy MQ, Hayman SR, Buadi FK, Zeldenrust SR, Dingli D, Russell SJ, Lust JA, Greipp PR, Kyle RA, Gertz MA. Improved survival in multiple myeloma and impact of novel therapies. Blood 2008;111(5): 2516-2520.

[3] Attal M, Lauwers-Cances V, Marit G, Caillot D, Moreau P, Facon T, Stoppa AM, Hulin C, Benboubker L, Garderet L, Decaux O, Leyvraz S, Vekemans MC, Voillat L, Michallet M, Pegourie B, Dumontet C, Roussel M, Leleu X, Mathiot C, Payen C, Avet-Loiseau H, Harousseau JL; IFM Investigators. Lenalidomide maintenance after stem-cell transplantation for multiple myeloma. New England Journal of Medicine 2012; 366(19):1782-91.

[4] Bjorkstrand BB,Lungjman P, Svensson H,Hermans J, Alegre A,Apperley J,Blade J, Carlson K,Cavo M, Ferrant A, Goldstone AH, Laurenzi A,Majolino I, Marcus R, Prentice HG, Remes K,Samson D,Sureda A,Verdonck LF,Volin L,Gahrton G.Allogeneic bone marrow transplantation versus autologus stem cell transplantation in multiple myeloma:a retrospective case matched study from the European group for Blood and Marrow Transplantation. Blood 1996:88(12);4711-18.

[5] Avet-Loiseau H, Attal M, Moreau P, Charbonnel C, Garban F, Hulin C, Leyvraz S, Michallet M, Yakoub-Agha I, Garderet L, Marit G, Michaux L, Voillat L, Renaud M,

Grosbois B, Guillerm G, Benboubker L, Monconduit M, Thieblemont C, Casassus P, Caillot D, Stoppa AM, Sotto JJ, Wetterwald M, Dumontet C, Fuzibet JG, Azais I, Dorvaux V, Zandecki M, Bataille R, Minvielle S, Harousseau JL, Facon T, Mathiot C. Avet-Loiseau H, Attal M, Campion L, Caillot D, Hulin C, Marit G, Stoppa AM, Voillat L, Wetterwald M, Pegourie B, Voog E, Tiab M, Banos A, Jaubert J, Bouscary D, Macro M, Kolb B, Traulle C, Mathiot C, Magrangeas F, Minvielle S, Facon T, Moreau P. Long-term analysis of the IFM 99 trials for myeloma: cytogenetic abnormalities [t(4;14), del(17p), 1q gains] play a major role in defining long-term survival. J Clin Oncol. 2012 30(16):1949-52.

[6] Zhou Y, Zhang Q, Stephens O, Heuck CJ, Tian E, Sawyer JR, Cartron-Mizeracki MA, Qu P, Keller J, Epstein J, Barlogie B, Shaughnessy JD Jr. Prediction of cytogenetic abnormalities with gene expression profiles. Blood 2012; 119(21):e148-50

[7] Roos-Weil D, Moreau P, Avet-Loiseau H, Golmard JL, Kuentz M, Vigouroux S, Socié G, Furst S, Soulier J, Le Gouill S, François S, Thiebaut A, Buzyn A, Maillard N, Yakoub-Agha I, Raus N, Fermand JP, Michallet M, Blaise D, Dhédin N; Société Française de Greffe de Moelle et de Thérapie Cellulaire (SFGM-TC). Impact of genetic abnormalities after allogeneic stem cell transplantation in multiple myeloma: a report of the Société Française de Greffe de Moelle et de Thérapie Cellulaire. Haematologica. 2011; 96(10):1504-11.

[8] Gahrton G, Tura S, Ljungman P, Belanger C, Brandt L, Cavo M, Facon T, Granena A, Gore M, Gratwohl A, Löwenberg B, Nikoskelainen J, Reiffers JJ, Samson D, Verdonck L,Volin L, and for the European Group for Bone Marrow Transplantation. Allogeneic bone marrow transplantation in multiple myeloma. European Group for Bone Marrow Transplantation. New England Journal of Medicine 1991;325(18):1267-73.

[9] Gahrton G, Tura S, Ljungman P, Bladé J, Brandt L, Cavo M, Façon T, Gratwohl A, Hagenbeek A, Jacobs P, et al. Prognostic factors in allogeneic bone marrow transplantation for multiple myeloma. Journal of Clinical Oncology 1995;13(6):1312-22.

[10] Bensinger WI, Buckner CD, Anasetti C, Clift R, Storb R, Barnett T, Chauncey T, Shulman H, Appelbaum FR. Allogeneic marrow transplantation for multiple myeloma: an analysis of risk factors on outcome. Blood 1996; 88(7):2787-93.

[11] Durie BGM, Gale RP, Klein JP, Pelz C, Nugent ML, Horowitz MM. Allogenic Bone Marrow Transplantation In Multiple Myeloma: An IBMTR Analysis. American Society of Clinical Oncology (ASCO). Proceedings- American Society of Clinical Oncolology 1995; 15:405 (abstr 1358)

[12] Barlogie B, Kyle RA, Anderson KC, Greipp PR, Lazarus HM, Hurd DD, McCoy J, Moore DF Jr, Dakhil SR, Lanier KS, Chapman RA, Cromer JN, Salmon SE, Durie B, Crowley JC. Standard chemotherapy compared with high-dose chemoradiotherapy for multiple myeloma: final results of phase III US Intergroup Trial S9321. Journal of Clinical Oncology 2006;24(6):929-936.

[13] Storb R, Raff RF, Appelbaum FR, Graham TC, Schuening FG, Sale G, Pepe M. Comparison of fractionated to single-dose total body irradiation in conditioning canine littermates for DLA-identical marrow grafts. Blood 1989; 74(3):1139-43.

[14] Storb R, Yu C, Wagner JL, Deeg HJ, Nash RA, Kiem HP, Leisenring W, Shulman H. Stable mixed hematopoietic chimerism in DLA-identical littermate dogs given sublethal total body irradiation before and pharmacological immunosuppression after marrow transplantation. Blood. 1997 Apr 15;89(8):3048-54.

[15] Maloney DG, Molina AJ, Sahebi F, Stockerl-Goldstein KE, Sandmaier BM, Bensinger W, Storer B, Hegenbart U, Somlo G, Chauncey T, Bruno B, Appelbaum FR, Blume KG, Forman SJ, McSweeney P, Storb R. Allografting with nonmyeloablative conditioning following cytoreductive autografts for the treatment of patients with multiple myeloma. Blood 2003; 102(9):3447-54.

[16] Kröger N, Schwerdtfeger R, Kiehl M, Sayer HG, Renges H, Zabelina T, Fehse B, Tögel F, Wittkowsky G, Kuse R, Zander AR. Autologous stem cell transplantation followed by a dose-reduced allograft induces high complete remission rate in multiple myeloma. Blood 2002; 100(3): 755-760.

[17] Giralt S, Aleman A, Anagnostopoulos A, Weber D, Khouri I, Anderlini P, Molldrem J, Ueno NT, Donato M, Korbling M, Gajewski J, Alexanian R, Champlin R. Fludarabine/melphalan conditioning for allogeneic transplantation in patients with multiple myeloma. Bone Marrow Transplantation 2002;30(6):367-73.

[18] Crawley C, Szydlo R, Lalancette M, Bacigalupo A, Lange A, Brune M, Juliusson G, Nagler A, Gratwohl A, Passweg J, Komarnicki M, Vitek A, Mayer J, Zander A, Sierra J, Rambaldi A, Ringden O, Niederwieser D, Apperley JF; Chronic Leukemia Working Party of the EBMT. Outcomes of reduced-intensity transplantation for chronic myeloid leukemia: an analysis of prognostic factors from the Chronic Leukemia Working Party of the EBMT. Blood;106(9):2969-76.

[19] Crawley C, Iacobelli S, Björkstrand B, Apperley JF, Niederwieser D, Gahrton G. Reduced intensity conditioning for myeloma:lower nonrelapse mortality but higher relapse rates compared with myeloablative conditioning. Blood 2007;109(8):3588-94.

[20] Rotta M, Storer BE, Sahebi F, Shizuru JA, Bruno B, Lange T, Agura ED, McSweeney PA, Pulsipher MA, Hari P, Maziarz RT, Chauncey TR, Appelbaum FR, Sorror ML, Bensinger W, Sandmaier BM, Storb RF, Maloney DG. Long-term outcome of patients with multiple myeloma after autologous hematopoietic cell transplantation and nonmyeloablative allografting. Blood. 2009;113(14):3383-91.

[21] Schimoni A,Hardan I,Ayuk E, Schilling G, Atanakovic D, ZellerW, Yerushalmi R, Zander A,Kroger N, Nagler A. Allogenic Hematopoietic Stem-Cell Transplantation With Reduced-Intensity Conditioning in Patients With Refractory and Recurrent Multiple Myeloma. Cancer 2010;116(15):3621-30.

[22] El-Cheikh J, Crocchiolo R, Boher JM, Furst S, Stoppa AM, Ladaique P, Faucher C, Calmels B, Castagna L, Lemarie C, De Colella JM, Coso D, Bouabdallah R, Chaban-

non C, Blaise D. Comparable outcomes between unrelated and related donors after reduced-intensity conditioning allogeneic hematopoietic stem cell transplantation in patients with high-risk multiple myeloma. European Journal of Haematology 2012;88(6):497-503.

[23] Bensinger W, Rotta M, Storer B, Chauncey T, Holmberg L, Becker P, Sandmaier BM, Storb R, Maloney D. Allo-SCT for multiple myeloma: a review of outcomes at a single transplant center. Bone Marrow Transplantation 2012 Feb 13. doi: 10.1038/bmt. 2012.1.

[24] Bruno B, Rotta M, Patriarca F, Mattei D, Allione B, Carnevale-Schianca F, Sorasio R, Rambaldi A, Casini M, Parma M, Bavaro P, Onida F, Busca A, Castagna L, Benedetti E, Iori AP, Giaccone L, Palumbo A, Corradini P, Fanin R, Maloney D, Storb R, Baldi I, Ricardi U, Boccadoro M. Nonmyeloablative allografting for newly diagnosed multiple myeloma: the experience of the Gruppo Italiano Trapianti di Midollo. Blood 2009;113(14):3375-82.

[25] Vesole DH, Zhang L, Flomenberg N, Greipp PR, Lazarus HM, Huff CA; ECOG Myeloma and BMT Committees. A Phase II Trial of Autologous Stem Cell Transplantation Followed by Mini-Allogeneic Stem Cell Transplantation for the Treatment of Multiple Myeloma: An Analysis of Eastern Cooperative Oncology Group ECOG E4A98 and E1A97. Biology of Blood and Marrow Transplantation 2009;15(1):83-91.

[26] Lokhorst HM, van der Holt B, Cornelissen JJ, Kersten MJ, van Oers M, Raymakers R, Minnema MC, Zweegman S, Janssen JJ, Zijlmans M, Bos G, Schaap N, Wittebol S, de Weerdt O, Ammerlaan R, Sonneveld P. Donor versus no-donor comparison of newly diagnosed myeloma patients included in the HOVON-50 multiple myeloma study. Blood 2012;119(26):6219-25.

[27] Garban F, Attal M, Michallet M, Hulin C, Bourhis JH, Yakoub-Agha I, Lamy T, Marit G, Maloisel F, Berthou C, Dib M, Caillot D, Deprijck B, Ketterer N, Harousseau JL, Sotto JJ, Moreau P. Prospective comparison of autologous stem cell transplantation followed by dose-reduced allograft (IFM99-03 trial) with tandem autologous stem cell transplantation (IFM99-04 trial) in high-risk de novo multiple myeloma. Blood 2006;107(9):3474-80.

[28] Moreau P, Garban F, Attal M, Michallet M, Marit G, Hulin C, Benboubker L, Doyen C, Mohty M, Yakoub-Agha I, Leyvraz S, Casassus P, Avet-Loiseau H, Garderet L, Mathiot C, Harousseau JL; IFM Group. Long-term follow-up results of IFM99-03 and IFM99-04 trials comparing nonmyeloablative allotransplantation with autologous transplantation in high-risk de novo multiple myeloma. Blood 2008;112(9):3914-5.

[29] Bruno B, Rotta M, Patriarca F, Mordini N, Allione B, Carnevale-Schianca F, Giaccone L, Sorasio R, Omedè P, Baldi I, Bringhen S, Massaia M, Aglietta M, Levis A, Gallamini A, Fanin R, Palumbo A, Storb R, Ciccone G, Boccadoro M. A comparison of allografting with autografting for newly diagnosed myeloma. New England Journal of Medicine 2007;356(11):1110-20.

[30] Rosiñol L, Pérez-Simón JA, Sureda A, de la Rubia J, de Arriba F, Lahuerta JJ, González JD, Díaz-Mediavilla J, Hernández B, García-Frade J, Carrera D, León A, Hernández M, Abellán PF, Bergua JM, San Miguel J, Bladé J; Programa para el Estudio y la Terapéutica de las Hemopatías Malignas y Grupo Español de Mieloma (PETHEMA/GEM). A prospective PETHEMA study of tandem autologous transplantation versus autograft followed by reduced-intensity conditioning allogeneic transplantation in newly diagnosed multiple myeloma. Blood 2008;112(9):3591-3.

[31] Krishnan A, Pasquini MC, Logan B, Stadtmauer EA, Vesole DH, Alyea E 3rd, Antin JH, Comenzo R, Goodman S, Hari P, Laport G, Qazilbash MH, Rowley S, Sahebi F, Somlo G, Vogl DT, Weisdorf D, Ewell M, Wu J, Geller NL, Horowitz MM, Giralt S, Maloney DG; Blood Marrow Transplant Clinical Trials Network (BMT CTN). Autologous haemopoietic stem-cell transplantation followed by allogeneic or autologous haemopoietic stem-cell transplantation in patients with multiple myeloma (BMT CTN 0102): a phase 3 biological assignment trial. Lancet Oncology 2011; 12(13): 1195-203.

[32] Giaccone L, Storer B, Patriarca F, Rotta M, Sorasio R, Allione B, Carnevale-Schianca F, Festuccia M, Brunello L, Omedè P, Bringhen S, Aglietta M, Levis A, Mordini N, Gallamini A, Fanin R, Massaia M, Palumbo A, Ciccone G, Storb R, Gooley TA, Boccadoro M, Bruno B. Long-term follow-up of a comparison of nonmyeloablative allografting with autografting for newly diagnosed myeloma. Blood 2011;117(24):6721-7.

[33] Roddie C&Peggs KS. Donor lymphocyte infusion following allogeneic hematopoietic stem cell transplantation. Expert Opinion on Biological Therapy 2011; 11(4): 473-487.

[34] Beitinjaneh A, Saliba R , Bashir Q , Shah N , Parmar S , Hosing C , Popat U, Anderlini P, Dinh Y , Qureshi S , Rondon G , Champlin R , Giralt S, Qazilbash M. Durable responses after donor lymphocyte infusion for patients with residual multiple myeloma following non-myeloablative allogeneic stem cell transplant. Leukemia & Lymphoma 2012; 53(8): 1525-1529

[35] van de Donk NW, Kröger N, Hegenbart U, Corradini P, San Miguel JF, Goldschmidt H, Perez-Simon JA, Zijlmans M, Raymakers RA, Montefusco V, Ayuk FA, van Oers MH, Nagler A, Verdonck LF, Lokhorst HM. Prognostic factors for donor lymphocyte infusions following non-myeloablative allogeneic stem cell transplantation in multiple myeloma. Bone Marrow Transplantation 2006;37(12):1135-41.

[36] Dazzi F, Szydlo RM, Craddock C, Cross NC, Kaeda J, Chase A, Olavarria E, van Rhee F, Kanfer E, Apperley JF, Goldman JM. Comparison of single-dose and escalating-dose regimens of donor lymphocyte infusion for relapse after allografting for chronic myeloid leukemia. Blood 2000;95(1):67-71

[37] Peggs KS, Thomson K, Hart DP, Geary J, Morris EC, Yong K, Goldstone AH, Linch DC, Mackinnon S. Dose-escalated donor lymphocyte infusions following reduced intensity transplantation:toxicity, chimerism, and disease responses. Blood 2004;103(4): 1548-56.

[38] Peggs KS, Mackinnon S, Williams CD, D'Sa S, Thuraisundaram D, Kyriakou C, Morris EC, Hale G, Waldmann H, Linch DC, Goldstone AH, Yong K. Reduced-intensity transplantation with in vivo T-cell depletion and adjuvant dose escalating donor lymphocyte infusions for chemotherapy-sensitive myeloma: limited efficacy of graft-versus-tumor activity. Biology of Blood and Marrow Transplantation 2003;9(4):257-65.

[39] Teo SK. Properties of thalidomide and its analogues: implications for anticancer therapy. The AAPS Journal 2005 22;7(1):E14-9.

[40] Mohty M,Attal M,Marit G,Bulobois CE,Garban F,Gratecos N,Rio B,Vernant JP,Sotto JJ, Cahn JY,Blaise D, Jouet JP,Facon T,Yakoub-Agha I. Thalidomide salvage therapy following allogeneic stem cell transplantation for multiple myeloma: a retrospective study from the Intergroupe Francophone du Myélome (IFM) and the Société Française de Greffe de Moelle et Thérapie Cellulaire (SFGM-TC). Bone Marrow Transplantation 2005;35(2):165-9.

[41] Kröger N, Shimoni A, Zagrivnaja M, Ayuk F, Lioznov M, Schieder H, Renges H, Fehse B, Zabelina T, Nagler A, Zander AR.Low-dose thalidomide and donor lymphocyte infusion as adoptive immunotherapy after allogeneic stem cell transplantation in patients with multiple myeloma. Blood 2004;104(10):3361-3.

[42] Cheikh J,Crocchiolo R,Furst S,Ladaique P,Castagna L,Faucher C,Granata A,Lemarie C,Calmel B,Stoppa AM,Coella JM Duran S,Chabannon C,Blaise D. Lenalidomide plus donor-lymphocytes infusion after allogeneic stem-cell transplantation with reduced-intensity conditioning in patients with high-risk multiple myeloma. Experimental Hematology 2012;40(7):521-7.

[43] Minnema MC, van der Veer MS, Aarts T, Emmelot M, Mutis T, Lokhorst HM. Lenalidomide alone or in combination with dexamethasone is highly effective in patientswith relapsed multiple myeloma following allogeneic stem cell transplantation and increases the frequency of CD4(+)Foxp3(+) T cells. Leukemia 2009;23(3):605-7.

[44] Sonneveld P, Lokhorst HM, Mutis T, Minnema MC. Lenalidomide maintenance after nonmyeloablative allogeneic stem cell transplantation in multiple myeloma is not feasible: results of the HOVON 76 Trial. Blood 2011;118(9):2413-9.

[45] Koreth J, Stevenson KE, Kim HT, Garcia M, Ho VT, Armand P, Cutler C, Ritz J, Antin JH, Soiffer RJ, Alyea EP 3rd. Bortezomib, tacrolimus, and methotrexate for prophylaxis of graft-versus-host disease after reduced-intensity conditioning allogeneic stem cell transplantation from HLA-mismatched unrelated donors. Blood 2009;114(18): 3956-9.

[46] El-Cheikh J, Michallet M, Nagler A, de Lavallade H, Nicolini FE, Shimoni A, Faucher C, Sobh M, Revesz D, Hardan I, Fürst S, Blaise D, Mohty M. High response rate and improved graft-versus-host disease following bortezomib as salvage therapy after reduced intensity conditioning allogeneic stem cell transplantation for multiple myeloma. Haematologica 2008; 93(3):455-8.

Chapter 9

Cellular Immunotherapy Using Dendritic Cells in Multiple Myeloma: New Concept to Enhance Efficacy

Je-Jung Lee, Youn-Kyung Lee, Hyun Ju Lee,
Sung-Hoon Jung and Thanh-Nhan Nguyen-Pham

Additional information is available at the end of the chapter

http://dx.doi.org/10.5772/54100

1. Introduction

Multiple myeloma (MM) is a clonal B-cell malignancy that is currently incurable with conventional chemotherapy, even if high-dose chemotherapy with autologous or allogeneic hematopoietic stem cell transplantation (HSCT) and the development of novel molecular target agents have resulted in a marked improvement in overall survival [1, 2]. Allogeneic HSCT, which induces a clinically significant immune-mediated allogeneic graft-versus-myeloma (GVM) effect, has provided the framework for the development of immunotherapeutic strategies [3, 4]. To prolong the survival of patients with MM, who are undergoing allogeneic HSCT, a donor lymphocyte infusion can be used successfully as a salvage therapy, which is based on the GVM effect in some cases of MM that relapse after allogeneic HSCT [5, 6]. A clinically significant immune-mediated GVM effect provides the framework for the development of immune-based therapeutic options that use antigen-presenting cells (APCs) with increased potency, such as dendritic cells (DCs), in MM [6].

DCs are the most potent APCs for initiating cellular immune responses through the stimulation of naive T cells. Because of their ability to stimulate T cells, DCs act as links between innate immunity and adaptive immunity in antitumor immune responses [7]. DCs orchestrate a variety of immune responses by stimulating the differentiation of naïve $CD4^+$ T cells into helper T effectors such as Th1, Th2 or Th17 type [8, 9]. Cytokines secreted by DCs at the time of initial T cell stimulation play an important role in the subsequent differentiation of effector T cells. Th1 cells, through interferon-gamma (IFN-γ) production, regulate antigen presentation and immunity against intracellular pathogens [8]. DC-based vaccines have become the most attractive tools for cancer immunotherapy and have been used in more than 20 malignancies; most commonly melanoma, renal cell carcinoma, prostate cancer and colorectal carcinoma

[10]. Cellular immunotherapy using DCs is emerging as a useful immunotherapeutic modality to treat MM [11]. While antigen-specific cytotoxic T lymphocytes (CTLs) and immune response can be induced by DC vaccination in MM patients, clinical responses so far have been largely unsatisfying to be observed only in a minority of treated patients with MM. Progress in understanding DC biology in cancer patients and the recruitment of suppressive cells of the adaptive and innate immune system in antitumor immunity of cellular immunotherapy is leading to new concept which aims at improved immune and clinical outcomes in MM. New concept is developing to generate novel therapeutic targets that could restore DC capacity to prime T cells and trigger effective anticancer responses in combination with other therapies to offset tumor-induced suppression in MM.

2. Dendritic cell in myeloma immunity

DCs have a potent antigen-specific T cell stimulatory capacity and therefore should be considered to the one of the promising antitumor immunotherapeutic options. In tumor-specific immunity, secreted products or fragments from tumor cells enter into DCs through the endosome and are processed and presented on MHC class molecules of DCs [12]. Processed antigens presented on these molecules of DCs are recognized by $CD4^+$ T helper cells, which not only enhance to the $CD8^+$ T cell response but also facilitate to develop a humoral immune response for surface antigens expressed on the tumor cells. The antigens presented on MHC class I are recognized by $CD8^+$ CTLs, which have a direct cytotoxic effect on tumor cells. Unfortunately, patients with MM have basically dysfunctional DCs that are functionally defective, evidenced by the decreased number of circulating precursors of DCs as well as the impaired T cell stimulatory capacities compared with normal controls [13, 14]. The defective functions of DCs in patients with MM are partially attributed to the production of IL-6 and other tumor-derived factors. DCs in MM patients are a target of tumor-associated suppressive factors, such as IL-10, transforming growth factor- beta (TGF-β), vascular endothelial growth factor (VEGF), and IL-6, resulting in their aberrant functions and impaired development of effector functions in tumor-specific lymphocytes [15]. There were only few patients with MM who responded clinically to vaccination with antigen-loaded autologous DCs. There may be several reasons for this failure from MM patients itself. MM is believed to induce immunoparesis that interferes with DC function and hence affects the effective antitumor immune responses in these patients. They are able to escape immune surveillance by down-regulation of immune markers as well as through the production of immunosuppressive cytokines by the tumor cells or by activation of suppressor cells such as regulatory T cells and myeloid cells. Myeloma cells can produce immuno-inhibitory cytokines, such as IL-10, TGF-β, VEGF, and IL-6, which play major roles in the pathogenesis of MM [15]. In addition, the survival and proliferation of myeloma cells are partially facilitated by impaired endogenous immune surveillance against tumor antigens, including the abrogation of DC function, by constitutive activation of the signal transducer and activator of transcription 3 (STAT3) [13]. Impairment in both humoral and cellular immunity in MM is associated with impaired B cell responses; decreased T cell numbers including $CD4^+$ T cells and impaired CTL responses; and dysfunction of natural killer (NK) cells and NKT cells responses [16-19]. In addition, the recruitment and expansion of $CD4^+CD25^+$ regulatory T cells (Tregs) in the suppression of tumor immunity has been reported in MM patients [20, 21]. More recently, the proportion of $CD14^+HLA\text{-}DR^{-/low}$ myeloid-derived suppressor cells (MDSCs) and $CD4^+$ forkhead box P3 $(FoxP3)^+$ Tregs cells was increased in MM patients at diagnosis, resulting in a significant impediment of immune cells related to cancer immunotherapy [22].

3. Current DC vaccination research in MM

Usually, *ex vivo* DCs were generated from circulating blood precursors (i.e. monocytes) or bone marrow progenitor cells and educated them with myeloma-associated antigens prior to vaccination to patients with MM.

3.1. Idiotype-pulsed DCs

Immunoglobulin idiotype (Id) is a tumor-specific antigen that is produced by each B cell tumor clone. Id protein has been used for immunotherapy in patients with MM [23, 24]. Id vaccination could induce immune responses by both antibodies and Id-specific T cells, including $CD4^+$ and $CD8^+$ T cells, through the presentation of Id protein on the surface of professional APCs [24]. Id-specific CTL lines that kill autologous primary myeloma cells *in vitro* have been generated [25, 26]. Autologous DCs that were generated from MM patients have been shown to efficiently endocytose different classes of Id proteins, and autologous Id-specific CTLs that were generated by Id-pulsed DCs were able to recognize and kill autologous primary myeloma cells *in vitro* [25, 26]. Various studies of DC-based Id vaccination in MM have been reported [27-34]. Although Id-specific CTLs and immune responses could be induced in some patients, clinical responses have rarely been observed after vaccination possibly because Id protein is a weak antigen and immature DCs have been used in some studies [27].

3.2. Myeloma-associated antigens-based DC immunotherapy

In general, the production of DC vaccines using whole tumor antigens has become a promising tool for immunotherapy against MM. There are several types of myeloma-associated antigen for loading onto DCs: loading with myeloma lysates [35, 36], loading with dying myeloma cells [37-39], transfection with myeloma-derived RNA [40], pulsing with myeloma-derived heat shock protein (HSP) gp96 [41, 42], and hybridization with myeloma cells [43, 44]. These techniques have the advantage of allowing the presentation of multiple epitopes to MHC on DCs, therefore inducing polyclonal T cell responses from many potentially unknown tumor-associated antigens (TAAs) and reducing the probability of immune escape by a single TAA.

Various myeloma-associated antigens that may induce immune responses from DC-based vaccines have been identified in MM patients. MUC1-specific CTLs that were induced *in vitro* using peptide-pulsed DCs or plasma cell RNA-loaded DCs efficiently killed not only target cells pulsed with the antigenic peptide but also MM cells [40, 45]. DCs transfected with PTD-NY-ESO-1 protein can induce $CD8^+$ cellular antitumor immunity superior to that achieved with NY-ESO-1 protein alone [46]. Sp17-specific HLA class I-restricted CTLs were successfully generated by DCs that had been loaded with recombinant Sp17 protein and were able to kill autologous tumor cells that expressed Sp17 [47]. The overexpression of hTERT on MM compared to the expression levels in normal cells indicated that this telomerase also could be used as a myeloma-associated antigen. hTERT was capable of triggering antitumor-CTL responses and killing $hTERT^+$ tumor cells [48]. Recently, a report demonstrated that activated T lymphocytes were able to successfully kill myeloma cells after stimulation by DCs loaded with hTERT- and MUC1-derived nonapeptides [49]. DKK1, a novel protein that is not expressed in most normal tissues but is expressed in almost all myeloma cells, may be an important antigenic target for anti-myeloma immunotherapy. DKK1-specific CTLs that were generated by DCs pulsed with DKK1 peptides were specifically lysed by autologous primary myeloma cells and DKK1-positive cell lines [50].

4. New concepts to enhance the efficacy of cellular immunotherapy in MM

4.1. How to enhance the efficacy of DC vaccinations

Because of unsatisfied clinical response of DC vaccination trials in MM, a number of groups have looked at whether the DC vaccination may be more effective if better cytokine combinations are used to enhance DC function, effective tumor antigens are investigated to use, suppressive signal transcriptions are blocked to overcome defective DC function, the interaction with immunosuppressor cells is interrupted to avoid the effect of these suppressor cells, or DC vaccines need to be combined with other therapies.

4.2. The next generation of DCs

To improve DC vaccination, the investigators exploit to the microbial activation signals leading to generate potent DCs with high secretion of cytokines such as IL-12p70, which generate strong tumor-specific Th1 response and helper function for the generation of memory T cells, high production of polarizing signals, which help the generation of high avidity in CTLs that may be resistant to tumor microenvironment, and strong costimulation mediated via several costimulatory molecular pathways [51, 52]. This induces to eliminate Tregs and block tumor microenvironment results in the full activity of elicited CTLs and tumor rejection.

The initial phase of DC-based vaccines involving immature or partially-mature "first-generation" DCs has been reported [53, 54]. However, such DCs express suboptimal levels of costimulatory molecules and constitute weaker immunogens than subsequently implemented mature DCs, the "second-generation" of clinically applied standard DCs (sDCs), which induced by cytokine cocktails containing IL-1β/TNF-α/IL-6/prostaglandin E_2 (PGE_2) [55]. However, to date, sDC vaccines still have some drawbacks, including the mediation of Th2 polarization by increased secretion of the immunosuppressive cytokine IL-10 from DCs and high activity in activating Tregs [56, 57]. Therefore, several investigators, including our group, have tried to develop new generation of potent DC that possess all required features for inducing effective tumor-specific immune responses. We demonstrated the feasibility of

http://dx.doi.org/10.5772/54100

inducing potent α-type 1-polarizing DCs (αDC1s) by exposing immature DCs to α-type 1-polarizing cytokine cocktail containing IL-1β, TNF-α, IFN-α, IFN-γ, and polyinosinic:polycytidylic acid [poly(I:C)] to generate strong functional CTLs on average 20-fold higher than sDCs [58-62]. Recently, we successfully generated αDC1s from MM patients with high expression of costimulatory molecules, significant production of IL-12p70, and potent generation of myeloma-specific CTLs [37, 38]. Such a novel strategy would provide improved potency of *ex vivo*-generated DCs for cancer immunotherapy.

The other strategy to induce new potent DCs from patients with MM was the use of helper cells to promote type 1-polarization of DCs. Indeed, it has been demonstrated that NK cells play a major immunoregulatory role in the development of protective T cell-mediated immunity against intracellular pathogens and cancers [63]. Such helper activity of NK cells is at least partially mediated by the functional modulation of DCs. This phenomenon depended on the production of IFN-γ and TNF-α from the activated NK cells [63] and was associated with enhanced cross-presentation of tumor antigen and the induction of Th1 and CTL responses [39, 64, 65]. Recent data from our laboratory and other groups has demonstrated that NK-DC interactions promote the subsequent induction of tumor-specific responses in $CD4^+$ and $CD8^+$ T cells, allowing NK cells to act as helper cells in the development of type 1-polarized DCs in responses against cancer [39, 64, 65]. Resting NK cells that are activated in the presence of toll-like receptor (TLR) agonists, IL-2, and IFN-α can induce potent DCs with enhanced IL-12p70 production *in vitro*, generating strong antigen-specific CTLs against myeloma cells [39].

We also found that the selected combinations of TLR agonists synergistically triggered a Th1-polarizing capacity through production of high amounts of IL-12p70 [66]. However, the major limitation of this combination was the decreased ability of these cells to migrate into lymph nodes compared to that of conventional sDCs. When DCs are activated by individual TLR agonists, such as lipopolysaccharide (LPS) or poly(I:C), or by a combination of 2 TLR agonists, all cells mature and produce high levels of bioactive IL-12p70 in early phase of maturation and after subsequent stimulation with T cell-related DC activating signal CD40L. In addition, the phenotyes of these matured DCs were markedly enhanced when a combination of type I and type II IFN was added. These combinations of stimuli also regulated the expression of CD38 and CD74, markers related to the full activation of DCs [67, 68]. We demonstrated that, at the optimal concentration used to stimulate DCs, the combination of 2 TLR agonists with type I and II IFNs can be used to generate fully mature DCs that have high migratory capacity and can maintain IL-12p70-producing capacity. The regulation of CD38 and CD74 in DCs could in turn enhance the migratory activity of DCs in the presence of a combination of 2 TLR agonists and IFNs [69].

Ursolic acid (URC) is isolated from *Uncaria rhynchophylla* and phytochemically classified as a triterpene. Triterpene compounds have been identified as a unique class of natural products possessing diverse biological activities. Recently, we reported that URC activates human DCs in a fashion that favors Th1 polarization via the activation of TLR2- and/or TLR4-dependent IL-12p70 and induces the production of IFN-γ by $CD4^+$ naïve T cells [70]. In addition, combination URC and IFN-γ enhanced the activation of DCs via promotion of IFN-γ-induced Th1 cell polarization that was dependent on the activation of IL-12p70 and independent of TLR4 [71, 72]. The potential of natural products to enhance DC maturation and activation has important implications for the use of DCs as a cancer vaccine.

4.3. New sources of myeloma-associated antigens for DC vaccines

Another important consideration to improve the efficacy of DC vaccination in patients with MM is an effective tumor antigen, instead of using idiotype proteins with a weak antigenicity. The use of whole tumor cells, instead of single antigen, may help to enhance antitumor effects to target multiple tumor variants. It is necessary to use purified, optimized myeloma cells, if possible, as a source of tumor antigens for loading onto DCs to generate potent myeloma-specific CTLs [35]. However, it is not only impractical to obtain sufficient amounts of purified autologous myeloma cells for tumor antigens in the clinical setting from patients with MM and it is also unsuitable for those with a lower tumor burden status. As an alternative source of tumor-relevant antigens, allogeneic tumor cells or established cancer cell lines have been used to overcome the limitation in various tumors [37, 38]. DCs loaded with tumor antigens derived from allogeneic myeloma cells could generate myeloma-specific CTLs against autologous myeloma cells in patients with MM [37, 39]. The success of using an allogeneic myeloma cell line as tumor antigens led to the possibility that allogeneic myeloma cells could also be used as a viable source of tumor antigens in the context of appropriate major MHC alleles to autologous CTLs. In addition, autologous DCs loaded with dying myeloma cells of allogeneic matched monoclonal immunoglobulin subtype showed to generate potent myeloma-specific CTLs against autologous myeloma cells in MM patients [38] These findings suggested that allogeneic myeloma cell lines and allogeneic matched monoclonal immunoglobulin subtype of myeloma were effective tumor antigens capable of inducing functional CTLs against patients' own myeloma cells.

Improved understanding of which specific anticancer agents lead to immunogenic cell death and whether these process can enhance antitumor immunity may facilitate the mechanism how chemotherapy and immunotherapy combination can induce immune responses against cancer. Recently, we have worked to develop strategies that recover dysfunction of DCs caused from loading tumor antigens through treatment of myeloma cells with a combination of the selective JAK/STAT3 inhibitor, JSI-124, and a kind of proteasome inhibitor, bortezomib. We observed that production of inhibitory cytokines, such as IL-10, IL-23, and especially IL-6, which induces DC dysfunction in MM patients, was down-regulated in DCs loaded with dying myeloma tumor cells that induced by these agents. Furthermore, phospho-STAT3 was also down-regulated in the DCs. These DCs displayed a superior ability to induce myeloma-specific responses of CTLs. More recently, we are investigating whether chaetocin could be used to induce dying tumor cells for loading onto DCs to enhance myeloma-specific antitumor responses. We show that anti-myeloma drug-induced dying tumor cells can be used as the source of myeloma antigens to loading onto DCs that could elicit potent anti-myeloma activity of CTLs due to the expression of HSP and cancer testis antigens as a mechanism of immunogenic death of human MM cells.

http://dx.doi.org/10.5772/54100

4.4. Blocking immunosuppressive activity during the loading of tumor antigens for DC vaccines

The suppressive effects of tumor cells during DC generation have been explained previously by the ability of the tumor microenvironment to suppress DC differentiation [73]. This process can influence STAT3 and ERK phosphorylation, resulting in hyperactivation of STAT3 and ERK, which may be responsible for defective generation of DCs [74]. The immune-mediated antitumor effects of DCs are enhanced by inhibition of the JAK2/STAT3 pathway [75], inhibition of p38 or activation of the MEK/ERK or MAP kinase pathways, and neutralization of IL-6 [76]. Recently, we found that when MM-derived DCs were generated by loading tumor lysates from autologous myeloma cells, these DCs showed lower phenotypic maturation, less T cell stimulatory capacity, less CTL activity, and highly abnormal IL-6 and IL-12 secretion compared to the secretion by unloaded DCs. Moreover, the levels of VEGF, phospho-STAT3, and phospho-ERK1/2 in these DCs were significantly higher than in unloaded DCs. After neutralization of VEGF activity, DC functions, signal transduction, and cytokine production were returned to normal level. Therefore, inhibitory factors and abnormal signaling pathways during maturation with tumor antigens in DCs may be responsible for the defective activity of DCs in MM, and these abnormalities may be overcome by neutralizing the signaling that would lead to a suppressed immune response [77].

5. Combination therapy: New concept to enhance efficacy of DC vaccines

Many factors contribute to the limited clinical efficacy of DC vaccines. The tumor microenvironment contains different kinds of inhibitory cells, such as Tregs and MDSC, and inhibitory molecules, such as IL-10, IL-6, TGF-β, and VEGF, all of which prevent the activation of effector T cells in response to DC responses [16-21, 23, 78, 79]. Although DC vaccines showed effective antitumor effect in experimental *ex vivo* systems, they didn't effectively induce strong immune responses that were enough to kill tumors *in vivo*. Therefore, strategies to improve the efficacy of DC vaccines are to overcome the immune tolerance/suppression induced by these cells, which are involved in the use of a combination of DC vaccine with either stimulatory cytokines or the targeting elimination of inhibitory cells and molecules in tumor microenvironment.

5.1. DC vaccine and cytokine combination

Cytokines, such as GM-CSF or IL-2, known to enhance cell-mediated immune responses may be administered as adjuvants with the vaccines aiming to create an environment where specific immune responses are readily induced [80, 81]. To enhance the efficacy of DC vaccination, Id-pulsed DCs were combined with GM-CSF [80, 82-84], with immunogenic carrier molecules such as KLH [27, 28, 31-33, 82, 85], or cytokine IL-2 [80, 83] to improve the effectiveness of these DC vaccines in patients with MM. Recently, a phase I study was performed in patients with MM using autologous DCs/tumor cells fusion in combination with GM-CSF administration at the day of DC vaccination [86]. The expansion of circulating $CD4^+$ and $CD8^+$ T cells reactive with autologous myeloma cells were detected in 11 of 15 evaluable patients. A majority of patients with advanced disease demonstrated disease stabilization. In a murine myeloma model, mice were vaccinated with DC-plasmacytoma cell fusions and demonstrated that administration of IL-12 with the vaccine resulted in potentiation of *in vivo* T cell proliferation and cytotoxicity and eradication of established disease [87]. Therefore, the combination of DC vaccine with stimulatory cytokines is a feasible approach to provide a new source of DC-based vaccines for the development of immunotherapy against MM.

5.2. DC vaccine and chemotherapy combination

Chemotherapy can help to reverse the immunosuppression caused by cancers and also further enhance the capacity of DCs to trigger antitumor immunity [88]. Accumulating evidence indicates that conventional chemotherapy as well as radiotherapy selectively eliminates immunosuppressive cells, triggers the activation of DCs, and enhances antigen cross-presentation. Furthermore, specific anticancer agents lead to immunogenic cell death of tumor cells and these processes can enhance antitumor immunity.

Recent studies have shown that chemotherapeutic agents increase the efficacy of active or adoptive antitumor immunotherapies through beneficial immunomodulatory effects [89, 90]. Cyclophosphamide eliminates the activities of tumor-induced suppressor T cells in tumor-bearing hosts [90] and induces the production of immunostimulatory cytokines, such as type I IFN [91]. In addition, low-dose cyclophosphamide has been shown to down-regulate suppressor T cells and to decrease the production of TGF-β and IL-10 while inducing a Th2/Th1 shift in the cytokine profile [92-94]. Low-dose cyclophosphamide may enhance the antitumor efficacy of DC vaccines by increasing the proportion of IFN-γ secreting lymphocytes and suppressing the proportion of $CD4^{+}CD25^{+}FoxP3^{+}$ Tregs in tumor-bearing mice [95]. The result of a clinical trial using allogeneic DC vaccines combined with low-dose cyclophosphamide has revealed that the combination therapy could induce stronger antitumor responses compared to the DC vaccine alone [96]. Recently, we demonstrated that a single administration of low-dose cyclophosphamide before the first DC vaccination showed to augment antitumor effects of DC vaccines to completely eradicate the tumor and to prolong the survival of vaccinated mice [64].

Lenalidomide is a thalidomide analog that has more potent anti-myeloma effects and less adverse effects [97]. Lenalidomide can induce apoptosis of myeloma cells, inhibit the production of cytokines (IL-6, VEGF, and TNF-α) in bone marrow of myeloma patients, and stimulate T cell and NK cell proliferation, cytotoxicity, and cytokine (IL-2, IFN-γ) production [97]. In addition, lenalidomide can inhibit the frequency and function of Tregs, resulting in inhibition of Treg expansion and FoxP3 expression in cancer patients patients [98]. Interestingly, this drug can also induce the activation of APC function, resulting in upregulation of CD40, CD80, and CD86 in chronic lymphocytic leukemia [99]. Therefore, lenalidomide can be used as an immunomodulatory drug in order to enhance immune responses against cancer. Our *in vitro* study showed that lenalidomide enhanced the maturation and function of DCs in the presence of LPS, resulting in synergistic stimulation of DCs to increase phenotype expression, IL-12p70 production, T cell stimulation capacities, and CTL activities against myeloma cells, and to suppress the generation of Tregs. Moreover, our *in vivo* mouse myeloma model showed that a treatment combining the lenalidomide with DC vaccination markedly improved antitumor effect by inhibiting immunosuppressor cells, recovering effector cells, and inducing superior polarization of the Th1/Th2 balance in favor of the Th1 response. This immunomodulatory effect may be a crucial component of the enhancer-like properties of lenalidomide in the context of antitumor immunity against MM.

5.3. Chemotherapeutic agent can induce "immunogenic myeloma-cell death" to trigger activation of DCs and to enhance cross-presentation of DCs

Most of chemotherapeutic agents kill tumor cells by the induction of apoptosis. Previously, chemotherapy and immunotherapy have usually been regarded as unrelated therapy in the treatment of cancers because chemotherapy-induced apoptotic cell death has long been considered as non-immunogenic or inducing immune tolerance. Recently, apoptotic cell death when coupled with inflammatory signals, such as HSPs, is clearly known to induce the activation of DCs and triggers the immune response [100]. Some chemotherapeutic agents could induce a type of tumor cell death that activates efficient antitumor immunity, so it is called "immunogenic tumor-cell death". Immunogenic tumor-cell death expresses danger signals on the tumor cell surface or secretes immunostimulatory factors, such as HSPs, calreticulin, high mobility group box 1 protein (HMGB1), and ATP, into the tumor microenvironment, thereby promoting DC maturation and stimulating a powerful T cell immune response [88].

Cyclophosphamide is well known as a potent cytotoxic and lymphoablative drug in conventional and high dosages. However, more recent work highlighted as an immunostimulatory and/or antiangiogenic agent at low dosages, openning up novel indication in the field of cancer immunotherapy. In recent reports, cyclophosphamide administration in tumor-bearing mice induced pre-apoptotic surface translocation of calreticulin on tumor cells [101], which serves as an "eat-me" signal for phagocytes [102] and the release of high-mobility group box1 (HMGB1) protein in the extracellular milieu [101], which constitutes a "danger signal" triggering activation of the DC processing machinery [103]. These events are prerequisites for adequate engulfment of tumor apoptotic material and optimal $CD8^+$ T cell cross-priming by DCs [102, 103].

HSPs are intracellular chaperones for many proteins, but they can also be expressed on the cell surface or even be released under stress conditions [104, 105]. HSP acts as an adjuvant in initiating the activation of DCs or as protein vehicle to facilitate the presentation of antigen peptides to T cells. Spisek et al. [106] reported that uptake of myeloma cells by DCs after tumor cell death induced by bortezomib leads to the induction of antitumor immunity and enhances DC-mediated tumor immune response, indicating the probability mechanism due to the expression of HSP90 on the surface of dying cells, thereby facilitating the activation of DCs in response to dying tumor cells. Our study also found that HSPs released from dying tumor cells, which were induced by a combination of the selective JAK/STAT3 inhibitor JSI-124 and proteasome inhibitor bortezomib, act on tumor cells to recover DC dysfunction and to induce cytokine and chemokine production from DCs, resulting in generation of potent myeloma-specific CTL response against myeloma cells.

5.4. Possible combination DCs and other approaches

In the presence of regulatory and suppressive environment, it is very difficult to elicit or induce effective immune response after DC vaccination in cancer patients. To improve the clinical outcomes, DC vaccines need to be combined, in particular for patients at advanced stages, with other approaches that offset the suppressive tumor environment [107]. It has been known that the specific depletion of $CD4^+CD25^+$ Treg cells by anti-CD25 antibodies increases the efficiency of the anti-tumor immune response of tumor-bearing animals, although the tumors are not completely rejected [108]. An increased number of $CD4^+CD25^+FoxP3^+$ regulatory T cells have been demonstrated in patients with MM [22, 109]. Depletion of Treg may have resulted in improved response to tumor vaccine in animal models and a clinical study. In addition, blocking antibodies or soluble receptors were exploited for the blockade of suppressive cytokines in the tumor microenvironment, such as IL-10 [110], IL-13 [111], TGF-β [112] and VEGF [113]. Such strategies can be used to block immune-inhibitory signals in lymphocytes as illustrated by anti-CTLA-4 [114] and/or anti-PD1 [115] or to block their ligands expressed on tumors.

Another strategy to improve DC vaccination is combination approach with other immune cells, including adoptive T cells or NK cells. In adoptive T-cell transfer, one can seek to modulate the number of regulatory T cells, and transfer a population of activated effector cells. The combination of DC vaccination and adoptive T-cell transfer led to a more robust antitumor response than the use of each treatment modality [116]. These findings illuminate a new potential application for DC vaccination in the *in vivo* stimulation of adoptively transferred T cells. Therefore, combining active and passive immunotherapies in the treatment of MM may enhance the efficacy of tumor vaccine in the future.

6. Future perspectives

Progress in understanding DC biology in MM patients and the recruitment of suppressive cells of the adaptive and innate immune system in antitumor immunity of cellular immunotherapy is leading to new concept which aims at improved immune and clinical outcomes in MM. The new generation of DCs may be a potential vaccine therapy for inducing the rate of tumor responses and prolonging survival of patients with MM. Furthermore, information from studies that combine DC vaccine with other therapies, including chemotherapy, radiation therapy, molecular target agents, other immunotherapy (adaptive T cells or NK cells), or adjuvants will have high impact on enhancing therapeutic immunity in MM by simultaneously enhancing the potency of immune responses and offsetting immunoregulatory pathways.

Acknowledgements

This study was financially supported by grant no. 2011-0005285 from General Researcher Program Type II of the National Research Foundation of Korea; grant no. RTI05-01-01 from

http://dx.doi.org/10.5772/54100

the Regional Technology Innovation Program of the Ministry of Commerce, Industry and Energy; grant no. A000200058 from the Regional Industrial Technology Development program of the Ministry of Knowledge and Economy; grant no. 1120390 from the National R&D Program for Cancer Control, Ministry for Health and Welfare; grant no. 2011-0030034 from Leading Foreign Research Institute Recruitment Program through the National Research Foundation of Korea (NRF) funded by the Ministry of Education, Science and Technology (MEST), Republic of Korea.

Author details

Je-Jung Lee[1,2,3], Youn-Kyung Lee[3], Hyun Ju Lee[1,2], Sung-Hoon Jung[1,2] and Thanh-Nhan Nguyen-Pham[1,2]

1 Research Center for Cancer Immunotherapy, Chonnam National University Hwasun Hospital, Jeollanamdo, Republic of Korea

2 Department of Hematology-Oncology, Chonnam National University Hwasun Hospital, Jeollanamdo, Republic of Korea

3 Vaxcell-Bio Therapeutics, Hwasun, Jeollanamdo, Republic of Korea

References

[1] Kyle RA, Rajkumar SV. Multiple myeloma. N Engl J Med 2004; 351: 1860-1873.

[2] Sirohi B, Powles R. Multiple myeloma. Lancet 2004; 363: 875-887.

[3] Attal M, Harousseau JL. The role of high-dose therapy with autologous stem cell support in the era of novel agents. Semin Hematol 2009; 46: 127-132.

[4] Lonial S, Cavenagh J. Emerging combination treatment strategies containing novel agents in newly diagnosed multiple myeloma. Br J Haematol 2009; 145: 681-708.

[5] Perez-Simon JA, Martino R, Alegre A et al. Chronic but not acute graft-versus-host disease improves outcome in multiple myeloma patients after non-myeloablative allogeneic transplantation. Br J Haematol 2003; 121: 104-108.

[6] Harrison SJ, Cook G, Nibbs RJ, Prince HM. Immunotherapy of multiple myeloma: the start of a long and tortuous journey. Expert Rev Anticancer Ther 2006; 6: 1769-1785.

[7] Banchereau J, Steinman RM. Dendritic cells and the control of immunity. Nature 1998; 392: 245-252.

[8] O'Garra A. Cytokines induce the development of functionally heterogeneous T helper cell subsets. Immunity 1998; 8: 275-283.

[9] Wynn TA. T(H)-17: a giant step from T(H)1 and T(H)2. Nat Immunol 2005; 6: 1069-1070.

[10] Ridgway D. The first 1000 dendritic cell vaccinees. Cancer Invest 2003; 21: 873-886.

[11] Banchereau J, Palucka AK. Dendritic cells as therapeutic vaccines against cancer. Nat Rev Immunol 2005; 5: 296-306.

[12] Albert ML, Sauter B, Bhardwaj N. Dendritic cells acquire antigen from apoptotic cells and induce class I-restricted CTLs. Nature 1998; 392: 86-89.

[13] Brown RD, Pope B, Murray A et al. Dendritic cells from patients with myeloma are numerically normal but functionally defective as they fail to up-regulate CD80 (B7-1) expression after huCD40LT stimulation because of inhibition by transforming growth factor-beta1 and interleukin-10. Blood 2001; 98: 2992-2998.

[14] Ratta M, Fagnoni F, Curti A et al. Dendritic cells are functionally defective in multiple myeloma: the role of interleukin-6. Blood 2002; 100: 230-237.

[15] Yu H, Kortylewski M, Pardoll D. Crosstalk between cancer and immune cells: role of STAT3 in the tumour microenvironment. Nat Rev Immunol 2007; 7: 41-51.

[16] Ogawara H, Handa H, Yamazaki T et al. High Th1/Th2 ratio in patients with multiple myeloma. Leuk Res 2005; 29: 135-140.

[17] Maecker B, Anderson KS, von Bergwelt-Baildon MS et al. Viral antigen-specific CD8+ T-cell responses are impaired in multiple myeloma. Br J Haematol 2003; 121: 842-848.

[18] Dhodapkar MV, Geller MD, Chang DH et al. A reversible defect in natural killer T cell function characterizes the progression of premalignant to malignant multiple myeloma. J Exp Med 2003; 197: 1667-1676.

[19] Jarahian M, Watzl C, Issa Y et al. Blockade of natural killer cell-mediated lysis by NCAM140 expressed on tumor cells. Int J Cancer 2007; 120: 2625-2634.

[20] Prabhala RH, Neri P, Bae JE et al. Dysfunctional T regulatory cells in multiple myeloma. Blood 2006; 107: 301-304.

[21] Banerjee DK, Dhodapkar MV, Matayeva E et al. Expansion of FOXP3high regulatory T cells by human dendritic cells (DCs) in vitro and after injection of cytokine-matured DCs in myeloma patients. Blood 2006; 108: 2655-2661.

[22] Brimnes MK, Vangsted AJ, Knudsen LM et al. Increased level of both CD4+FOXP3+ regulatory T cells and CD14+HLA-DR/low myeloid-derived suppressor cells and decreased level of dendritic cells in patients with multiple myeloma. Scand J Immunol 2010; 72: 540-547.

[23] Kwak LW, Taub DD, Duffey PL et al. Transfer of myeloma idiotype-specific immunity from an actively immunised marrow donor. Lancet 1995; 345: 1016-1020.

[24] Li Y, Bendandi M, Deng Y et al. Tumor-specific recognition of human myeloma cells by idiotype-induced CD8(+) T cells. Blood 2000; 96: 2828-2833.

[25] Butch AW, Kelly KA, Munshi NC. Dendritic cells derived from multiple myeloma patients efficiently internalize different classes of myeloma protein. Exp Hematol 2001; 29: 85-92.

[26] Wen YJ, Barlogie B, Yi Q. Idiotype-specific cytotoxic T lymphocytes in multiple myeloma: evidence for their capacity to lyse autologous primary tumor cells. Blood 2001; 97: 1750-1755.

[27] Lim SH, Bailey-Wood R. Idiotypic protein-pulsed dendritic cell vaccination in multiple myeloma. Int J Cancer 1999; 83: 215-222.

[28] Liso A, Stockerl-Goldstein KE, Auffermann-Gretzinger S et al. Idiotype vaccination using dendritic cells after autologous peripheral blood progenitor cell transplantation for multiple myeloma. Biol Blood Marrow Transplant 2000; 6: 621-627.

[29] Titzer S, Christensen O, Manzke O et al. Vaccination of multiple myeloma patients with idiotype-pulsed dendritic cells: immunological and clinical aspects. Br J Haematol 2000; 108: 805-816.

[30] Yi Q, Desikan R, Barlogie B, Munshi N. Optimizing dendritic cell-based immunotherapy in multiple myeloma. Br J Haematol 2002; 117: 297-305.

[31] Reichardt VL, Milazzo C, Brugger W et al. Idiotype vaccination of multiple myeloma patients using monocyte-derived dendritic cells. Haematologica 2003; 88: 1139-1149.

[32] Bendandi M, Rodriguez-Calvillo M, Inoges S et al. Combined vaccination with idiotype-pulsed allogeneic dendritic cells and soluble protein idiotype for multiple myeloma patients relapsing after reduced-intensity conditioning allogeneic stem cell transplantation. Leuk Lymphoma 2006; 47: 29-37.

[33] Yi Q, Szmania S, Freeman J et al. Optimizing dendritic cell-based immunotherapy in multiple myeloma: intranodal injections of idiotype-pulsed CD40 ligand-matured vaccines led to induction of type-1 and cytotoxic T-cell immune responses in patients. Br J Haematol 2010; 150: 554-564.

[34] Rollig C, Schmidt C, Bornhauser M et al. Induction of cellular immune responses in patients with stage-I multiple myeloma after vaccination with autologous idiotype-pulsed dendritic cells. J Immunother 2011; 34: 100-106.

[35] Lee JJ, Choi BH, Kang HK et al. Induction of multiple myeloma-specific cytotoxic T lymphocyte stimulation by dendritic cell pulsing with purified and optimized myeloma cell lysates. Leuk Lymphoma 2007; 48: 2022-2031.

[36] Wen YJ, Min R, Tricot G et al. Tumor lysate-specific cytotoxic T lymphocytes in multiple myeloma: promising effector cells for immunotherapy. Blood 2002; 99: 3280-3285.

[37] Yang DH, Kim MH, Hong CY et al. Alpha-type 1-polarized dendritic cells loaded with apoptotic allogeneic myeloma cell line induce strong CTL responses against autologous myeloma cells. Ann Hematol 2010; 89: 795-801.

[38] Yang DH, Kim MH, Lee YK et al. Successful cross-presentation of allogeneic myeloma cells by autologous alpha-type 1-polarized dendritic cells as an effective tumor antigen in myeloma patients with matched monoclonal immunoglobulins. Ann Hematol 2011; 90: 1419-1426.

[39] Nguyen-Pham TN, Im CM, Nguyen TA et al. Induction of myeloma-specific cytotoxic T lymphocytes responses by natural killer cells stimulated-dendritic cells in patients with multiple myeloma. Leuk Res 2011; 35: 1241-1247.

[40] Milazzo C, Reichardt VL, Muller MR et al. Induction of myeloma-specific cytotoxic T cells using dendritic cells transfected with tumor-derived RNA. Blood 2003; 101: 977-982.

[41] Qian J, Wang S, Yang J et al. Targeting heat shock proteins for immunotherapy in multiple myeloma: generation of myeloma-specific CTLs using dendritic cells pulsed with tumor-derived gp96. Clin Cancer Res 2005; 11: 8808-8815.

[42] Qian J, Hong S, Wang S et al. Myeloma cell line-derived, pooled heat shock proteins as a universal vaccine for immunotherapy of multiple myeloma. Blood 2009; 114: 3880-3889.

[43] Hao S, Bi X, Xu S et al. Enhanced antitumor immunity derived from a novel vaccine of fusion hybrid between dendritic and engineered myeloma cells. Exp Oncol 2004; 26: 300-306.

[44] Vasir B, Borges V, Wu Z et al. Fusion of dendritic cells with multiple myeloma cells results in maturation and enhanced antigen presentation. Br J Haematol 2005; 129: 687-700.

[45] Brossart P, Schneider A, Dill P et al. The epithelial tumor antigen MUC1 is expressed in hematological malignancies and is recognized by MUC1-specific cytotoxic T-lymphocytes. Cancer Res 2001; 61: 6846-6850.

[46] Batchu RB, Moreno AM, Szmania SM et al. Protein transduction of dendritic cells for NY-ESO-1-based immunotherapy of myeloma. Cancer Res 2005; 65: 10041-10049.

[47] Chiriva-Internati M, Wang Z, Salati E et al. Sperm protein 17 (Sp17) is a suitable target for immunotherapy of multiple myeloma. Blood 2002; 100: 961-965.

[48] Vonderheide RH, Hahn WC, Schultze JL, Nadler LM. The telomerase catalytic subunit is a widely expressed tumor-associated antigen recognized by cytotoxic T lymphocytes. Immunity 1999; 10: 673-679.

[49] Ocadlikova D, Kryukov F, Mollova K et al. Generation of myeloma-specific T cells using dendritic cells loaded with MUC1- and hTERT- drived nonapeptides or myeloma cell apoptotic bodies. Neoplasma 2010; 57: 455-464.

[50] Qian J, Xie J, Hong S et al. Dickkopf-1 (DKK1) is a widely expressed and potent tumor-associated antigen in multiple myeloma. Blood 2007; 110: 1587-1594.

[51] Palucka K, Ueno H, Zurawski G et al. Building on dendritic cell subsets to improve cancer vaccines. Curr Opin Immunol 2010; 22: 258-263.

[52] Palucka K, Ueno H, Banchereau J. Recent developments in cancer vaccines. J Immunol 2011; 186: 1325-1331.

[53] Hsu FJ, Benike C, Fagnoni F et al. Vaccination of patients with B-cell lymphoma using autologous antigen-pulsed dendritic cells. Nat Med 1996; 2: 52-58.

[54] Nestle FO, Alijagic S, Gilliet M et al. Vaccination of melanoma patients with peptide- or tumor lysate-pulsed dendritic cells. Nat Med 1998; 4: 328-332.

[55] Jonuleit H, Kuhn U, Muller G et al. Pro-inflammatory cytokines and prostaglandins induce maturation of potent immunostimulatory dendritic cells under fetal calf serum-free conditions. Eur J Immunol 1997; 27: 3135-3142.

[56] Kalinski P, Vieira PL, Schuitemaker JH et al. Prostaglandin E(2) is a selective inducer of interleukin-12 p40 (IL-12p40) production and an inhibitor of bioactive IL-12p70 heterodimer. Blood 2001; 97: 3466-3469.

[57] Yamazaki S, Inaba K, Tarbell KV, Steinman RM. Dendritic cells expand antigen-specific Foxp3+ CD25+ CD4+ regulatory T cells including suppressors of alloreactivity. Immunol Rev 2006; 212: 314-329.

[58] Mailliard RB, Wankowicz-Kalinska A, Cai Q et al. alpha-type-1 polarized dendritic cells: a novel immunization tool with optimized CTL-inducing activity. Cancer Res 2004; 64: 5934-5937.

[59] Lee JJ, Foon KA, Mailliard RB et al. Type 1-polarized dendritic cells loaded with autologous tumor are a potent immunogen against chronic lymphocytic leukemia. J Leukoc Biol 2008; 84: 319-325.

[60] Wesa A, Kalinski P, Kirkwood JM et al. Polarized type-1 dendritic cells (DC1) producing high levels of IL-12 family members rescue patient TH1-type antimelanoma CD4+ T cell responses in vitro. J Immunother 2007; 30: 75-82.

[61] Giermasz AS, Urban JA, Nakamura Y et al. Type-1 polarized dendritic cells primed for high IL-12 production show enhanced activity as cancer vaccines. Cancer Immunol Immunother 2009; 58: 1329-1336.

[62] Okada H, Kalinski P, Ueda R et al. Induction of CD8+ T-cell responses against novel glioma-associated antigen peptides and clinical activity by vaccinations with {alpha}-type 1 polarized dendritic cells and polyinosinic-polycytidylic acid stabilized by lysine and carboxymethylcellulose in patients with recurrent malignant glioma. J Clin Oncol 2011; 29: 330-336.

[63] Gerosa F, Baldani-Guerra B, Nisii C et al. Reciprocal activating interaction between natural killer cells and dendritic cells. J Exp Med 2002; 195: 327-333.

[64] Pham TN, Hong CY, Min JJ et al. Enhancement of antitumor effect using dendritic cells activated with natural killer cells in the presence of Toll-like receptor agonist. Exp Mol Med 2010; 42: 407-419.

[65] Mailliard RB, Son YI, Redlinger R et al. Dendritic cells mediate NK cell help for Th1 and CTL responses: two-signal requirement for the induction of NK cell helper function. J Immunol 2003; 171: 2366-2373.

[66] Napolitani G, Rinaldi A, Bertoni F et al. Selected Toll-like receptor agonist combinations synergistically trigger a T helper type 1-polarizing program in dendritic cells. Nat Immunol 2005; 6: 769-776.

[67] Frasca L, Fedele G, Deaglio S et al. CD38 orchestrates migration, survival, and Th1 immune response of human mature dendritic cells. Blood 2006; 107: 2392-2399.

[68] Faure-Andre G, Vargas P, Yuseff MI et al. Regulation of dendritic cell migration by CD74, the MHC class II-associated invariant chain. Science 2008; 322: 1705-1710.

[69] Nguyen-Pham TN, Lim MS, Nguyen TA et al. Type I and II interferons enhance dendritic cell maturation and migration capacity by regulating CD38 and CD74 that have synergistic effects with TLR agonists. Cell Mol Immunol 2011; 8: 341-347.

[70] Jung TY, Pham TN, Umeyama A et al. Ursolic acid isolated from Uncaria rhynchophylla activates human dendritic cells via TLR2 and/or TLR4 and induces the production of IFN-gamma by CD4+ naive T cells. Eur J Pharmacol 2010; 643: 297-303.

[71] Bae WK, Umeyama A, Chung IJ et al. Uncarinic acid C plus IFN-gamma generates monocyte-derived dendritic cells and induces a potent Th1 polarization with capacity to migrate. Cell Immunol 2010; 266: 104-110.

[72] Kim KS, Pham TN, Jin CJ et al. Uncarinic Acid C Isolated from Uncaria rhynchophylla Induces Differentiation of Th1-Promoting Dendritic Cells Through TLR4 Signaling. Biomark Insights 2011; 6: 27-38.

[73] Savill J, Dransfield I, Gregory C, Haslett C. A blast from the past: clearance of apoptotic cells regulates immune responses. Nat Rev Immunol 2002; 2: 965-975.

[74] Kitamura H, Kamon H, Sawa S et al. IL-6-STAT3 controls intracellular MHC class II alphabeta dimer level through cathepsin S activity in dendritic cells. Immunity 2005; 23: 491-502.

[75] Nefedova Y, Gabrilovich DI. Targeting of Jak/STAT pathway in antigen presenting cells in cancer. Curr Cancer Drug Targets 2007; 7: 71-77.

[76] Wang S, Hong S, Yang J et al. Optimizing immunotherapy in multiple myeloma: Restoring the function of patients' monocyte-derived dendritic cells by inhibiting p38 or activating MEK/ERK MAPK and neutralizing interleukin-6 in progenitor cells. Blood 2006; 108: 4071-4077.

[77] Yang DH, Park JS, Jin CJ et al. The dysfunction and abnormal signaling pathway of dendritic cells loaded by tumor antigen can be overcome by neutralizing VEGF in multiple myeloma. Leuk Res 2009; 33: 665-670.

[78] Ostrand-Rosenberg S, Sinha P. Myeloid-derived suppressor cells: linking inflammation and cancer. J Immunol 2009; 182: 4499-4506.

[79] Bergenbrant S, Yi Q, Osterborg A et al. Modulation of anti-idiotypic immune response by immunization with the autologous M-component protein in multiple myeloma patients. Br J Haematol 1996; 92: 840-846.

[80] Massaia M, Borrione P, Battaglio S et al. Idiotype vaccination in human myeloma: generation of tumor-specific immune responses after high-dose chemotherapy. Blood 1999; 94: 673-683.

[81] Shimizu K, Fields RC, Giedlin M, Mule JJ. Systemic administration of interleukin 2 enhances the therapeutic efficacy of dendritic cell-based tumor vaccines. Proc Natl Acad Sci U S A 1999; 96: 2268-2273.

[82] Coscia M, Mariani S, Battaglio S et al. Long-term follow-up of idiotype vaccination in human myeloma as a maintenance therapy after high-dose chemotherapy. Leukemia 2004; 18: 139-145.

[83] Rasmussen T, Hansson L, Osterborg A et al. Idiotype vaccination in multiple myeloma induced a reduction of circulating clonal tumor B cells. Blood 2003; 101: 4607-4610.

[84] Cull G, Durrant L, Stainer C et al. Generation of anti-idiotype immune responses following vaccination with idiotype-protein pulsed dendritic cells in myeloma. Br J Haematol 1999; 107: 648-655.

[85] Reichardt VL, Okada CY, Liso A et al. Idiotype vaccination using dendritic cells after autologous peripheral blood stem cell transplantation for multiple myeloma--a feasibility study. Blood 1999; 93: 2411-2419.

[86] Rosenblatt J, Vasir B, Uhl L et al. Vaccination with dendritic cell/tumor fusion cells results in cellular and humoral antitumor immune responses in patients with multiple myeloma. Blood 2011; 117: 393-402.

[87] Gong J, Koido S, Chen D et al. Immunization against murine multiple myeloma with fusions of dendritic and plasmacytoma cells is potentiated by interleukin 12. Blood 2002; 99: 2512-2517.

[88] Lake RA, Robinson BW. Immunotherapy and chemotherapy--a practical partnership. Nat Rev Cancer 2005; 5: 397-405.

[89] Mihalyo MA, Doody AD, McAleer JP et al. In vivo cyclophosphamide and IL-2 treatment impedes self-antigen-induced effector CD4 cell tolerization: implications for adoptive immunotherapy. J Immunol 2004; 172: 5338-5345.

[90] North RJ. Cyclophosphamide-facilitated adoptive immunotherapy of an established tumor depends on elimination of tumor-induced suppressor T cells. J Exp Med 1982; 155: 1063-1074.

[91] Proietti E, Greco G, Garrone B et al. Importance of cyclophosphamide-induced bystander effect on T cells for a successful tumor eradication in response to adoptive immunotherapy in mice. J Clin Invest 1998; 101: 429-441.

[92] Berd D, Maguire HC, Jr., Mastrangelo MJ. Potentiation of human cell-mediated and humoral immunity by low-dose cyclophosphamide. Cancer Res 1984; 44: 5439-5443.

[93] Matar P, Rozados VR, Gervasoni SI, Scharovsky GO. Th2/Th1 switch induced by a single low dose of cyclophosphamide in a rat metastatic lymphoma model. Cancer Immunol Immunother 2002; 50: 588-596.

[94] Matar P, Rozados VR, Gonzalez AD et al. Mechanism of antimetastatic immunopotentiation by low-dose cyclophosphamide. Eur J Cancer 2000; 36: 1060-1066.

[95] Liu JY, Wu Y, Zhang XS et al. Single administration of low dose cyclophosphamide augments the antitumor effect of dendritic cell vaccine. Cancer Immunol Immunother 2007; 56: 1597-1604.

[96] Holtl L, Ramoner R, Zelle-Rieser C et al. Allogeneic dendritic cell vaccination against metastatic renal cell carcinoma with or without cyclophosphamide. Cancer Immunol Immunother 2005; 54: 663-670.

[97] Quach H, Ritchie D, Stewart AK et al. Mechanism of action of immunomodulatory drugs (IMiDS) in multiple myeloma. Leukemia 2010; 24: 22-32.

[98] Galustian C, Meyer B, Labarthe MC et al. The anti-cancer agents lenalidomide and pomalidomide inhibit the proliferation and function of T regulatory cells. Cancer Immunol Immunother 2009; 58: 1033-1045.

[99] Ramsay AG, Gribben JG. Immune dysfunction in chronic lymphocytic leukemia T cells and lenalidomide as an immunomodulatory drug. Haematologica 2009; 94: 1198-1202.

http://dx.doi.org/10.5772/54100

[100] Restifo NP. Building better vaccines: how apoptotic cell death can induce inflammation and activate innate and adaptive immunity. Curr Opin Immunol 2000; 12: 597-603.

[101] Schiavoni G, Sistigu A, Valentini M et al. Cyclophosphamide synergizes with type I interferons through systemic dendritic cell reactivation and induction of immunogenic tumor apoptosis. Cancer Res 2011; 71: 768-778.

[102] Obeid M, Tesniere A, Ghiringhelli F et al. Calreticulin exposure dictates the immunogenicity of cancer cell death. Nat Med 2007; 13: 54-61.

[103] Apetoh L, Ghiringhelli F, Tesniere A et al. Toll-like receptor 4-dependent contribution of the immune system to anticancer chemotherapy and radiotherapy. Nat Med 2007; 13: 1050-1059.

[104] Chen T, Cao X. Stress for maintaining memory: HSP70 as a mobile messenger for innate and adaptive immunity. Eur J Immunol 2010; 40: 1541-1544.

[105] Srivastava P. Interaction of heat shock proteins with peptides and antigen presenting cells: chaperoning of the innate and adaptive immune responses. Annu Rev Immunol 2002; 20: 395-425.

[106] Spisek R, Charalambous A, Mazumder A et al. Bortezomib enhances dendritic cell (DC)-mediated induction of immunity to human myeloma via exposure of cell surface heat shock protein 90 on dying tumor cells: therapeutic implications. Blood 2007; 109: 4839-4845.

[107] Dougan M, Dranoff G. Immune therapy for cancer. Annu Rev Immunol 2009; 27: 83-117.

[108] Javia LR, Rosenberg SA. CD4+CD25+ suppressor lymphocytes in the circulation of patients immunized against melanoma antigens. J Immunother 2003; 26: 85-93.

[109] Beyer M, Kochanek M, Giese T et al. In vivo peripheral expansion of naive CD4+CD25high FoxP3+ regulatory T cells in patients with multiple myeloma. Blood 2006; 107: 3940-3949.

[110] Moore KW, de Waal Malefyt R, Coffman RL, O'Garra A. Interleukin-10 and the interleukin-10 receptor. Annu Rev Immunol 2001; 19: 683-765.

[111] Terabe M, Matsui S, Noben-Trauth N et al. NKT cell-mediated repression of tumor immunosurveillance by IL-13 and the IL-4R-STAT6 pathway. Nat Immunol 2000; 1: 515-520.

[112] Terabe M, Ambrosino E, Takaku S et al. Synergistic enhancement of CD8+ T cell-mediated tumor vaccine efficacy by an anti-transforming growth factor-beta monoclonal antibody. Clin Cancer Res 2009; 15: 6560-6569.

[113] Rabinovich GA, Gabrilovich D, Sotomayor EM. Immunosuppressive strategies that are mediated by tumor cells. Annu Rev Immunol 2007; 25: 267-296.

[114] Peggs KS, Quezada SA, Korman AJ, Allison JP. Principles and use of anti-CTLA4 antibody in human cancer immunotherapy. Curr Opin Immunol 2006; 18: 206-213.

[115] Pilon-Thomas S, Mackay A, Vohra N, Mule JJ. Blockade of programmed death ligand 1 enhances the therapeutic efficacy of combination immunotherapy against melanoma. J Immunol 2010; 184: 3442-3449.

[116] Lou Y, Wang G, Lizee G et al. Dendritic cells strongly boost the antitumor activity of adoptively transferred T cells in vivo. Cancer Res 2004; 64: 6783-6790.

Chapter 10

Novel Prognostic Modalities in Multiple Myeloma

Mariam Boota, Joshua Bornhorst, Zeba Singh and
Saad Z. Usmani

Additional information is available at the end of the chapter

http://dx.doi.org/10.5772/55965

1. Introduction

The therapy for multiple myeloma has made major strides over the last 15 years, by and large due to the advances in molecular biology and the focus on patient-oriented translational investigations. Although the survival outcomes have improved significantly, clinical features such as older age, renal insufficiency at diagnosis, primary plasma cell leukemia and extra-medullary disease remain major therapeutic challenge. The explosion of data from all the clinical, genomic and proteomic investigations has also made it difficult to assimilate all the information and translate it effectively for clinical practice. Although multiple myeloma is still considered by most though leaders as an incurable but treatable disease, the development of novel diagnostic and therapeutic modalities are bringing optimism of potential curability dream of being curable. Over the last decade, new biologic markers and novel imaging modalities have been explored in the context of clinical trials. The present chapter will attempt to summarize these data and propose how to incorporate this knowledge in current clinical practice.

2. Laboratory & pathology tools

2.1. Durie-Salmon staging and the international staging system

The Durie-Salmon Staging (DSS) system [1] was developed as a prognostic model almost four decades ago when the standard of care for myeloma was oral melphalan and prednisone. Over the years, DSS has stood the test of time as a reasonable assessor of disease burden even in the era of novel agents. The major the drawback of the DSS was that it does not account for the biologic variability of disease even in patients with comparable disease burden. The International Staging System (ISS) [2] was developed to include some biologic information by incorporating serum albumin as a markers of disease burden and host risk, whereas serum beta-2 microglobulin (β2M) levels was included as marker of biologic behavior. Both DSS and ISS stratify patients in to stages I, II and III. Although ISS was tested and validated on patient data-set from the pre-novel drug era, ISS III disease remains a major challenge even in intensive treatment approaches such the Arkansas Total Therapy program (See Figures 1A-C).

Incorporating cytogenetic data in prognostication

Like most cancers, multiple myeloma has both inter-patient and intra-patient heterogeneity. The last 15 years have seen major progress in both the understanding of MM disease biology and development of biologically relevant MM therapies. Even with such advances, there are several prominent biologic factors that play a major role in overall prognosis. MM patients can be categorized into genomically defined low risk or high risk depending upon underlying molecular cytogenetic abnormalities identified using either fluorescent in situ hybridization (FISH) and gene expression profiling (GEP). In transplant eligible patients, presence of any cytogenetic abnormality portends poorer PFS and OS as observed in the two Total Therapy 3 trials [3], [4] by the Arkansas Myeloma group (Figure 2 A, unpublished data), whereas there were no difference in cumulative incidence of achieved a partial or complete response (Figure 2 B, unpublished data). The poor prognostic cytogenetic abnormalities include translocation (4; 14), translocation (14; 16), translocation (6; 14), translocation (14; 20), hyperdiploidy, amplification of chromosome 1q21 and deletion 17p, and their presence is associated with shorter overall survival and duration of response to therapy.

Translocation (4; 14) can be found in roughly 10-15% of newly diagnosed MM patients and results in an overexpression of fibroblast growth factor receptor 3 (FGFR3) that in turn drives cellular proliferation and survival. Although it can be argued that bortezomib can now overcome the adverse prognosis associated with translocation (4; 14), it remains a poor prognostic markers in geographic areas where either socioeconomics or medical economics dictate initial choice of therapy for newly diagnosed MM [5]. Translocations (14;16) and (14;20) [6], [7] occur in less than 5% of newly diagnosed MM cases and lead to overexpression of MAF and MAF-B proto-oncogenes, respectively. Deletion 17p results in deletion of the tumor suppressor gene p53 and occurs in ~10% new MM cases [8]. It has been reported that bortezomib may overcome adverse prognosis associated with deletion 17p [9], but it appears that this benefit only happens in "low-risk" MM patients as defined by the Arkansas 70-gene expression profiling risk model [10]. Lastly, amplification of chromosome 1q21 has not only been associated with MGUS to MM progression [11] but also with poor prognosis in MM regardless of therapeutic era [12]. Amongst the many genes over-expressed by 1q21 amplification, are the proteasome genes which appear to portend poor durability of response and may be partly responsible for resistance to bortezomib [12]. In an effort to incorporate biologic information in upfront staging, there have several attempts to combine cytogenetic data with ISS in prognostic models. Neben et al [13] demonstrated that newly diagnosed MM patients with high burden of disease (ISS stages II/III) when presenting with either t (4; 14) or del17p have overall shorter PFS and OS (Figure 2 C).

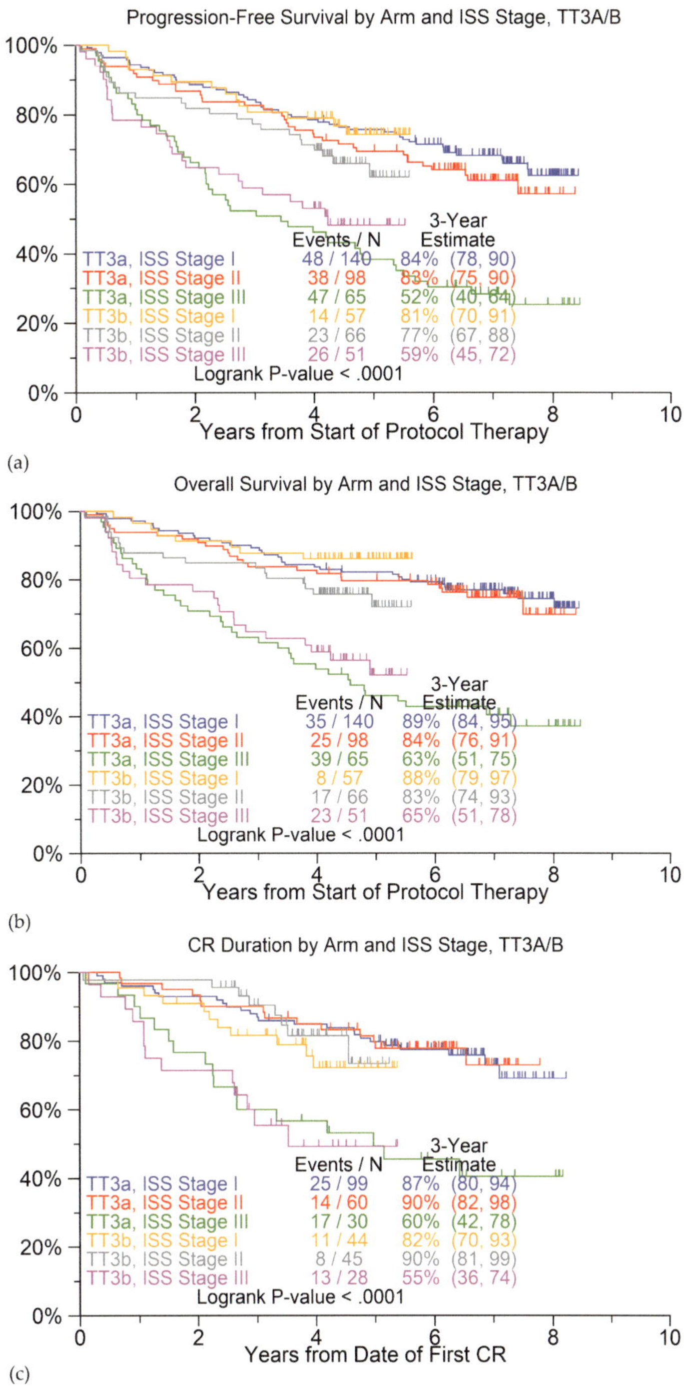

Figure 1. Impact of ISS Stage in Total Therapy 3 trials on progression free survival (a), overall survival (b), and complete response (CR) duration (c).

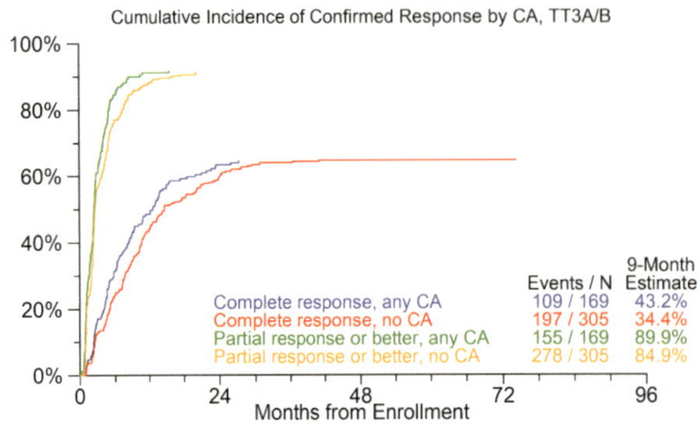

(a)

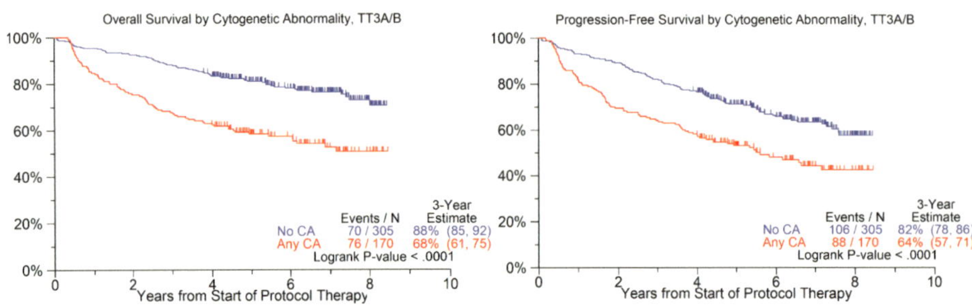

(b)

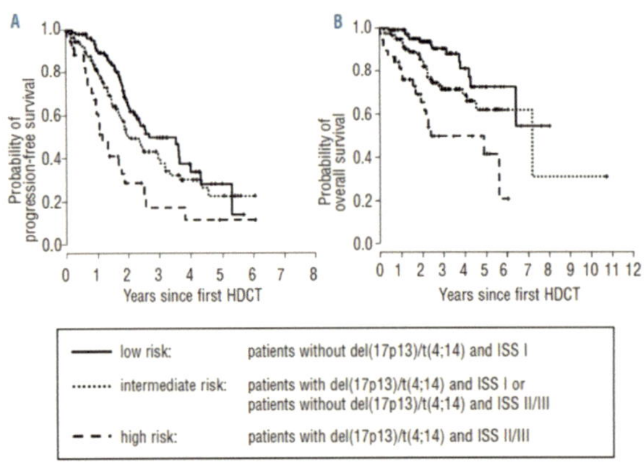

(c)

Figure 2. Impact of cytogenetic abnormalities to achieving response (a), overall and progression free survival (b). Combined ISS staging and cytogenetic risk stratification in newly diagnosed MM (c).

2.2. Serum light chain and heavy chain assays

The measurement of biological markers for multiple myeloma serum and urine specimen has proven to be invaluable in detection and monitoring of disease progression. In fact, the observation of association of multiple myeloma with the presence of Bence Jones proteins in the urine 150 years ago consisting of immunoglobulin free light chains represents one of the first widely utilized tumor marker assays. Since that time a great deal of effort has gone into the development of new markers for multiple myeloma, as well as more efficient use of existing markers. These include nephlometric determination of serum free light chains (FLC) and more recently intact Ig subsets; IgGκ, IgGλ, IgAκ and IgAλ (heavy/light chain immunoassays or HLC). Both of these markers have exhibited apparent value as diagnostic and prognostic indicators.

As our understanding of the utility of these markers deepens, we achieve better understanding in how to most effectively use these markers in combination with other methods for monoclonal protein detection (See Figure 3). Current international guidelines for identifying monoclonal gammopathies (MG) include serum protein electrophoresis (SPEP), immunofixation electrophoresis (IFE) and serum free light chain (FLC) immunoassays with derived kappa/lambda (κ/λ) ratios [14], [15]. As a first step, Immunofixation (IFE) is typically the assay utilized to identify the clonal isotype and is also generally utilized to provide a qualitative assessment of monoclonal (MC) Igs and light chain proteins, although alternate algorithms have been evaluated [16].

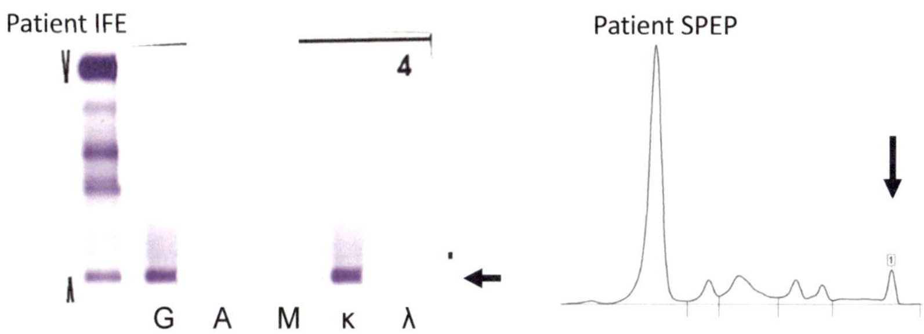

Test	Patient	Reference Interval
Original Clone by IFE	IgGκ	None
SPEP M-protein determination	3.0 g/L	Negative
Total IgG	4.82 g/L	7.14 - 13.94 g/L
HLC IgGκ	4.39 g/L	4.03-9.78 g/L
HLC IgGλ	0.47g/L	1.97-5.71 g/L
HLCr (IgGκ/IgGλ ratio)	9.36	0.98-2.75
FLCκ	2.57 mg/dL	0.33-1.94 mg/dL
FLCλ	0.33 mg/dL	0.57-2.63 mg/dL
FLCr (κ/λ ratio)	7.79	0.26-1.65

Figure 3. Combining serum protein electrophoresis, immunofixation, the free light chain assay and heavy chain assay to profile a patient with newly diagnosed MM.

Free light chain assays

Although monoclonal serum free light chains (FLC) can be quantified by SPEP in some cases, the use of sFLC nephelopmetric or turbidimetric immunoassay has become standard practice for measuring free kappa (κ) and frees lambda (λ) light chains in monoclonal gammopathies and other patient specimens [17]- [19]. These assays measure free light chains and do not react to light chains bound to heavy chain [20]. In addition to high sensitivity and specificity, advantages of the use of serum FLC nephelometric assays involves the use of numerical κ/λ ratios as a clinically sensitive marker of monoclonal FLC production as it also includes suppression of the non-tumor FLC in its calculation [21].

In the decade since introduction of the free light chain serum assay a great deal has been elucidated regarding the clinical value of these assays. The value of serum free light chains in the detection and screening for disease has been well established, culminating in the inclusion of the free light chain measurements into the International Myeloma working group guidelines. The vast majority of multiple myeloma symptomatic patients (95%) exhibit abnormal free light chain ratios [22]. The use of a combination of serum IFE and sFLC chain is proposed to be sufficient to screen/detect disease in new multiple myeloma patients. Furthermore, in contrast to M-spike, the κ/λ ratio (FLCr) has been reported to be a superior prognostic marker for active multiple myeloma, smoldering multiple myeloma and MGUS [24]- [26].

Heavy light chain assays

The observed utility of sFLC κ/λ ratios has prompted interest in the analysis of intact Ig'κ, Ig'λ and Ig'κ/Ig' λ ratios, which has been made possible with the recent availability of HLC or Hevylite™ immunoassays which have been recently made available from the Binding Site [27], [28]. These assays utilize epitopes which span specific intact heavy and light chain pairings. Thus they can be used to quantitatively measure concentrations of specific antibody species such as IgG κ, IgG λ, IgA κ and IgA λ. It should be noted that the Hevylite assay is not specific to a monoclonal protein but the presence of monoclonal protein is often indicated by an abnormal HLC kappa/lambda ratio. Although the clinical utility of these Heavy Light Chain measurements are still being explored, there is indication that HLC Ig'κ/Ig'λ ratios may have diagnostic value for multiple myeloma and may also have utility in the monitoring of disease state [27]- [29]. Following identification by IFE, monoclonal immunoglobulins are typically quantified by serum protein electrophoresis (SPEP) and total immunoglobulin determinations, although the results of these assays do not always agree [30]. The clinical utility of the HLC assay could be particularly beneficial when measurements of monoclonal immunoglobulins may be adversely affected as a result of procedural challenges associated with electrophoresis and biological variances typically observed in myeloma patients. Finally, recent reports have also suggested that measurement of the HLC ratios and suppression of concentrations of non-clonal HLC proteins of the same class are of prognostic significance in monoclonal gammopathies of undetermined significance (MGUS) [31] and MM [32]. Further work continues to elucidate the degree and clinical prognostic role of HLC measurements.

http://dx.doi.org/10.5772/55965

2.3. Flow cytometry

The diagnosis of multiple myeloma and determining the response to therapy has traditionally been done by morphological evaluation of the bone marrow for neoplastic plasma cells, and protein studies including serum protein electrophoresis, and immunofixation. Flow cytometry (FCM) for plasma cell enumeration in the bone marrow or peripheral blood has not been popular, in part due to the lower yield of plasma cells by FCM [33], [34]. With advent of multicolor flow cytometers, FCM is now recognized as a fast, cheap and sensitive tool to get multiparametric information on the plasma cells in MM. FCM has a distinct advantage over morphological, immunohistochemical, or even molecular tests in distinguishing normal from neoplastic plasma cells when the plasma cell numbers are very low. The availability of standardized consensus guidelines from the European Myeloma Network [33] regarding methodology, antibody panels and combinations, and absolute numbers required for assessment to obtain reliable results for small numbers of neoplastic plasma cells by FCM has improved confidence in using FCM as a diagnostic and prognostic tool in MM.

The main prognostic uses of multiparametric flow cytometry (MFC) in MM include antigenic profile of malignant plasma cells and detection of minimal residual disease detection. Several antigens are differentially expressed on normal and neoplastic plasma cells. These include CD38, CD138, CD45, CD56, CD19, CD117, CD20, CD27, CD28, CD33, CD39, CD40, CD44, CD81, Cyclin C1, and CD34 [34]- [37]. The expression of these antigens is on a continuum; therefore no single antigen can distinguish a normal from neoplastic PC. Results from several large consensus studies have shown that a minimum panel of CD19 and CD56 in addition to the basic CD38, CD138, and CD45 can discriminate neoplastic PC in more than 90% of the instances, and the discriminatory power increases to more than 95% on addition of CD117, CD20, CD28, and CD27 to the panel [35], [36]. In addition to enumeration of neoplastic plasma cells in the bone marrow, several studies have demonstrated the prognostic value of the residual normal plasma cell population in the bone marrow [37] demonstrated that in nearly 80% of patients with MGUS, >5% plasma cells out of the total bone marrow plasma cells are normal (benign, reactive), as opposed to <15% of patients with MM who may have >5% normal plasma cells; a distinction of MGUS from smoldering myeloma can thus be made by assessing the proportion of residual normal PC. The authors further demonstrated that patients with MGUS and SMM with a marked predominance of aberrant plasma cells/ total bone marrow plasma cells (> or = 95%) at diagnosis had a significantly higher risk of progression to symptomatic MM, and in multivariate analysis the percentage of aberrant plasma cells to total bone marrow plasma cells was the most important independent variable together with DNA aneuploidy for progression free survival in both MGUS and SMM [37]. Furthermore, MM patients with >5% normal plasma cells constitute a biologically distinct group with low tumor burden and a better response to HDT/autologous HSCT [38].

Prognostic value of individual antigens

The prognostic significance of individual antigens expressed by the neoplastic plasma cells is less clear. A correlation of CD20 expression with cyclin D1 positivity and presence of t(11;14) and a better outcome has been reported; not all CD20 expressing myelomas express cyclin D1 or t(11;14), and vice versa [39]. The importance of CD20 expression lies in the potential for use of Rituxumab in these patients. Neural adhesion molecule or CD56 is an aberrant marker expressed in 75% of MM cases. Loss of CD56 is described in plasma cell leukemia and myeloma cells in extramedullary locations [40]; a correlation of CD56 negativity with plasma cell leukemia or circulating myeloma cells and decreased osteolysis is reported [41], but no definite association with aggressive disease is established [42]. Syndecan-1 (CD138), a molecule belonging to the heparin sulphate family, is a universal marker for normal and neoplastic plasma cells [43]. CD138 mediates myeloma cell adhesion, and interaction with the extracellular matrix. CD138 may be shed from the cell surface. Soluble CD138 is a marker of plasma cell apoptosis and some studies have shown soluble CD138 level is a powerful independent prognostic factor both at diagnosis and at plateau phase [44], [45]. Shed CD138 accumulates in the fibrotic stroma; its presence on intravascular and intrasinusoidal plasma cells indicates that its loss is not associated with extramedullary disease [46]. CD45 expression is observed in plasma cells with higher proliferative index and as such may be associated with high-grade myeloma. Recent studies have shown that CD19, CD28, and CD117 provide clinically significant prognostic information; positivity for CD19 and CD28 and lack of expression of CD117 correlate with shorter overall and progression-free survival [46]. Many of these immunophenotypic-clincal outcome associations may be due to the associated genetic abnormalities and not the antigen expression per say– CD28+/CD117- myelomas are often non-hyperdiploid and associated with a higher frequency of t(4;14); CD28 positivity also with 17(p) deletion, and CD20 expression with t(11;14). These –immunophenotypic and genetic correlations need further investigation for validation [46].

Detection of minimal residual disease and prognosis

According to the IMWG response criteria [25], [47], complete remission (CR) in MM requires absence of demonstrable monoclonal protein by serum electrophoresis or immunofixation, disappearance of soft tissue plasmacyomas, and <5% bone marrow plasma cells. Since morphological evaluation of the bone marrow has limited sensitivity, the IMWG proposed additional criteria including absence of clonal plasma cells based on immunohistochemical staining of bone marrow sections, and a normalized free light chain ratio to further define stringent CR. We (unpublished observation) and others [48] have observed that oligoclonal plasma cell proliferations are common after auto HSCT and may disturb the free light chain ratios and limit interpretation of plasma cell clonality by immunohistochemical or in-situ hybridization studies on the bone marrow biopsies. Figure 4 show an example of MFC performed in on a 6-color instrument. Simultaneous analysis of multiple discriminatory antigens allows separation of a small proportion of aberrant plasma cells within a background of reactive plasma cells. The predictive prognostic role of MRD by MFC of plasma cells has been demonstrated both in the pre- and post transplant setting. Dingli et al [49] demonstrated that detection of circulating myeloma cells in the peripheral blood by FCM prior to auto-HSCT is an independent prognostic factor for overall survival and time to disease progression in multivariate analysis. In a prospective study of MRD assessment by MFC of plasma cells in 295 newly diagnosed MM patients uniformly treated in the GEM2000 protocol, both the progression-free survival ($p<1.001$) and overall survival ($p=0.002$) were longer in patients who were MRD negative by MFC of plasma cells on day 100 following auto-HSCT [50]. The predictive value of MFC persists even in patients who are negative for MM by immunofixation.

Population	#Events	%Parent	%Total	CD38 FITC-A Mean	CD81 PE-A Mean	CD27 PerCP... Mean
All Events	1,708,386	####	100.0	457	657	584
P1	1,600,611	93.7	93.7	479	675	698
P2	26,867	1.7	1.6	9,016	1,087	2,711
P3	23,724	88.3	1.4	8,481	1,230	2,232
56-	23,409	98.7	1.4	8,416	1,199	2,179
56+	314	1.3	0.0	12,916	4,316	6,085
38/19-	16,236	68.4	1.0	4,568	765	793
38/19+	7,631	31.7	0.4	16,940	2,227	6,325
CD19	9,227	0.6	0.5	628	3,888	422

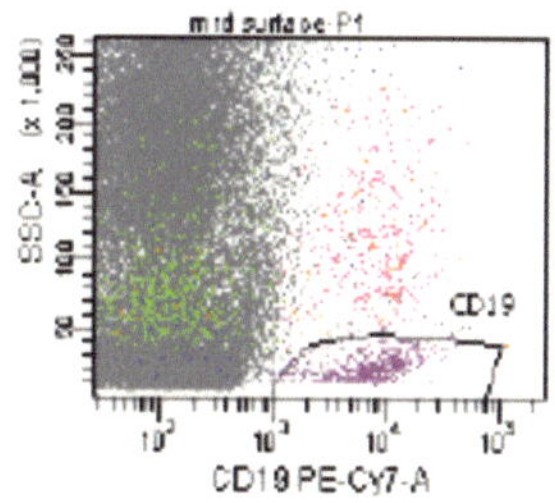

Figure 4. Dot plots showing cell gating strategies to evaluate minimal residual disease in Note that the selected cells in green are CD45-, CD38 (low), CD27-, CD19-, CD81(weak to negative), and CD56- in contrast to the normal residual plasma cells (red) that are CD45+, CD38(bright), CD27+, CD19+, CD81+, and CD56-, and normal B- cells (purple) that are CD45+, CD19+, and CD81+, but negative for CD38, and CD27. Total 1.7 million events are analyzed. The abnormal/normal plasma cell ratio can be calculated from the numbers in the table (2.38%).

2.4. Gene expression profiling

GEP was first used to study MM by De Vos and colleagues in 2001 [51]. In these early experiments, human myeloma cell lines and plasma cell leukemia patient samples were analyzed on small-scale, filter-based complementary DNA arrays to identify genes involved in intercellular signalling. Subsequently, Stewart et al used a combination of high-throughput DNA sequencing and microarrays using DNA samples from several cases of plasma cell leukemia to establish a comprehensive list of genes that are expressed in MM [52]. GEP analyses in MM have evolved tremendously over the last decade and helped with getting a global biologic understanding of the disease.

GEP also helps identify different signatures that confer an adverse outcome as shown by the University of Arkansas for Medical Sciences (UAMS) 70-gene signature (GEP-70) as proof of concept that identifies 13-20% "high risk" newly diagnosed patients with short progression free and overall survival even when with the Total Therapy approach[3],[4], [53]. The GEP-70 model has 30% of the informative genes mapped to chromosome 1 and poor prognosis is associated with 1q21 amplified genes. A UAMS 17-gene signature has also been reported, primarily using the 1q21 amplified genes, which could predict outcome as well as the 70-gene signature [54] but has not replaced the GEP-70. The UAMS GEP-80 gene signature [12] was discovered when comparing pre- and post-bortezomib GEP studies in newly diagnosed MM treated on the Total Therapy 3 trials[3],[4]. This signature was used to identify patients who may be resistant to bortezomib therapy and it showed both higher PSMD4 expression levels and higher 1q21 copy numbers affecting clinical outcome adversely. The UAMS GEP-80 high risk signature provides additive and complimentary information to the UAMS GEP-70 signature.

The prognostic validity of the GEP-70 high risk signature has been confirmed in several independent patient cohorts (IFM 99 trial [55], ECOG E4A03 trial [55], HOVON-65 trial [57]). The Intergroupe Francophone du Myélome (IFM) have developed a 15-gene model [55], which described a set of genes that control proliferation and chromosomal instability. This model was able to identify high risk group in UAMS population but with less statistical significance. It was also interesting to note that IFM-15 and UAMS GEP-70 gene models do not share any common genes, which likely reflects the redundancy in the genes and pathways with prognostic significance in MM. Recently, the EMC-92 gene model has been reported on the HOVON65 clinical trial patients, with no overlapping genes compared with UAMS 70-gene signature and it identifies an additional 3-4% high risk MM patients to the existing GEP signatures [57].

Patients with low risk disease usually survive on a median about 6-7 years or longer when compared to those with high risk disease, who survive on a median ~ 3 years. On the other hand those with intermediate risk have been shown to have comparable survival to low risk patients in studies where there was early use of bortezomib plus ASCT [58]. The disease subset with GEP70 high risk signature, translocation (14; 16), translocation (14; 20), and deletion 17p remains a challenge. Clinical trials addressing this difficult group of newly diagnosed patients are now being conducted, such as the SWOG-1211(NCT01668719) study [59], to establish guiding posts for future trials.

3. Emerging role of magnetic resonance imaging & 18-Flouro-Deoxy-Glucose (FDG) positron emission tomography

Imaging techniques are also considered as important prognostic tools. The metastatic bone survey (MBS), a whole body x-ray, has been used as a standard for evaluating bone disease (osteolytic lesions or osteopenia). Unfortunately, the MBS does not detect bone destruction until more than 70% of the bone has decalcified [60]. The DSS[1] has associated poor prognosis to patients with > 2 MBS osteolytic lesions, a feature seen in 33% of newly diagnosed MM patients [61]. It also appears that the MBS related poor prognosis still holds true in the era of novel agents [62], [63].

Magnetic resonance imaging (MRI) and more recently, positron emission tomography integrated with computed tomography (PET/CT) using radionuclide18F labeled with fluoro-deoxyglucose (18F-FDG) have demonstrated effective detection of bone lesions, marrow involvement and in the case of the latter; demonstrating active or inactive disease and their use can provide vital prognostic information (See Figure 5). Studies utilizing the PET/CT and MRI by the Arkansas group [61]- [63] and the Italian group [64] have looked at the prognostic implications of the number of focal lesions (FL), the uptake of FDG expressed as standardized uptake value (SUV), presence of extramedullary disease (EMD), at baseline and after treatment in previously untreated myeloma patients. The results from these studies showed that FL number adversely affected over survival (OS) and event free survival (EFS) independently, as did presence of EMD and failure of FDG suppression. Higher SUV of the most active FL (SUV^{max}) on PET/CT is also associated with poor outcomes(SUV^{max} >3.9 [62] or SUV^{max} >4.2 [64]).

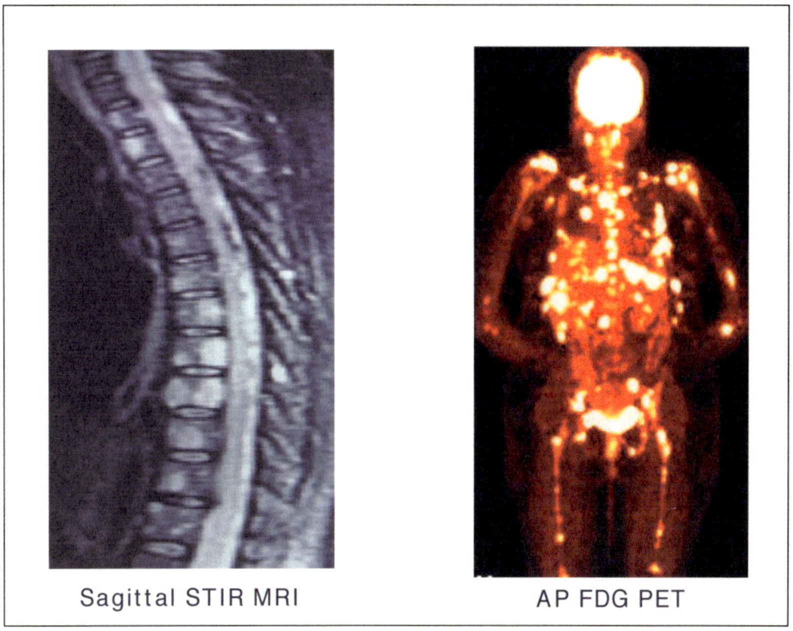

Figure 5. Left panel shows MRI focal lesion on sagittal STIR images; right panel shows AP FDG uptake on PET

Specifically, baseline PET focal lesions > 3 (32% of newly diagnosed MM) and baseline MRI focal lesions > 7 (36% of newly diagnosed MM) were associated with shorter EFS and OS in Total Therapy 3 trials. It was also observed seen that complete suppression of FDG before the first autologous stem cell transplant (ASCT) conferred a favorable affect on outcome especially seen in the GEP 70 – defined high risk patients [61], [62]. More recently, it has also shown that absence of PET suppression by Day 7 of first induction cycle in MM patients treated on the Total therapy 3 trials have shorter progression free survival (PFS) and OS [65]. These observations have important implications and would need further validation in the era of novel therapy induction regimens. One could potentially identification of high risk patients based on imaging response that would require change in therapeutic strategy, similar in fashion to how PET is employed in aggressive lymphomas.

PET/CT and MRI are not yet established as a standard for diagnosis and disease evaluation, as concerns have arisen due to heterogeneity of visual criteria and inconsistency in interpretation of results [66]. In current practice, the PET/CT can be employed in patients presenting with solitary plasmacytomas where the clinical suspicion for systemic disease is high, or when patients are relapsing biochemically but bone marrow biopsy provides ambiguous results. The use of MRI and PET/CT is presently limited to clinical investigations, partly due to the economic implications of broader usage in clinical practice. These concerns may be alleviated may be in the future with development of more efficient and cost-effective technologies.

4. Conclusion and future directions

Our understanding of MM has grown many folds over the last 2 decades with a better understanding of the genomic heterogeneity associated with this disease. We are just beginning to combine the clinical and biologic prognostic markers in newly diagnosed multiple myeloma patients in efforts to better stratify patients and choosing appropriate therapies. There are multinational efforts, such as the CoMMpass study, aiming to provide for a comprehensive understanding of the disease in the era of novel agents [66]. With the advances in drug development, we are getting closer to developing a risk-adaptive therapeutic strategy for majority of MM patients. There is a robust pipeline of novel targeted agents on the horizon for MM. It appears that there will be enough effective and tolerable therapeutic agents in the oncologist's armamentarium that the treatment strategy will take in to account both the clinical and biologic risk factors for a truly personalized medicine experience. The advances in diagnostic and prognostic tools will also provide impetus for a response-adaptive strategy which will likely be incorporated in the therapeutic matrix as the data emerges over the next decade.

Author details

Mariam Boota[1], Joshua Bornhorst[2], Zeba Singh[2] and Saad Z. Usmani[1*]

*Address all correspondence to: susmani@uams.edu

1 Myeloma Institute for Research & Therapy, University of Arkansas for Medical Sciences, Little Rock, AR, USA

2 Department of Pathology, University of Arkansas for Medical Sciences, Little Rock, AR, USA

References

[1] Durie, B. G, & Salmon, S. E. A clinical staging system for multiple myeloma. Correlation of measured myeloma cell mass with presenting clinical features, response to treatment, and survival. Cancer. (1975). Sep;, 36(3), 842-54.

[2] Greipp, P. R. San Miguel J, Durie BG, et al. International staging system for multiple myeloma. J Clin Oncol. (2005). May 20;, 23(15), 3412-20.

[3] Nair, B, Van Rhee, F, Shaughnessy, J. D, et al. Superior results of Total Therapy 3 (2003-33) in gene expression profiling-defined low-risk multiple myeloma confirmed in subsequent trial 2006-66 with VRD maintenance. Blood. (2010). , 115(21), 4168-73.

[4] Barlogie, B, Anaissie, E, Van Rhee, F, et al. Incorporating bortezomib into upfront treatment for multiple myeloma: early results of total therapy 3. Br J Haematol. (2007). , 138(2), 176-85.

[5] Avet-loiseau, H, Attal, M, Campion, L, et al. Long-term analysis of the IFM 99 trials for myeloma: cytogenetic abnormalities [t(4;14), del(17gains] play a major role in defining long-term survival.J Clin Oncol. (2012). Jun 1;30(16):1949-52., 1q.

[6] Ross, F. M, Chiecchio, L, Dagrada, G, et al. The t(14;20) is a poor prognostic factor in myeloma but is associated with long-term stable disease in monoclonal gammopathies of undetermined significance. Haematologica.(2010). , 95(7), 1221-5.

[7] Fonseca, R, Blood, E, Rue, M, et al. Clinical and biologic implications of recurrent genomic aberrations in myeloma. Blood (2003). , 101(11), 4569-75.

[8] Reece, D, Song, K. W, Fu, T, et al. Influence of cytogenetics in patients with relapsed or refractory multiple myeloma treated with lenalidomide plus dexamethasone: adverse effect of deletion 17Blood. 114:522-525, (2009). , 13.

[9] Neben, K, Lokhorst, H. M, Jauch, A, et al. Administration of bortezomib before and after autologous stem cell transplantation improves outcome in multiple myeloma patients with deletion 17p. Blood. (2012). Jan 26;, 119(4), 940-8.

[10] Shaughnessy, J. D, Zhou, Y, & Haessler, J. vet al. TP53 deletion is not an adverse feature in multiple myeloma treated with total therapy 3. Br J Haematol. (2009). Nov;, 147(3), 347-51.

[11] Hanamura, I, Stewart, J. P, Huang, Y, Zhan, F, Santra, M, Sawyer, J. R, et al. Frequent gain of chromosome band 1q21 in plasma-cell dyscrasias detected by fluorescence in situ hybridization: incidence increases from MGUS to relapsed myeloma and is related to prognosis and disease progression following tandem stem-cell transplantation. Blood. (2006). , 108(5), 1724-32.

[12] Shaughnessy JD JrQu P, Usmani S, et al. Pharmacogenomics of bortezomib test-dosing identifies hyperexpression of proteasome genes, especially PSMD4, as novel high-risk feature in myeloma treated with Total Therapy 3. Blood (2011). , 118(13), 3512-24.

[13] Neben, K, Jauch, A, Bertsch, U, et al. Combining information regarding chromosomal aberrations t(4;14) and del(17with the International Staging System classification allows stratification of myeloma patients undergoing autologous stem cell transplantation. Haematologica. (2010). Jul;95(7):1150-7., 13.

[14] Dispenzieri, A, Kyle, R, Merlini, G, et al. International Myeloma Working Group guidelines for serum-free light chain analysis in multiple myeloma and related disor-

ders. Leukemia : official journal of the Leukemia Society of America, Leukemia Research Fund, UK. (2009). Epub 2008/11/21., 23(2), 215-24.

[15] Anderson, K. C, Alsina, M, Bensinger, W, et al. NCCN clinical practice guidelines in oncology: multiple myeloma J Natl Compr Canc Netw. (2010).

[16] Katzmann, J. A. Screening panels for monoclonal gammopathies: time to change. The Clinical biochemist Reviews / Australian Association of Clinical Biochemists. (2009). Epub 2009/10/21., 30(3), 105-11.

[17] Katzmann, J. A, Clark, R. J, Abraham, R. S, et al. Serum reference intervals and diagnostic ranges for free kappa and free lambda immunoglobulin light chains: relative sensitivity for detection of monoclonal light chains. Clinical chemistry. (2002)., 48(9), 1437-44.

[18] Bradwell, A. R. Serum free light chain measurements move to center stage. Clinical chemistry. (2005)., 51(5), 805-7.

[19] Katzmann, J. A, Kyle, R. A, Benson, J, et al. Screening Panels for Detection of Monoclonal Gammopathies. Clinical chemistry. (2009)., 55(8), 1517-22.

[20] Bradwell, A. R, Carr-smith, H. D, Mead, G. P, et al. Highly sensitive, automated immunoassay for immunoglobulin free light chains in serum and urine. Clinical chemistry. (2001)., 47(4), 673-80.

[21] Drayson, M, Tang, L. X, Drew, R, et al. Serum free light-chain measurements for identifying and monitoring patients with nonsecretory multiple myeloma. Blood. (2001)., 97(9), 2900-2.

[22] Snozek, C. L, Katzmann, J. A, Kyle, R. A, et al. Prognostic value of the serum free light chain ratio in newly diagnosed myeloma: proposed incorporation into the international staging system. Leukemia : official journal of the Leukemia Society of America, Leukemia Research Fund, UK. (2008)., 22(10), 1933-7.

[23] Dingli, D, Pacheco, J. M, Dispenzieri, A, et al. Serum M-spike and transplant outcome in patients with multiple myeloma. Cancer Sci. (2007)., 98(7), 1035-40.

[24] Dispenzieri, A, Kyle, R, Katzmann, J. A, et al. Immunoglobulin free light chain ratio is an independent risk factor for progression of smoldering multiple myeloma. Blood. (2007). a.

[25] Durie, B. G, Harousseau, J. L, Miguel, J. S, et al. International uniform response criteria for multiple myeloma. Leukemia : official journal of the Leukemia Society of America, Leukemia Research Fund, UK. (2006)., 20(12), 1467-73.

[26] Bradwell, A. R, Harding, S. J, Fourrier, N. J, et al. Assessment of monoclonal gammopathies by nephelometric measurement of individual immunoglobulin kappa/lambda ratios. Clinical chemistry. (2009). Epub 2009/07/21., 55(9), 1646-55.

[27] Keren, D. F. Heavy/Light-chain analysis of monoclonal gammopathies. Clinical chemistry. (2009). Epub 2009/07/11., 55(9), 1606-8.

[28] Ludwig, H, Milosavljevic, D, Zojer, N, et al. Immunoglobulin heavy/light chain ratios improve paraprotein detection and monitoring, identify residual disease and correlate with survival in multiple myeloma patients. Leukemia : official journal of the Leukemia Society of America, Leukemia Research Fund, UK. (2012). Epub 2012/09/08.

[29] Murray, D. L, Ryu, E, Snyder, M. R, et al. Quantitation of Serum Monoclonal Proteins: Relationship between Agarose Gel Electrophoresis and Immunonephelometry. Clinical chemistry. (2009). , 55(8), 1523-9.

[30] Katzmann, J. A, Clark, R, Kyle, R. A, et al. Suppression of uninvolved immunoglobulins defined by heavy/light-chain pair suppression is a risk factor for progression of MGUS. Leukemia : official journal of the Leukemia Society of America, Leukemia Research Fund, UK. (2012). Epub 2012/07/12.

[31] Bradwell, A, Harding, S, Fourrier, N, et al. Prognostic utility of intact immunoglobulin Ig'kappa/Ig'lambda ratios in multiple myeloma patients. Leukemia : official journal of the Leukemia Society of America, Leukemia Research Fund, UK. (2012). Epub 2012/06/16.

[32] Rawstron, A. C, Orfao, A, Beksac, M, et al. European Myeloma Network. Report of the European Myeloma Network on multiparametric flow cytometry in multiple myeloma and related disorders. Haematologica. (2008). Mar;, 93(3), 431-8.

[33] Bataille, T, Jégo, R, & Robillard, G. N, et al. The phenotype of normal, reactive and malignant plasma cells. Identification of "many and multiple myelomas" and of new targets for myeloma therapy. Haematologica. (2006). Sep;, 91(9), 1234-40.

[34] Rawstron, A. C, & Davies, F. E. DasGupta R, et al. Flow cytometric disease monitoring in multiple myeloma: the relationship between normal and neoplastic plasma cells predicts outcome after transplantation. Blood. (2002). Nov 1;, 100(9), 3095-100.

[35] Mateo, G, Montalbán, M. A, Vidriales, M. B, et al. PETHEMA Study Group; GEM Study Group. Prognostic value of immunophenotyping in multiple myeloma: a study by the PETHEMA/GEM cooperative study groups on patients uniformly treated with high-dose therapy. J Clin Oncol. (2008). Jun 1;, 26(16), 2737-44.

[36] Pérez-persona, E, Vidriales, M. B, Mateo, G, et al. New criteria to identify risk of progression in monoclonal gammopathy of uncertain significance and smoldering multiple myeloma based on multiparameter flow cytometry analysis of bone marrow plasma cells. Blood. (2007). Oct 1;, 110(7), 2586-92.

[37] Paiva, B, Vidriales, M. B, Mateo, G, et al. GEM (Grupo Español de MM)/PETHEMA (Programa para el Estudio de la Terapéutica en Hemopatías Malignas) Cooperative Study Groups. The persistence of immunophenotypically normal residual bone mar-

row plasma cells at diagnosis identifies a good prognostic subgroup of symptomatic multiple myeloma patients. Blood. (2009). Nov 12;, 114(20), 4369-72.

[38] Kapoor, P, Greipp, P. T, Morice, W. G, et al. Anti-CD20 monoclonal antibody therapy in multiple myeloma. Br J Haematol. (2008). Apr;, 141(2), 135-48.

[39] Chang, H, Bartlett, E. S, Patterson, B, et al. The absence of CD56 on malignant plasma cells in the cerebrospinal fluid is the hallmark of multiple myeloma involving central nervous system. Br J Haematol. (2005). May;, 129(4), 539-41.

[40] Ely, S. A, & Knowles, D. M. Expression of CD56/neural cell adhesion molecule correlates with the presence of lytic bone lesions in multiple myeloma and distinguishes myeloma from monoclonal gammopathy of undetermined significance and lymphomas with plasmacytoid differentiation. Am J Pathol. (2002). Apr;, 160(4), 1293-9.

[41] Harrington, A. M, Hari, P, & Kroft, S. H. Utility of CD56 immunohistochemical studies in follow-up of plasma cell myeloma. Am J Clin Pathol. (2009). Jul;, 132(1), 60-6.

[42] Kambham, N, Kong, C, Longacre, T. A, et al. Utility of syndecan-1 (CD138) expression in the diagnosis of undifferentiated malignant neoplasms: a tissue microarray study of 1,754 cases. Appl Immunohistochem Mol Morphol. (2005). Dec;, 13(4), 304-10.

[43] Aref, S, Goda, T, & Sherbiny, M. Syndecan-1 in multiple myeloma: relationship to conventional prognostic factors. Hematology. (2003). Aug;, 8(4), 221-8.

[44] Lovell, R, Dunn, J. A, Begum, G, et al. Working Party on Leukaemia in Adults of the National Cancer Research Institute Haematological Oncology Clinical Studies Group. Soluble syndecan-1 level at diagnosis is an independent prognostic factor in multiple myeloma and the extent of fall from diagnosis to plateau predicts for overall survival. Br J Haematol. (2005). Aug;, 130(4), 542-8.

[45] Bayer-garner, I. B, Sanderson, R. D, Dhodapkar, M. V, et al. Syndecan-1 (CD138) immunoreactivity in bone marrow biopsies of multiple myeloma: shed syndecan-1 accumulates in fibrotic regions. Mod Pathol. (2001). Oct;, 14(10), 1052-8.

[46] Mateo, G, Montalbán, M. A, Vidriales, M. B, et al. PETHEMA Study Group; GEM Study Group. Prognostic value of immunophenotyping in multiple myeloma: a study by the PETHEMA/GEM cooperative study groups on patients uniformly treated with high-dose therapy. J Clin Oncol. (2008). Jun 1;, 26(16), 2737-44.

[47] Kyle, R. A, & Rajkumar, S. V. Criteria for diagnosis, staging, risk stratification and response assessment of multiple myeloma. Leukemia. (2009). Jan;, 23(1), 3-9.

[48] De Larrea, C. F, Cibeira, M. T, Elena, M, et al. Abnormal serum free light chain ratio in patients with multiple myeloma in complete remission has strong association with the presence of oligoclonal bands: implications for stringent complete remission definition. Blood. (2009). Dec 3;, 114(24), 4954-6.

[49] Dingli, D, Nowakowski, G. S, Dispenzieri, A, et al. Flow cytometric detection of circulating myeloma cells before transplantation in patients with multiple myeloma: a simple risk stratification system. Blood. (2006). , 107(8), 3384-8.

[50] Paiva, B, Vidriales, M. B, Cerveró, J, et al. GEM (Grupo Español de MM)/PETHEMA (Programa para el Estudio de la Terapéutica en Hemopatías Malignas) Cooperative Study Groups. Multiparameter flow cytometric remission is the most relevant prognostic factor for multiple myeloma patients who undergo autologous stem cell transplantation. Blood. (2008). Nov 15;, 112(10), 4017-23.

[51] De Vos, J, Couderc, G, Tarte, K, et al. Identifying intercellular signaling genes expressed in malignant plasma cells by using complementary DNA arrays. Blood. (2001). , 98(3), 771-780.

[52] Claudio, J. O, Masih-khan, E, Tang, H, et al. A molecular compendium of genes expressed in multiple myeloma. Blood. (2002). , 100(6), 2175-2186.

[53] Zhou, Y, Barlogie, B, & Shaughnessy, J. D. Jr. The molecular characterization and clinical management of multiple myeloma in the post-genome era. Leukemia (2009). , 23, 1941-56.

[54] Shaughnessy JD JrZhan F, Burington B, et al. A validated gene expression model of high-risk multiple myeloma is defined by deregulated expression of genes mapping to chromosome 1. Blood (2007). , 109, 2276-2284.

[55] Decaux, O, Lode, L, Magrangeas, F, et al. Prediction of survival in multiple myeloma based on gene-expression profiles revealed cell cycle and chromosomal instability signatures in high-risk patients and hyperdiploid signatures in low-risk patients. J Clin Oncol. (2008). , 26, 4798-805.

[56] Kumar, S. K, Uno, H, Jacobus, S. J, et al. Impact of gene expression profiling-based risk stratification in patients with myeloma receiving initial therapy with lenalidomide and dexamethasone. Blood. (2011). , 118(16), 4359-62.

[57] Kuiper, R, Broyl, A, De Knegt, Y, et al. A gene expression signature for high-risk multiple myeloma. Leukemia. (2012). , 26(11), 2406-13.

[58] Rajkumar, S. V. Treatment of multiple myeloma. Nat Rev Clin Oncol. (2011). , 8, 479-491.

[59] http://clinicaltrials gov/ct2/show/NCT01668719

[60] Edelstyn, G. A, Gillespie, P. J, & Grebbell, F. S. The radiological demonstration of osseous metastases. Experimental observations. Clin Radiol. (1967). , 18(2), 158-62.

[61] Waheed, S, Mitchell, A, Usmani, S, Epstein, J, Yaccoby, S, Nair, B, et al. Standard and novel imaging methods for multiple myeloma: correlates with prognostic laboratory variables including gene expression profiling data. Haematologica. (2012). Jun 24. [Epub ahead of print]

[62] Bartel, T. B, Haessler, J, Brown, T. L, et al. F18-fluorodeoxyglucose positron emission tomography in the context of other imaging techniques and prognostic factors in multiple myeloma. Blood (2009). , 114, 2068-2076.

[63] Walker, R, Barlogie, B, Haessler, J, et al. Magnetic resonance imaging in multiple myeloma: diagnostic and clinical implications. J Clin Oncol. (2007). , 25(9), 1121-8.

[64] Zamagni, E, Patriarca, F, Nanni, C, Zannetti, B, Englaro, E, Pezzi, A, et al. Prognostic relevance of 18-F FDG PET/CT in newly diagnosed multiple myeloma patients treated with up-front autologous transplantation. Blood (2011). , 118, 5989-5995.

[65] Usmani, S. Z, Mitchell, A, Waheed, S, et al. Prognostic implications of serial fluorodeoxyglucose emission tomography in multiple myeloma treated with Total Therapy 3. Blood. (2013). Jan 10. [Epub ahead of print], 18.

[66] Moreau, P. PET-CT in MM: a new definition of CR. Blood (2011). , 118, 5984-5985.

[67] http://www.themmrf.org/research-programs/commpass-study/

Chapter 11

Bone Disease in Multiple Myeloma

Maja Hinge, Thomas Lund, Jean-Marie Delaisse and Torben Plesner

Additional information is available at the end of the chapter

http://dx.doi.org/10.5772/55190

1. Introduction

Osteolytic bone disease in multiple myeloma (MM) is a common event. Already at diagnosis, approximately eighty percent of patients present with abnormal bone structure [1;2]. During disease progression a large proportion of patients will develop ostelytic lesions [3]. MM bone disease not only results in a reduced quality of life due to pain, pathological fractures, or symptomatic hypercalcaemia [4]; but may also be *the* deciding factor that determines if a patient requires anti-myeloma treatment or if a watch and wait strategy can be applied [5]. In this chapter we will discuss the normal bone remodelling process, and how it is affected in MM. During the last decades, increased knowledge about bone pathophysiology in general has led to an improved understanding of MM bone disease. The description of the receptor activator of nuclear factor kappa B (RANK) and its ligand in the nineties was one of the most significant steps. We will also address how biochemical markers may be used to monitor the velocity of the different processes in bone remodelling. The next part of the chapter will be dedicated to the treatment of MM bone disease. For many years, bisphosphonates have been a cornerstone in the treatment of MM bone disease and despite the occurrence of osteonecrosis of the jaw that was first reported as a result of the of bisphosphonate treatment in the early part of this century, these agents remain the most important components of treatment for MM bone disease. Lastly, we will discuss how various anti-myeloma treatments may influence bone turnover. During the last decade a number of novel drugs have been approved for the treatment of MM and especially proteasome inhibitors seems to have a positive effect on MM bone disease besides their anti-myleoma effect.

2. Pathogenesis of multiple myeloma bone disease

2.1. Introduction

The reason for the excessive loss of bone mass observed in MM is multi factorial. For many years attention was primarily focused on the increase in bone degradation which is observed in the majority of MM patients.

Over the last decade however, it has become increasingly evident that impaired bone formation also plays an important role in MM bone disease. In monoclonal gammopathy of unknown significance (MGUS) and early stage MM with preserved bone structure, normal or even increased bone formation may be observed. With disease progression and development of osteolytic lesions bone formation becomes impaired, and this may be an important contributing factor for the development of osteolytic lesions (see figure 1).

The interaction between the bone marrow microenvironment and the myeloma cells is also considered to be crucial. A large number of cytokines and chemokines, that regulate the activity of bone resorbing osteoclasts and bone forming osteoblasts, have been identified and studied in MM. Recently, a structure consisting of a flat layer of osteoblast lineage cells, that separates the bone surface from the bone marrow during bone remodelling, has been described. Disruption of this cell layer, called the bone remodelling compartment (BRC) canopy, allows direct contact between myeloma cells and the active bone remodelling cells, and this may affect both cell types. Osteocytes have been sparsely investigated in MM. However, a recent article illustrates that also this type of cell may be important for a better understanding of MM bone disease [6].

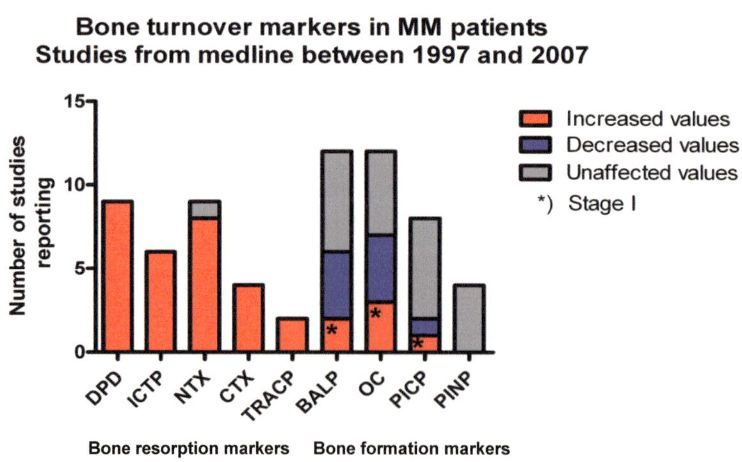

With permission from the author; Søndergaard T. The effect of simvastatin on bone markers in multiple myeloma and a description of the bone remodeling compartment. University of Southern Denmark, 2008.

Figure 1. Number of studies evaluating biochemical markers of bone turnover in MM patients in a ten year period. Bone resorption markers are uniformly elevated, while the bone formation markers are more divergent, with increased levels observed in early stages of MM.

3. Normal bone remodelling

Osteoclasts are the cells responsible for bone resorption. They originate from the monocyte-macrophage cell line. Differentiation of hematopoietic precursor cells into mature osteoclasts requires different environmental factors of which macrophage-colony stimulating factor (M-CSF) and receptor activator for NF-κB ligand (RANKL) play an essential role. The early step in osteoclastogenesis seems to be influenced by M-CSF [7], whereas RANKL initiates differentiation, cell fusion, and activation of mature osteoclasts [8]. During osteoclast development the cell replaces the nonspecific esterase activity with tartrate-resistant acid phosphatase isotype 5b (TRACP 5b), which is believed to be specific for osteoclasts. Osteoclastogenesis results in the formation of large multinucleated cells located on the bone surface where bone degradation takes place. Bone degradation is achieved by an active secretion of protons from the osteoclasts into the resorption pits. The protons decrease the pH and cause decalcification of the bone matrix [9]. After decalcification the collagen fibres are degraded mainly by the proteolytic enzymes cathepsin K and various matrix metalloproteinases [10].

Osteoblasts are responsible for the formation of new bone following osteoclast-mediated bone resorption. Osteoblasts originate from differentiated mesenchymal stem cells under the influence of Runt-related transcription factor (Runx2) and the wingless type signalling (Wnt) factors. Runx2 is required for the differentiation of mesenchymal cells into osteoblasts [11]. The Wnt-pathway mediates the formation of a complex, which in turn inhibits the proteasomal degradation of β-catenin. The increasing level of β-catenin has a stimulating effect on osteoblast differentiation and maturation [12]. The Wnt-pathway can be inhibited by Dickkopf 1 (DKK1), resulting in decreased bone formation.

Mature osteoblasts are lined in groups located along the newly resorbed bone. Placed on the resorption site, the osteoblasts secrete the components needed to generate bone matrix, mainly collagen type 1 [13]. The bone formation ends with calcification of the newly synthesized bone. During bone formation some osteoblasts are incorporated into the bone matrix and become osteocytes. Bone lining cells and the canopy cells are also of osteoblast lineage.

Activation of bone remodelling is not yet clearly understood. However, it is thought that osteocytes may, at least partly, be of importance for the activation of bone remodelling. Osteocytes in the bone matrix may respond to mechanical stimulation and via communication through their networks of canaliculli initiate bone resorption. Osteocyte death probably also plays a role in the recruitment of osteoclasts.

Bone remodelling takes place on bone surface where the osteoclasts and osteoblasts are covered by a canopy of flattened cells of osteoblast lineage [14;15]. The space between the canopy and the bone surface undergoing remodelling is named the bone remodelling compartment (BRC). Disruption of the BRC canopy may impair bone remodelling [16]. Several factors of importance for the regulation of bone remodelling have been identified during the last decades. Within this chapter, we will only review some of the most important. The RANKL, RANK, and the decoy receptor osteoprotegerin (OPG) are probably the most significant factors in the regulation of normal physiological bone remodelling. RANK is expressed on the surface of osteoclast precursor cells, and as mentioned above, stimulation with RANKL is essential for osteoclastogenesis [17]. RANKL is expressed by osteoblasts and bone marrow stromal cells. OPG has a high affinity for RANKL and functions as the physiological inhibitor of RANKL [18]. Since osteoblasts can stimulate osteoclast activity through the expression of RANKL and inhibit it through the secretion of OPG, osteoblasts hold a key position in the coupling between bone formation and bone degradation. Another interesting regulator of bone degradation is macrophage inflammatory protein 1-α (MIP-1α). MIP-1α has been shown to be a potent activator of osteoclasts [19]. MIP-1α stimulates the activity and formation of osteoclasts indirectly by increasing the stromal cell expression of RANKL on the one hand [20; 21], but it also stimulates osteoclast formation independently of the RANKL system, though binding to the CCR1 or the CCR5 osteoclast receptor [21].

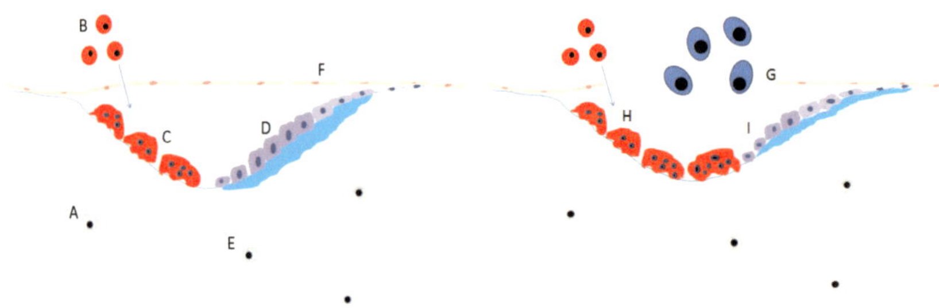

Figure 2. Normal bone remodelling and bone remodelling in multiple myeloma. A: Osteocytes sense mechanical stress and activate bone remodelling. B: Osteoclast precursors differentiate into mature multinucleated osteoclasts. C: The osteoclasts resorb bone matrix. D: Following bone resorption mononucleated osteoblasts lay down new bone in the resorbed area. E: During bone formation of new bone, osteoblasts are imbedded in the new bone matrix and differentiate into osteocytes. F: The bone remodelling takes place beneath a canopy of cells belonging to the osteoblast lineage G: Malignant plasma cells disrupt the bone remodelling compartment canopy and H: Increase osteoclastogenesis and I: Decrease osteoblastogenesis.

4. Abnormal bone remodelling in multiple myeloma

Increased bone degradation is an early event in MM. Retrospective studies using bone histomorphometry on bone marrow biopsies from patients diagnosed with MGUS harvested three to twelve months before these patients developed MM, were found to have increased bone degradation compared with MGUS patients who did not progress to MM during the first year after MGUS was diagnosed [22]. In MM both the number and the activity of the osteoclasts are found to be increased, and this may result in either focal or more diffuse loss of bone matrix when not compensated for by an equal increase in bone formation [23;24].

Several factors of importance for the development of MM bone disease have been identified during the last decades. The RANK/RANKL/OPG system is one of the most significant. In normal bone remodelling the RANKL/OPG ratio is tightly balanced. In MM the RANKL/OPG ratio is increased, both due to an elevated level of RANKL and as a result of a decrease in the level of OPG, thus resulting in increased bone resorption [25]. The increased soluble RANKL/OPG ratio has been shown to correlate with the extent of bone disease and even with overall survival [25;26]. In addition, myeloma cells stimulate bone degradation by the secretion of MIP-1α. In approximately 70% of MM patients, bone marrow serum levels of MIP-1α are elevated [27] and peripheral blood levels of MIP-1α have been found to correlate with bone disease and overall survival [28;29].

Vascular endothelial growth factor (VEGF) is known to be important for neovascularisation, but it probably also plays a role in the activation of osteoclasts in MM. VEGF has been demonstrated, in vitro, to act like macrophage colony-stimulating factor (M-CSF), thus inducing osteoclast differentiation [30]. Furthermore, a simultaneous blockade of VEGF and osteopontin has been shown to inhibit angiogenesis and bone resorption in co-cultures of myeloma cells and osteoclasts [31]. Taken together, these results indicate that VEGF could be of importance in bone resorption, and since the majority of myeloma cells can secrete VEGF it has been suggested that VEGF may support osteoclastic bone resorption in MM [32]. Interleukin-6 (IL-6), stromal-derived factor-1α, tumor necrosis factor-α, and interleukin-11 are other examples of cytokines known to stimulate osteoclasts, which are suggested to be of importance in the development of MM bone disease [33;34].

The myeloma cells do not only affect the osteoclasts indirectly through the secretion of cytokines into the bone marrow microenvironment, but a direct contact between myeloma cells and bone marrow stromal cells or osteoclasts also seems to be an important factor in the development of MM bone disease.

Disruption of the BRC canopy is a frequent finding in MM. This breakdown of the BRC canopy allows a direct contact between the myeloma cells and the osteoclasts and osteoblasts involved in bone remodelling. This event probably contributes to impaired bone formation and enhanced bone resorption [16]. The extent of BRC canopy disruption in a histomorphometric study of iliac crest biopsies was found to correlate with the magnitude of osteolytic lesions in patients with MM [16]. Direct contact between human myeloma cells and bone marrow stromal cells or pre-osteoblasts tested in a co-culture system resulted in a marked decrease in the production of OPG, and thereby an imbalance in the RANKL/OPG ratio resulting in increased bone degradation [35]. Cell to cell contact between myeloma cells and bone marrow stromal cells has also been demonstrated to induce the secretion of IL-6 by bone marrow stromal cells [31]. IL- 6 stimulates osteoclast formation and also has a promoting effect on myeloma cell proliferation [36]. It has also been suggested that myeloma cells can fuse with osteoclasts to create myeloma-osteoclast hybrid cells that may more aggressively erode bone than non-hybrid osteoclasts [16;37].

Co-cultures of myeloma cells and osteoclasts have demonstrated an increased viability of the myeloma cells caused by the direct cell to cell contact with osteoclasts [38]. Osteoclasts also produce factors capable of promoting myeloma cell growth, including IL-6 [39] and insulin-like-growth factor-1 (IGF-1) [40]. Osteoclasts can also support myeloma cell growth through the production of angiogenic factors, and the direct contact between myeloma cells and osteoclasts in co-cultures has been shown to enhance vascular tubule formation [41]. In animal models the inhibition of osteoclast activity with recombinant OPG or bisphosphonates has resulted in an increased in survival of mice inoculated with myeloma cells [42;43] but the clinical data from myeloma patients treated with bisphosphonates have been less consistent [44-48]. Nevertheless, the existence of a vicious cycle of bone resorption and tumour growth in patients with MM seems plausible and may be supported by the demonstration of a survival advantage in patients treated with zoledronic acid in the MRC IX trial [49].

Bone disease in MM is not only caused by an increased bone resorption, but the formation of new bone may also be affected. A reduced recruitment of osteoblasts, as well as reduced mineral deposition has been observed using histological methods in patients with MM [22]. In early stage of MM the number and activity of the osteoblasts can be increased but a marked decrease occurs as the plasma cell infiltration progresses [50]. Disruption of the BRC canopy in MM may be an important cause of the uncoupling of bone resorption and bone formation, with the result that bone resorption is not followed by bone formation or that the bone formation process is delayed or abolished [16]. Human plasma cells purified from bone marrow biopsies of MM patients have been found to express the gene for DKK1, and immunohistochemical analysis of bone marrow biopsies have shown that myeloma cells contain DKK1 [51]. In addition, blood and bone marrow serum levels of DKK1 have been demonstrated to be elevated in patients with MM bone disease [51]. Since DKK1 is believed to inhibit the stimulation of osteoblastogenesis via the Wnt-pathway this might cause impaired bone formation. Runx2 may also be affected by myeloma cells. Runx2 is required for osteoblast differentiation. The expression of Runx2 by mesenchymal cells has been found to decrease after direct cell to cell contact with myeloma cells in co-cultures [52].

Osteocytes have not been widely investigated, and their involvement in MM bone disease is unknown. Histological examination of compact bone from MM patients shows a significant change in the morphology of osteocytes and their lacunae [53]. Likewise, a major change in the gene expression profile of osteocytes in MM has also been observed. This indicates that osteocytes are markedly affected in MM. A recently published study showed that MM patients had significantly smaller numbers of viable osteocytes compared to healthy individuals [6]. Likewise MM patients with bone lesions were found to have a smaller number of viable osteocytes compared with MM patients without bone lesions. The amount of viable osteocytes was found to be negatively correlated with the number of osteoclasts and the authors suggest an involvement of the osteocytes in MM-induced osteoclast formation [6].

Futhermore, healing of bone lesions in MM bone disease does not occur frequently, even in patients who respond well to anti-myeloma treatment. It remains unclear why bone remodelling does not normalise when the influence from myeloma cells disappears after successful treatment. It may be due to irreversible damage of key elements in the bone formation process (i.e. the BRC).

5. Biochemical markers of bone turnover

Conventional radiography has for many years been the standard method for the diagnosis of myeloma bone disease. This modality, however, suffers from a low sensitivity, since 30% of the trabecular bone mass must be absent for a lesion to become detectable. Computed tomography can increase the sensitivity at the cost of higher radiation exposure. Both modalities, however, only provide static information concerning the accumulated bone disease. Biochemical markers of bone turnover can provide dynamic information concerning the velocity of bone turn-over at any given time point, and can be measured from either blood or urine samples. Furthermore, bone formation and bone resorption can be evaluated separately. Bone markers can be divided into two categories: they are either collagen fragments released during the formation or destruction of the collagen triple helix structure of which bone consists, or they are enzymes released form either osteoblasts or the osteoclasts (see figure 3). Bone resorption markers from the first group include the cross-linked telopeptides of type-1 collagen NTX, CTX, ICTP and DPD (Table 1). They are products of osteoclast-mediated degradation of collagen and therefore reflect bone resorption. Bone formation markers from this group include PINP and PINC (Table 1). These markers are products of the cleavage process of procollagen into collagen and therefore the measured levels will reflect the amount of newly formed bone matrix. The second group of bone markers include TRACP-5b, bALP and OC (Table 1). TRACP-5b is secreted by osteoclasts and used as a marker of osteoclast number and activity, whereas bALP and osteocalcin are produced by osteoblasts and used as markers of osteoblast number and activity. The levels of bone markers have been shown to correlate with the degree of bone resorption or bone formation using classical bone histomorphometry [54;55]. Furthermore, bone resorption markers decrease when treatment with anti-resorptive drugs is initiated [56]. Conversely, the discontinuation of anti-resorptive drugs leads to a rise in bone resorption markers [57]. However, when using biochemical markers it is important to be aware of the fact that the level of markers may be influenced by a number of factors, such as age, gender, drugs, renal- and liver function or diet. Especially the collagen-mediated markers are sensitive to food intake. Despite the interest in bone markers, there is still no consensus on how they should be used to monitor disease activity and response to treatment in MM [58].

Bone marker	**Abbreviation**	**Type**	**Analytical specimen**
C-terminal cross-linking telopeptide of type-1 collagen	CTX	Bone resorption marker	Serum, Urine
N-terminal cross-linking telopeptide of type-1 collagen	NTX	Bone resorption marker	Serum, Urine
C-terminal cross-linking telopeptide of type-1 collagen generated by metalloproteinase	ICTP	Bone resorption marker	Serum
Deoxypyridinoline	DPD	Bone resorption marker	Serum, Urine
Tartrate-resistant acid phosphatase isotype 5b	TRACP-5b	Bone resorption marker osteoclast activity	Serum
Bone-specific alkaline phosphatase	bALP	Bone formation marker	Serum
Osteocalcin	OC	Bone formation marker	Serum
Procollagen type-1 N-propeptide	PINP	Bone formation marker	Serum
Procollagen type-1 C-propeptide	PICP	Bone formation marker	Serum

Table 1. Biochemical markers of bone turnover

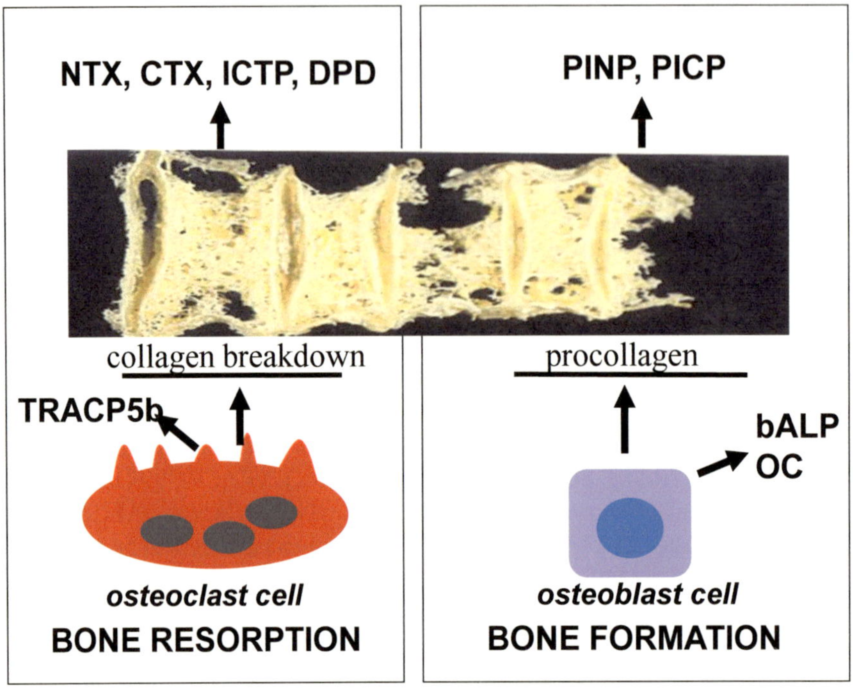

Figure 3. Biochemical markers of bone remodelling can be divided into markers reflecting bone resorption (left) and marker reflecting bone formation (right). They can also be divided in markers reflecting a change in the collagen matrix (upper part) or markers reflecting the activity of bone resorbing or bone forming cells (lower part).

6. Treatment of multiple myeloma bone disease

6.1. Anti-resorptive treatments:

Until now, bisphosphonates remain the only registered agents for the treatment of osteolytic bone disease in MM. Bisphosphonates are synthetic analogues of pyrophosphate with a high affinity for the hydroxyapatite in the bone. After administration, bisphosphonates are rapidly cleared from the blood and incorporated into the bone matrix or excreted through the kidneys. If imbedded in the bone matrix they remain incorporated for many years, or until the bone is degraded by the osteoclasts [59]. Three generations of bisphosphonates exist, and each is many fold more potent than the previous [60]. The different bisphosphonates can be distinguished by the absence or presences of a nitrogen atom in the R^2 position of the bisphosphonate, with the amino-bisphosphonates being the most potent. When the osteoclast degrades bone, the bisphosphonate is taken up through endocytosis and causes apoptosis either through the incorporation into non-functional adenosine triphosphate (non-nitrogen containing bisphosphonates), or through the inhibition of farnesyl pyrophosphate synthase (nitrogen containing bisphosphonates)[61]. Early studies, using the least potent bisphosphonate, etidronate, showed no clinical benefit on MM bone disease [62], whereas the slightly more potent clodronate could diminish progression of osteolysis, but had no effect on bone pain or pathological fractures [63]. In 1996 and 1998, Berenson *et al.* published two studies, in which patients were randomised to placebo or the amino-bisphosphonate pamidronate. A significant effect was observed with regard to reduced pain, fewer skeletal related events, and improved quality of life [64;65]. Initially, no effect could be observed in overall survival, however using a Cox multivariable regression analysis a slight increase in overall survival was observed for a subgroup of patients. A subsequent phase III trial, comparing the more potent bisphonate zoledronic acid with pamidronate in breast cancer patients with bone metastases and MM patients, demonstrated a superiority of zoledronic acid over pamidronate in reducing skeletal events in the breast cancer group but not in the MM sub-population. No difference was observed in overall survival [66]. Later publications indicated that there could be an effect on overall survival but only with the most potent bisphosphonates [67-70]. In 2010 a large meta-analysis concluded that there was no effect on overall survival in MM provided by bisphosphonates in general [71]. However, later the same year the large MRC IX trial, reported that zoledronic acid was superior to the non-nitrogen containing bisphosphonate clodronate, not only with regard to the control of bone disease, but zoledronic acid also increased overall survival by 5.5 months [49]. Because of the MRC IX data, an updated version of the meta-analysis was published in 2012. Still, no significant effect on overall survival was observed for bisphosphonates in general, but "meta regression analysis indicated that the beneficial effect of bisphosphonates on mortality in patients with MM may be a function of drug potency, with zoledronate being the most potent" [72].

Bisphosphonates are potential nephrotoxic compounds and dosage adjustment according to creatinine clearance are required [73].

In 2003, it was reported for the first time, that exposure to bisphosphonates could also cause osteonecrotic lesions, especially in the oral cavity. This complication was termed bisphosphonate-associated osteonecrosis of the jaw (BON) [74]. BON is commonly observed after surgical dental procedures, e.g. tooth extractions, but spontaneous cases do occur [75]. The incidence of BON increases with treatment duration [76], as well as with the potency of the bisphosphonate used [77]. The aetiology of BON remains controversial. One possible explanation could be that the profound suppression of osteoclast activity results in the accumulation of micro-fractures in the bone. This explanation is in accordance with the fact that BON incidence increases with treatment duration and potency of bisphosphonate type and that BON is also observed after treatment with denosumab, a monoclonal antibody that inhibits osteoclast activity by binding to RANKL. It has also been suggested that BON may occur because of the anti-angiogenic effects of bisphosphonates [78]. Indeed, BON seems to be more commonly observed in patients receiving other anti-angiogentic compounds such as thalidomide [77]. Thirdly, it has been speculated that the frequent findings of actinomycosis in the lesions may be part of the pathogenesis and not only a secondary event, especially since prophylactic antibiotics during dental procedures seem to reduce the incidence of BON [79]. Recently, osteomalacia, which in adults is often a consequence of vitamin D deficiency, has been suggested as a risk factor for BON [80]. Once established BON is difficult to cure, and surgical treatment may worsen the situation [75]. Case-reports suggest several treatment modalities, including low-level laser therapy [81;82], hyperbaric oxygen treatment [83], long-term administration of antibiotics [84], autologous bone marrow transplantation [85], and ozone therapy [86]. Because of the difficulties in treating BON, focus has mainly been on preventing the occurrence in the first place. This has been done partly by implementing preventive dental procedures prior to the initiation of therapy with bisphosphonates, but probably more importantly by reducing the exposure time to bisphosphonates. The oral microflora also seems to play a role in the development of BON and antibiotic prophylaxis before dental procedure may reduce the risk of developing BON [79]. Concerning the preventive procedures, there are data indicating a positive effect [87;88]. Concerning the reduced exposure time there are few supportive data, but recommendations based on expert opinion do exist [89-92]. Corso *et al.* demonstrated that monthly infusions for one year followed by four infusions the following year offered equal bone protection but reduced BON incidence compared to the monthly infusions for two years [93]. Lund *et al.* have provided evidence that one year of monthly infusions offers inferior anti-resorptive protection after discontinuation compared with two years of monthly infusions based on consecutive measurement of markers of bone turnover [57]. A more rational approach to reduce the bisphosphonate load without increasing the risk of osteolysis, could be to monitor the patient´s ongoing bone remodelling using biochemical markers of bone turnover in order to provide individualized treatment. Data now exist which indicate that bone remodelling markers may predict osteolysis before it becomes manifest by X-ray or CT-scan [94].

Denosumab is a humanized antibody with high affinity for RANKL. By targeting RANKL, denosumab mimics physiological OPG and thus blocks the stimulation of the osteoclasts through the NF-κB receptor. Denosumab could be expected to have a favourable impact on MM bone disease due to its effect on the increased RANKL/OPG ratio observed in MM patients. In 2006 Body *et al.* published a study investigating the effect of a single dose of subcutaneous denosumab compared with a single dose of intravenous pamidronate on the urinary and serum levels of the bone resorption marker NTX. The study population consisted of 54 patients with bone lesions and either MM (n=25) or breast cancer (n=29). The study reported that the compounds were well-tolerated and to a similar extent decreased the investigated bone resorption marker NTX [95]. A phase II study including 96 MM patients, in either relapse or plateau phase, where denosumab was administered every fourth week also demonstrated a decrease in bone resorption markers, even in patients previously treated with bisphosphonates, with an acceptable safety profile [96]. In a phase III trial patients (n=1776) with cancer bone metastases (excluding breast and prostate cancer) or MM (10% of the study population) were randomized to treatment with either zoledronic acid or denosumab. Denosumab was found to be equivalent to zoledronic acid in delaying time to first on-study skeletalrelated event. Noteworthy, in a subgroup analysis of the MM patients (n=180), mortality appeared to be increased in those treated with denosumab with a hazard ratio of 2.26 (95% CI: 1.13-4.50) [97]. Recently, new data from this trial has been published. Results of patient-reported outcomes of pain and health-related quality of life were reported to be equal in the two treatments arms [98]. The frequency of osteonecrosis of the jaw seemed to be equal for treatment with denosumab or zoledronic acid [97;99]. Denosumab is currently not registered for the treatment of MM bone disease by US Food and Drug Administration or the European Medicines Agency. [100;101], but it could perhaps in the future be used for the treatment of bone disease in patients with renal failure who are not suitable for treatment with bisphosphonates due to the risk of aggravation of renal function.

6.2. Possible future anti-resorptive drug treatments

Several drugs targeting MM bone disease are under development e.g. the CCR1-inhibitor (MLN3897) that blocks the CCR1 receptor on osteoclasts and thereby prevents stimulation by MIP-1α [102]. Another candidate for the treatment of MM bone disease is the anti-DKK1 human antibody BHQ880. The agent has been shown to increase osteoblast differentiation in vivo and in animal models to significantly increase the number of osteoblasts and trabecular thickness [103]. Whether this bone anabolic effect will be found in humans will be of interest because it raises the possibility for not only preventing bone loss, but also supporting new bone formation. Clinical trials with BHQ880 are ongoing [104].

6.3. Anti-myeloma treatments

Treatment of MM using conventional chemotherapy usually does not induce healing of osteolytic lesions even if patients respond well to the anti-myeloma treatment and obtain long progression free periods [105-107]. Although markers of bone resorption may decrease [55] serum levels of bone formation markers remain suppressed as a sign of continuously impaired bone formation even in patients who have obtained complete response after treatment with conventional chemotherapy [56;108].

Proteasome inhibitors have a well-documented anti-myeloma effect and they may also have an impact on MM bone disease through the inhibition of osteoclasts and stimulation of osteoblasts.

In vitro studies have demonstrated that proteasome inhibitors inhibit osteoclast differentiation and resorptive activity by reducing the activity of NF-κB [109;110]. In vivo studies of the effect of bortezomib on bone resorption markers show a rapid and significant decrease in CTX and urinary NTX, but it has also been observed that the levels begin to increase again already 2-3 days after the intravenous injection of bortezomib [111]. The levels of the bone resorption markers CTX and TRACP-5b and the RANKL/OPG ratio were also found to decrease after four cycles of treatment with bortezomib in a clinical study including 34 myeloma patients [112]. The ubiquitin-proteolytic pathway is a regulator of bone formation [113] and by blocking this pathway proteasome inhibitors can stimulate osteoblast differentiation. Suggestions of the underlying mechanism have been that proteasome inhibitors may increase the level of bone morphogenetic protein 2 [114] and prevent the proteolytic degradation of RUNX-2 [115]. In an in vitro study, it has been suggested the bortezomib may enhance bone formation through the inhibition of DKK1 expression in osteogenic cells [116]. More studies have provided evidence that proteasome inhibitors stimulate osteoblasts and bone formation in vitro as well as in animals models [114;116-118], and histological investigations have demonstrated increased numbers of osteoblasts in bone marrow sections from MM patient treated with bortezomib [115]. Clinical studies have demonstrated that anti-myeloma treatment with bortezomib induces an increased level of biochemical markers of bone formation both with regard to markers of osteoblast activation and also bone matrix deposition [118;119]. Alkaline phosphatase was found to be significantly increased in patients who responded to bortezomib treatment [119]. In another clinical study bone-specific alkaline phophatase (bALP) and osteocalcin were found to be increased not only in responding patients, but also in patients who did not achieve an anti-myeloma response to treatment with bortezomib [120]. This result supports the assumption that bortezomib may have a bone anabolic effect independent of its anti-myeloma effect. Enhancement of bone matrix deposition after mono-therapy with bortezomib, has also been shown by the demonstration of increased serum levels of PINP (Procollagen Type-I N-terminal propeptide) [118]. Both bALP and osteocalcin were found to be increased after treatment with bortezomib in a clinical study of 34 relapsed myeloma patients in non-responders and responders but the increase was highest in responding patients. However no radiographic signs of healing of the baseline osteolytic lesions were observed six month post-treatment [112]. Radiologic evidence of healing of lytic lesions was observed in six out of 11 patients who responded to combination treatment with bortezomib, melphalan, and prednisone while none of the evaluated patients who had achieved a response to treatment with melphalan and prednisone without bortezomib showed radiological signs of healing [121].

Pomalidomide (originally CC-4047), is a derivative of thalidomide that is anti-angiogenic and acts as an immunomodulator. Pomalidomide is now tested in Phase III clinical trials and will hopefully soon become available treatment of patients with relapsed or refractory MM. The drug has been granted orphan status for the treatment of MM by the European Medicines Agency [122]. Pomalidomide has been shown to inhibit osteoclasts differentiation in bone marrow cultures which leads to a strong inhibition of bone resorption [123]. The inhibition of osteoclast formation seems to occur through a reduction of the PU.1 expression. PU.1 is a critical transcription factor in the development of mature osteoclasts. Lenalidomide, another thalidomide derivative, has been shown to inhibit both an early step in osteoclastogenesis through reduction of PU.1 expression and to reduce secretion of RANKL from bone marrow stroma cells derived from patients with MM [124]. In a clinical study including 20 MM patients with bone disease Breitkreuts *et al.* found a significant decrease in the serum levels of the RANKL/OPG ratio after two cycles of treatment with lenalidomide [124]. Likewise, treatment with thalidomide in combination with dexamethasone has a favourable effect on the RANKL/OPG ratio [125]. Treatment with thalidomide in combination with dexamethasone can also decrease the levels of the bone resorption markers CTX, NTX and TRACP-5b, however the treatment does not increase the bone formation marker bALP or osteocalcin [126]. The failure to increase bone formations markers in serum, correlates with the observation that none of the responding patients in a clinical study of patients treated with a thalidomide/dexamethasone combination, showed any radiological signs of healing of osteolytic lesions [125].

7. Conclusion

The pathophysiology in multiple myeloma bone disease is complex. There is evidence that not only osteoclast activity but also other cells and structures responsible for normal bone metabolism are affected in different ways, suggesting that different targets for treatment may be identified. The notion that myeloma-induced stimulation of osteoclast may promote growth of myeloma cells and thus create a vicious circle emphasise the importance of improved understanding as well as development of more efficient treatment of myeloma-induced bone disease. Bisphosphonates remain so far the only registered drugs for treatment of multiple myeloma bone disease. Due to risk of renal damage and bisphosphonate-associated osteonecrosis of the jaw after treatment with the potent amino-bisphosphonates, alternatives are wanted and several new drugs are under investigation. Furthermore, the optimal duration of treatment with bisphosphonates remains unknown.

Treatment with conventional chemotherapy does not induce healing of osteolytic lesion even in patients who have obtained complete response. However, novel drugs used for treatment of multiple myeloma seem to affect bone metabolism besides their anti-myeloma effect and cases with radiological signs of healing following treatment with bortezomib have been reported.

The last decade has brought the understanding of multiple myeloma bone disease to a higher level, new anti-myeloma drugs with positive effect on bone disease have been registered and more are undergoing investigation. Still many questions regarding the pathophysiology and treatment of multiple myeloma bone disease remain to be answered.

Author details

Maja Hinge[1*], Thomas Lund[2], Jean-Marie Delaisse[1] and Torben Plesner[3]

*Address all correspondence to: maja.hinge@slb.regionsyddanmark.dk

1 Department of Clinical Cell Biology, Vejle/Lillebælt Hospital, University of Southern Denmark, Vejle, Denmark

2 Department of Haematology, Odense University Hospital, Odense, Denmark

3 Department of Internal Medicine, Division of Haematology, Vejle/Lillebælt Hospital, University of Southern Denmark, Denmark

References

[1] Kyle RA, Therneau TM, Rajkumar SV, Larson DR, Plevak MF, Melton LJ, III. Incidence of multiple myeloma in Olmsted County, Minnesota: Trend over 6 decades. Cancer 2004 Dec 1;101(11):2667-74.

[2] Kyle RA, Gertz MA, Witzig TE, Lust JA, Lacy MQ, Dispenzieri A, Fonseca R, Rajkumar SV, Offord JR, Larson DR, et al. Review of 1027 patients with newly diagnosed multiple myeloma. Mayo Clin.Proc. 2003 Jan;78(1):21-33.

[3] Melton LJ, III, Kyle RA, Achenbach SJ, Oberg AL, Rajkumar SV. Fracture risk with multiple myeloma: a population-based study. J.Bone Miner.Res. 2005 Mar;20(3): 487-93.

[4] Wisloff F, Hjorth M. Health-related quality of life assessed before and during chemotherapy predicts for survival in multiple myeloma. Nordic Myeloma Study Group. Br.J.Haematol. 1997 Apr;97(1):29-37.

[5] Kyle RA, Rajkumar SV. Criteria for diagnosis, staging, risk stratification and response assessment of multiple myeloma. Leukemia 2009 Jan;23(1):3-9.

[6] Giuliani N, Ferretti M, Bolzoni M, Storti P, Lazzaretti M, Dalla PB, Bonomini S, Martella E, Agnelli L, Neri A, et al. Increased osteocyte death in multiple myeloma patients: role in myeloma-induced osteoclast formation. Leukemia 2012 Jun;26(6): 1391-401.

[7] Roodman GD. Cell biology of the osteoclast. Exp.Hematol. 1999 Aug;27(8):1229-41.

[8] Wada T, Nakashima T, Hiroshi N, Penninger JM. RANKL-RANK signaling in osteoclastogenesis and bone disease. Trends Mol.Med. 2006 Jan;12(1):17-25.

[9] Baron R, Neff L, Louvard D, Courtoy PJ. Cell-mediated extracellular acidification and bone resorption: evidence for a low pH in resorbing lacunae and localization of a 100-kD lysosomal membrane protein at the osteoclast ruffled border. J.Cell Biol. 1985 Dec;101(6):2210-22.

[10] Delaisse JM, Andersen TL, Engsig MT, Henriksen K, Troen T, Blavier L. Matrix metalloproteinases (MMP) and cathepsin K contribute differently to osteoclastic activities. Microsc.Res.Tech. 2003 Aug 15;61(6):504-13.

[11] Datta HK, Ng WF, Walker JA, Tuck SP, Varanasi SS. The cell biology of bone metabolism. J.Clin.Pathol. 2008 May;61(5):577-87.

[12] Gavriatopoulou M, Dimopoulos MA, Christoulas D, Migkou M, Iakovaki M, Gkotzamanidou M, Terpos E. Dickkopf-1: a suitable target for the management of myeloma bone disease. Expert.Opin.Ther.Targets. 2009 Jul;13(7):839-48.

[13] Khosla S, Westendorf JJ, Oursler MJ. Building bone to reverse osteoporosis and repair fractures. J.Clin.Invest 2008 Feb;118(2):421-8.

[14] Andersen TL, Sondergaard TE, Skorzynska KE, gnaes-Hansen F, Plesner TL, Hauge EM, Plesner T, Delaisse JM. A physical mechanism for coupling bone resorption and formation in adult human bone. Am.J.Pathol. 2009 Jan;174(1):239-47.

[15] Hauge EM, Qvesel D, Eriksen EF, Mosekilde L, Melsen F. Cancellous bone remodeling occurs in specialized compartments lined by cells expressing osteoblastic markers. J.Bone Miner.Rcs. 2001 Sep;16(9):1575-82.

[16] Andersen TL, Soe K, Sondergaard TE, Plesner T, Delaisse JM. Myeloma cell-induced disruption of bone remodelling compartments leads to osteolytic lesions and generation of osteoclast-myeloma hybrid cells. Br.J.Haematol. 2010 Feb;148(4):551-61.

[17] Boyle WJ, Simonet WS, Lacey DL. Osteoclast differentiation and activation. Nature 2003 May 15;423(6937):337-42.

[18] Hofbauer LC, Schoppet M. Clinical implications of the osteoprotegerin/RANKL/RANK system for bone and vascular diseases. JAMA 2004 Jul 28;292(4):490-5.

[19] Uneda S, Hata H, Matsuno F, Harada N, Mitsuya Y, Kawano F, Mitsuya H. Macrophage inflammatory protein-1 alpha is produced by human multiple myeloma (MM) cells and its expression correlates with bone lesions in patients with MM. Br.J.Haematol. 2003 Jan;120(1):53-5.

[20] Han JH, Choi SJ, Kurihara N, Koide M, Oba Y, Roodman GD. Macrophage inflammatory protein-1alpha is an osteoclastogenic factor in myeloma that is independent of receptor activator of nuclear factor kappaB ligand. Blood 2001 Jun 1;97(11):3349-53.

[21] Oba Y, Lee JW, Ehrlich LA, Chung HY, Jelinek DF, Callander NS, Horuk R, Choi SJ, Roodman GD. MIP-1alpha utilizes both CCR1 and CCR5 to induce osteoclast formation and increase adhesion of myeloma cells to marrow stromal cells. Exp.Hematol. 2005 Mar;33(3):272-8.

[22] Bataille R, Chappard D, Marcelli C, Rossi JF, Dessauw P, Baldet P, Sany J, Alexandre C. Osteoblast stimulation in multiple myeloma lacking lytic bone lesions. Br.J.Haematol. 1990 Dec;76(4):484-7.

[23] Taube T, Beneton MN, McCloskey EV, Rogers S, Greaves M, Kanis JA. Abnormal bone remodelling in patients with myelomatosis and normal biochemical indices of bone resorption. Eur.J.Haematol. 1992 Oct;49(4):192-8.

[24] Valentin-Opran A, Charhon SA, Meunier PJ, Edouard CM, Arlot ME. Quantitative histology of myeloma-induced bone changes. Br.J.Haematol. 1982 Dec;52(4):601-10.

[25] Pearse RN, Sordillo EM, Yaccoby S, Wong BR, Liau DF, Colman N, Michaeli J, Epstein J, Choi Y. Multiple myeloma disrupts the TRANCE/ osteoprotegerin cytokine axis to trigger bone destruction and promote tumor progression. Proc.Natl.Acad.Sci.U.S.A 2001 Sep 25;98(20):11581-6.

[26] Terpos E, Szydlo R, Apperley JF, Hatjiharissi E, Politou M, Meletis J, Viniou N, Yataganas X, Goldman JM, Rahemtulla A. Soluble receptor activator of nuclear factor kappaB ligand-osteoprotegerin ratio predicts survival in multiple myeloma: proposal for a novel prognostic index. Blood 2003 Aug 1;102(3):1064-9.

[27] Choi SJ, Cruz JC, Craig F, Chung H, Devlin RD, Roodman GD, Alsina M. Macrophage inflammatory protein 1-alpha is a potential osteoclast stimulatory factor in multiple myeloma. Blood 2000 Jul 15;96(2):671-5.

[28] Terpos E, Politou M, Szydlo R, Goldman JM, Apperley JF, Rahemtulla A. Serum levels of macrophage inflammatory protein-1 alpha (MIP-1alpha) correlate with the extent of bone disease and survival in patients with multiple myeloma. Br.J.Haematol. 2003 Oct;123(1):106-9.

[29] Hashimoto T, Abe M, Oshima T, Shibata H, Ozaki S, Inoue D, Matsumoto T. Ability of myeloma cells to secrete macrophage inflammatory protein (MIP)-1alpha and MIP-1beta correlates with lytic bone lesions in patients with multiple myeloma. Br.J.Haematol. 2004 Apr;125(1):38-41.

[30] Niida S, Kaku M, Amano H, Yoshida H, Kataoka H, Nishikawa S, Tanne K, Maeda N, Nishikawa S, Kodama H. Vascular endothelial growth factor can substitute for macrophage colony-stimulating factor in the support of osteoclastic bone resorption. J.Exp.Med. 1999 Jul 19;190(2):293-8.

[31] Tanaka Y, Abe M, Hiasa M, Oda A, Amou H, Nakano A, Takeuchi K, Kitazoe K, Kido S, Inoue D, et al. Myeloma cell-osteoclast interaction enhances angiogenesis together with bone resorption: a role for vascular endothelial cell growth factor and osteopontin. Clin.Cancer Res. 2007 Feb 1;13(3):816-23.

[32] Edwards CM, Zhuang J, Mundy GR. The pathogenesis of the bone disease of multiple myeloma. Bone 2008 Jun;42(6):1007-13.

[33] Lentzsch S, Ehrlich LA, Roodman GD. Pathophysiology of multiple myeloma bone disease. Hematol.Oncol.Clin.North Am. 2007 Dec;21(6):1035-49, viii.

[34] Edwards CM, Zhuang J, Mundy GR. The pathogenesis of the bone disease of multiple myeloma. Bone 2008 Jun;42(6):1007-13.

[35] Giuliani N, Bataille R, Mancini C, Lazzaretti M, Barille S. Myeloma cells induce imbalance in the osteoprotegerin/osteoprotegerin ligand system in the human bone marrow environment. Blood 2001 Dec 15;98(13):3527-33.

[36] Cheung WC, Van NB. Distinct IL-6 signal transduction leads to growth arrest and death in B cells or growth promotion and cell survival in myeloma cells. Leukemia 2002 Jun;16(6):1182-8.

[37] Andersen TL, Boissy P, Sondergaard TE, Kupisiewicz K, Plesner T, Rasmussen T, Haaber J, Kolvraa S, Delaisse JM. Osteoclast nuclei of myeloma patients show chromosome translocations specific for the myeloma cell clone: a new type of cancer-host partnership? J.Pathol. 2007 Jan;211(1):10-7.

[38] Yaccoby S, Wezeman MJ, Henderson A, Cottler-Fox M, Yi Q, Barlogie B, Epstein J. Cancer and the microenvironment: myeloma-osteoclast interactions as a model. Cancer Res. 2004 Mar 15;64(6):2016-23.

[39] Abe M, Hiura K, Wilde J, Shioyasono A, Moriyama K, Hashimoto T, Kido S, Oshima T, Shibata H, Ozaki S, et al. Osteoclasts enhance myeloma cell growth and survival via cell-cell contact: a vicious cycle between bone destruction and myeloma expansion. Blood 2004 Oct 15;104(8):2484-91.

[40] Sprynski AC, Hose D, Caillot L, Reme T, Shaughnessy JD, Jr., Barlogie B, Seckinger A, Moreaux J, Hundemer M, Jourdan M, et al. The role of IGF-1 as a major growth factor for myeloma cell lines and the prognostic relevance of the expression of its receptor. Blood 2009 May 7;113(19):4614-26.

[41] Tanaka Y, Abe M, Hiasa M, Oda A, Amou H, Nakano A, Takeuchi K, Kitazoe K, Kido S, Inoue D, et al. Myeloma cell-osteoclast interaction enhances angiogenesis together with bone resorption: a role for vascular endothelial cell growth factor and osteopontin. Clin.Cancer Res. 2007 Feb 1;13(3):816-23.

[42] Vanderkerken K, De LE, Shipman C, Asosingh K, Willems A, Van CB, Croucher P. Recombinant osteoprotegerin decreases tumor burden and increases survival in a murine model of multiple myeloma. Cancer Res. 2003 Jan 15;63(2):287-9.

[43] Yaccoby S, Pearse RN, Johnson CL, Barlogie B, Choi Y, Epstein J. Myeloma interacts with the bone marrow microenvironment to induce osteoclastogenesis and is dependent on osteoclast activity. Br.J.Haematol. 2002 Feb;116(2):278-90.

[44] Brincker H, Westin J, Abildgaard N, Gimsing P, Turesson I, Hedenus M, Ford J, Kandra A. Failure of oral pamidronate to reduce skeletal morbidity in multiple myeloma: a double-blind placebo-controlled trial. Danish-Swedish co-operative study group. Br.J.Haematol. 1998 May;101(2):280-6.

[45] Menssen HD, Sakalova A, Fontana A, Herrmann Z, Boewer C, Facon T, Lichinitser MR, Singer CR, Euller-Ziegler L, Wetterwald M, et al. Effects of long-term intravenous ibandronate therapy on skeletal-related events, survival, and bone resorption markers in patients with advanced multiple myeloma. J.Clin.Oncol. 2002 May 1;20(9):2353-9.

[46] Berenson JR, Lichtenstein A, Porter L, Dimopoulos MA, Bordoni R, George S, Lipton A, Keller A, Ballester O, Kovacs M, et al. Long-term pamidronate treatment of advanced multiple myeloma patients reduces skeletal events. Myeloma Aredia Study Group. J.Clin.Oncol. 1998 Feb;16(2):593-602.

[47] Mhaskar R, Redzepovic J, Wheatley K, Clark OA, Miladinovic B, Glasmacher A, Kumar A, Djulbegovic B. Bisphosphonates in multiple myeloma: a network meta-analysis. Cochrane.Database.Syst.Rev. 2012;5:CD003188.

[48] Modi ND, Lentzsch S. Bisphosphonates as antimyeloma drugs. Leukemia 2012 Apr; 26(4):589-94.

[49] Morgan GJ, Davies FE, Gregory WM, Cocks K, Bell SE, Szubert AJ, Navarro-Coy N, Drayson MT, Owen RG, Feyler S, et al. First-line treatment with zoledronic acid as

compared with clodronic acid in multiple myeloma (MRC Myeloma IX): a randomised controlled trial. Lancet 2010 Dec 11;376(9757):1989-99.

[50] Taube T, Beneton MN, McCloskey EV, Rogers S, Greaves M, Kanis JA. Abnormal bone remodelling in patients with myelomatosis and normal biochemical indices of bone resorption. Eur.J.Haematol. 1992 Oct;49(4):192-8.

[51] Tian E, Zhan F, Walker R, Rasmussen E, Ma Y, Barlogie B, Shaughnessy JD, Jr. The role of the Wnt-signaling antagonist DKK1 in the development of osteolytic lesions in multiple myeloma. N.Engl.J.Med. 2003 Dec 25;349(26):2483-94.

[52] Giuliani N, Colla S, Morandi F, Lazzaretti M, Sala R, Bonomini S, Grano M, Colucci S, Svaldi M, Rizzoli V. Myeloma cells block RUNX2/CBFA1 activity in human bone marrow osteoblast progenitors and inhibit osteoblast formation and differentiation. Blood 2005 Oct 1;106(7):2472-83.

[53] Eisenberger S, Ackermann K, Voggenreiter G, Sultmann H, Kasperk C, Pyerin W. Metastases and multiple myeloma generate distinct transcriptional footprints in osteocytes in vivo. J.Pathol. 2008 Apr;214(5):617-26.

[54] Abildgaard N, Glerup H, Rungby J, dix-Hansen K, Kassem M, Brixen K, Heickendorff L, Nielsen JL, Eriksen EF. Biochemical markers of bone metabolism reflect osteoclastic and osteoblastic activity in multiple myeloma. Eur.J.Haematol. 2000 Feb; 64(2):121-9.

[55] Abildgaard N, Brixen K, Eriksen EF, Kristensen JE, Nielsen JL, Heickendorff L. Sequential analysis of biochemical markers of bone resorption and bone densitometry in multiple myeloma. Haematologica 2004 May;89(5):567-77.

[56] Terpos E, Palermos J, Tsionos K, Anargyrou K, Viniou N, Papassavas P, Meletis J, Yataganas X. Effect of pamidronate administration on markers of bone turnover and disease activity in multiple myeloma. Eur.J.Haematol. 2000 Nov;65(5):331-6.

[57] Lund T, Abildgaard N, Delaisse JM, Plesner T. Effect of withdrawal of zoledronic acid treatment on bone remodelling markers in multiple myeloma. Br.J.Haematol. 2010 Oct;151(1):92-3.

[58] Terpos E, Dimopoulos MA, Sezer O, Roodman D, Abildgaard N, Vescio R, Tosi P, Garcia-Sanz R, Davies F, Chanan-Khan A, et al. The use of biochemical markers of bone remodeling in multiple myeloma: a report of the International Myeloma Working Group. Leukemia 2010 Oct;24(10):1700-12.

[59] Khan SA, Kanis JA, Vasikaran S, Kline WF, Matuszewski BK, McCloskey EV, Beneton MN, Gertz BJ, Sciberras DG, Holland SD, et al. Elimination and biochemical responses to intravenous alendronate in postmenopausal osteoporosis. J.Bone Miner.Res. 1997 Oct;12(10):1700-7.

[60] Ramaswamy B, Shapiro CL. Bisphosphonates in the prevention and treatment of bone metastases. Oncology (Williston.Park) 2003 Sep;17(9):1261-70.

[61] Drake MT, Clarke BL, Khosla S. Bisphosphonates: mechanism of action and role in clinical practice. Mayo Clin.Proc. 2008 Sep;83(9):1032-45.

[62] Belch AR, Bergsagel DE, Wilson K, O'Reilly S, Wilson J, Sutton D, Pater J, Johnston D, Zee B. Effect of daily etidronate on the osteolysis of multiple myeloma. J.Clin.Oncol. 1991 Aug;9(8):1397-402.

[63] Lahtinen R, Laakso M, Palva I, Virkkunen P, Elomaa I. Randomised, placebo-controlled multicentre trial of clodronate in multiple myeloma. Finnish Leukaemia Group. Lancet 1992 Oct 31;340(8827):1049-52.

[64] Berenson JR, Lichtenstein A, Porter L, Dimopoulos MA, Bordoni R, George S, Lipton A, Keller A, Ballester O, Kovacs M, et al. Long-term pamidronate treatment of advanced multiple myeloma patients reduces skeletal events. Myeloma Aredia Study Group. J.Clin.Oncol. 1998 Feb;16(2):593-602.

[65] Berenson JR, Lichtenstein A, Porter L, Dimopoulos MA, Bordoni R, George S, Lipton A, Keller A, Ballester O, Kovacs MJ, et al. Efficacy of pamidronate in reducing skeletal events in patients with advanced multiple myeloma. Myeloma Aredia Study Group. N.Engl.J.Med. 1996 Feb 22;334(8):488-93.

[66] Rosen LS, Gordon D, Kaminski M, Howell A, Belch A, Mackey J, Apffelstaedt J, Hussein MA, Coleman RE, Reitsma DJ, et al. Long-term efficacy and safety of zoledronic acid compared with pamidronate disodium in the treatment of skeletal complications in patients with advanced multiple myeloma or breast carcinoma: a randomized, double-blind, multicenter, comparative trial. Cancer 2003 Oct 15;98(8):1735-44.

[67] Attal M, Harousseau JL, Leyvraz S, Doyen C, Hulin C, Benboubker L, Yakoub A, I, Bourhis JH, Garderet L, Pegourie B, et al. Maintenance therapy with thalidomide improves survival in patients with multiple myeloma. Blood 2006 Nov 15;108(10): 3289-94.

[68] Aviles A, Nambo MJ, Neri N, Castaneda C, Cleto S, Huerta-Guzman J. Antitumor effect of zoledronic acid in previously untreated patients with multiple myeloma. Med.Oncol. 2007;24(2):227-30.

[69] Berendson J DMCY-M. Improved survival in patients wiht multiple myeloma and high bALP levels treated wiht zoledronic acid compared wiht pamidronate: univariate and multivariate models of hazard ratios. 48th ASH, Annual Meeting and Exposion 2006 December 9-12, Orlando, FL.Abstract 3589 . 2006. Ref Type: Abstract

[70] McCloskey EV, Dunn JA, Kanis JA, MacLennan IC, Drayson MT. Long-term follow-up of a prospective, double-blind, placebo-controlled randomized trial of clodronate in multiple myeloma. Br.J.Haematol. 2001 Jun;113(4):1035-43.

[71] Mhaskar R, Redzepovic J, Wheatley K, Clark OA, Miladinovic B, Glasmacher A, Kumar A, Djulbegovic B. Bisphosphonates in multiple myeloma. Cochrane.Database.Syst.Rev. 2010;(3):CD003188.

[72] Mhaskar R, Redzepovic J, Wheatley K, Clark OA, Miladinovic B, Glasmacher A, Kumar A, Djulbegovic B. Bisphosphonates in multiple myeloma: a network meta-analysis. Cochrane.Database.Syst.Rev. 2012;5:CD003188.

[73] Terpos E, Sezer O, Croucher PI, Garcia-Sanz R, Boccadoro M, San MJ, Ashcroft J, Blade J, Cavo M, Delforge M, et al. The use of bisphosphonates in multiple myeloma: recommendations of an expert panel on behalf of the European Myeloma Network. Ann.Oncol. 2009 Aug;20(8):1303-17.

[74] Marx RE. Pamidronate (Aredia) and zoledronate (Zometa) induced avascular necrosis of the jaws: a growing epidemic. J.Oral Maxillofac.Surg. 2003 Sep;61(9):1115-7.

[75] Badros A, Weikel D, Salama A, Goloubeva O, Schneider A, Rapoport A, Fenton R, Gahres N, Sausville E, Ord R, et al. Osteonecrosis of the jaw in multiple myeloma patients: clinical features and risk factors. J.Clin.Oncol. 2006 Feb 20;24(6):945-52.

[76] Bamias A, Kastritis E, Bamia C, Moulopoulos LA, Melakopoulos I, Bozas G, Koutsoukou V, Gika D, Anagnostopoulos A, Papadimitriou C, et al. Osteonecrosis of the jaw in cancer after treatment with bisphosphonates: incidence and risk factors. J.Clin.Oncol. 2005 Dec 1;23(34):8580-7.

[77] Zervas K, Verrou E, Teleioudis Z, Vahtsevanos K, Banti A, Mihou D, Krikelis D, Terpos E. Incidence, risk factors and management of osteonecrosis of the jaw in patients with multiple myeloma: a single-centre experience in 303 patients. Br.J.Haematol. 2006 Sep;134(6):620-3.

[78] Dimopoulos MA, Kastritis E, Anagnostopoulos A, Melakopoulos I, Gika D, Moulopoulos LA, Bamia C, Terpos E, Tsionos K, Bamias A. Osteonecrosis of the jaw in patients with multiple myeloma treated with bisphosphonates: evidence of ncreased risk after treatment with zoledronic acid. Haematologica 2006 Jul;91(7):968-71.

[79] Montefusco V, Gay F, Spina F, Miceli R, Maniezzo M, Teresa AM, Farina L, Piva S, Palumbo A, Boccadoro M, et al. Antibiotic prophylaxis before dental procedures may reduce the incidence of osteonecrosis of the jaw in patients with multiple myeloma treated with bisphosphonates. Leuk.Lymphoma 2008 Nov;49(11):2156-62.

[80] Bedogni A, Saia G, Bettini G, Tronchet A, Totola A, Bedogni G, Tregnago P, Valenti MT, Bertoldo F, Ferronato G, et al. Osteomalacia: the missing link in the pathogenesis of bisphosphonate-related osteonecrosis of the jaws? Oncologist. 2012;17(8):1114-9.

[81] Scoletta M, Arduino PG, Reggio L, Dalmasso P, Mozzati M. Effect of low-level laser irradiation on bisphosphonate-nduced osteonecrosis of the jaws: preliminary results of a prospective study. Photomed.Laser Surg. 2010 Apr;28(2):179-84.

[82] Vescovi P, Merigo E, Meleti M, Manfredi M, Fornaini C, Nammour S. Surgical Approach and Laser Applications in BRONJ Osteoporotic and Cancer Patients. J.Osteoporos. 2012;2012:585434.

[83] Freiberger JJ. Utility of hyperbaric oxygen in treatment of bisphosphonate-related osteonecrosis of the jaws. J.Oral Maxillofac.Surg. 2009 May;67(5 Suppl):96-106.

[84] Montebugnoli L, Felicetti L, Gissi DB, Pizzigallo A, Pelliccioni GA, Marchetti C. Biphosphonate-associated osteonecrosis can be controlled by nonsurgical management. Oral Surg.Oral Med.Oral Pathol.Oral Radiol.Endod. 2007 Oct;104(4):473-7.

[85] Cella L, Oppici A, Arbasi M, Moretto M, Piepoli M, Vallisa D, Zangrandi A, Di NC, Cavanna L. Autologous bone marrow stem cell intralesional transplantation repairing bisphosphonate related osteonecrosis of the jaw. Head Face.Med. 2011;7:16.

[86] Agrillo A, Petrucci MT, Tedaldi M, Mustazza MC, Marino SM, Gallucci C, Iannetti G. New therapeutic protocol in the treatment of avascular necrosis of the jaws. J.Craniofac.Surg. 2006 Nov;17(6):1080-3.

[87] Ripamonti CI, Maniezzo M, Campa T, Fagnoni E, Brunelli C, Saibene G, Bareggi C, Ascani L, Cislaghi E. Decreased occurrence of osteonecrosis of the jaw after implementation of dental preventive measures in solid tumour patients with bone metastases treated with bisphosphonates. The experience of the National Cancer Institute of Milan. Ann.Oncol. 2009 Jan;20(1):137-45.

[88] Dimopoulos MA, Kastritis E, Bamia C, Melakopoulos I, Gika D, Roussou M, Migkou M, Eleftherakis-Papaiakovou E, Christoulas D, Terpos E, et al. Reduction of osteonecrosis of the jaw (ONJ) after implementation of preventive measures in patients with multiple myeloma treated with zoledronic acid. Ann.Oncol. 2009 Jan;20(1):117-20.

[89] Terpos E, Sezer O, Croucher PI, Garcia-Sanz R, Boccadoro M, San MJ, Ashcroft J, Blade J, Cavo M, Delforge M, et al. The use of bisphosphonates in multiple myeloma: recommendations of an expert panel on behalf of the European Myeloma Network. Ann.Oncol. 2009 Aug;20(8):1303-17.

[90] Durie BG. Use of bisphosphonates in multiple myeloma: IMWG response to Mayo Clinic consensus statement. Mayo Clin.Proc. 2007 Apr;82(4):516-7.

[91] Kyle RA, Yee GC, Somerfield MR, Flynn PJ, Halabi S, Jagannath S, Orlowski RZ, Roodman DG, Twilde P, Anderson K. American Society of Clinical Oncology 2007 clinical practice guideline update on the role of bisphosphonates in multiple myeloma. J.Clin.Oncol. 2007 Jun 10;25(17):2464-72.

[92] Lacy MQ, Dispenzieri A, Gertz MA, Greipp PR, Gollbach KL, Hayman SR, Kumar S, Lust JA, Rajkumar SV, Russell SJ, et al. Mayo clinic consensus statement for the use of bisphosphonates in multiple myeloma. Mayo Clin.Proc. 2006 Aug;81(8):1047-53.

[93] Corso A, Varettoni M, Zappasodi P, Klersy C, Mangiacavalli S, Pica G, Lazzarino M. A different schedule of zoledronic acid can reduce the risk of the osteonecrosis of the jaw in patients with multiple myeloma. Leukemia 2007 Jul;21(7):1545-8.

[94] Lund T, Abildgaard N, Andersen TL, Delaisse JM, Plesner T. Multiple myeloma: changes in serum C-terminal telopeptide of collagen type I and bone-specific alkaline

phosphatase can be used in daily practice to detect imminent osteolysis. Eur.J.Haematol. 2010 May;84(5):412-20.

[95] Body JJ, Facon T, Coleman RE, Lipton A, Geurs F, Fan M, Holloway D, Peterson MC, Bekker PJ. A study of the biological receptor activator of nuclear factor-kappaB ligand inhibitor, denosumab, in patients with multiple myeloma or bone metastases from breast cancer. Clin.Cancer Res. 2006 Feb 15;12(4):1221-8.

[96] Vij R, Horvath N, Spencer A, Taylor K, Vadhan-Raj S, Vescio R, Smith J, Qian Y, Yeh H, Jun S. An open-label, phase 2 trial of denosumab in the treatment of relapsed or plateau-phase multiple myeloma. Am.J.Hematol. 2009 Oct;84(10):650-6.

[97] Henry DH, Costa L, Goldwasser F, Hirsh V, Hungria V, Prausova J, Scagliotti GV, Sleeboom H, Spencer A, Vadhan-Raj S, et al. Randomized, double-blind study of denosumab versus zoledronic acid in the treatment of bone metastases in patients with advanced cancer (excluding breast and prostate cancer) or multiple myeloma. J.Clin.Oncol. 2011 Mar 20;29(9):1125-32.

[98] Vadhan-Raj S, von MR, Fallowfield LJ, Patrick DL, Goldwasser F, Cleeland CS, Henry DH, Novello S, Hungria V, Qian Y, et al. Clinical benefit in patients with metastatic bone disease: results of a phase 3 study of denosumab versus zoledronic acid. Ann.Oncol. 2012 Jul 31.

[99] Stopeck AT, Lipton A, Body JJ, Steger GG, Tonkin K, de Boer RH, Lichinitser M, Fujiwara Y, Yardley DA, Viniegra M, et al. Denosumab compared with zoledronic acid for the treatment of bone metastases in patients with advanced breast cancer: a randomized, double-blind study. J.Clin.Oncol. 2010 Dec 10;28(35):5132-9.

[100] http://www.cancer.gov/cancertopics/druginfo/fda-denosumab. 2012 Aug 8.

[101] http://www.ema.europa.eu/docs/en_GB/document_library/EPAR_-_Summary_for_the_public/human/002173/WC500110385.pdf. 2012 Aug 28.

[102] Morgan GJ, Wu P. Targeting bone in myeloma. Recent Results Cancer Res. 2012;192:127-43.

[103] Fulciniti M, Tassone P, Hideshima T, Vallet S, Nanjappa P, Ettenberg SA, Shen Z, Patel N, Tai YT, Chauhan D, et al. Anti-DKK1 mAb (BHQ880) as a potential therapeutic agent for multiple myeloma. Blood 2009 Jul 9;114(2):371-9.

[104] http://www.clinicaltrials.gov/.. 2012 Aug 29.

[105] Callander NS, Roodman GD. Myeloma bone disease. Semin.Hematol. 2001 Jul;38(3):276-85.

[106] Wahlin A, Holm J, Osterman G, Norberg B. Evaluation of serial bone X-ray examination in multiple myeloma. Acta Med.Scand. 1982;212(6):385-7.

[107] Epstein J, Walker R. Myeloma and bone disease: "the dangerous tango". Clin.Adv.Hematol.Oncol. 2006 Apr;4(4):300-6.

[108] Diamond T, Levy S, Day P, Barbagallo S, Manoharan A, Kwan YK. Biochemical, histomorphometric and densitometric changes in patients with multiple myeloma: effects of glucocorticoid therapy and disease activity. Br.J.Haematol. 1997 Jun;97(3):641-8.

[109] Zavrski I, Krebbel H, Wildemann B, Heider U, Kaiser M, Possinger K, Sezer O. Proteasome inhibitors abrogate osteoclast differentiation and osteoclast function. Biochem.Biophys.Res.Commun. 2005 Jul 22;333(1):200-5.

[110] von M, I, Krebbel H, Hecht M, Manz RA, Fleissner C, Mieth M, Kaiser M, Jakob C, Sterz J, Kleeberg L, et al. Bortezomib nhibits human osteoclastogenesis. Leukemia 2007 Sep;21(9):2025-34.

[111] Boissy P, Andersen TL, Lund T, Kupisiewicz K, Plesner T, Delaisse JM. Pulse treatment with the proteasome inhibitor bortezomib inhibits osteoclast resorptive activity in clinically relevant conditions. Leuk.Res. 2008 Nov;32(11):1661-8.

[112] Terpos E, Heath DJ, Rahemtulla A, Zervas K, Chantry A, Anagnostopoulos A, Pouli A, Katodritou E, Verrou E, Vervessou EC, et al. Bortezomib reduces serum dickkopf-1 and receptor activator of nuclear factor-kappaB ligand concentrations and normalises indices of bone remodelling in patients with relapsed multiple myeloma. Br.J.Haematol. 2006 Dec;135(5):688-92.

[113] Zhao M, Qiao M, Oyajobi BO, Mundy GR, Chen D. E3 ubiquitin ligase Smurf1 mediates core-binding factor alpha1/Runx2 degradation and plays a specific role in osteoblast differentiation. J.Biol.Chem. 2003 Jul 25;278(30):27939-44.

[114] Garrett IR, Chen D, Gutierrez G, Zhao M, Escobedo A, Rossini G, Harris SE, Gallwitz W, Kim KB, Hu S, et al. Selective nhibitors of the osteoblast proteasome stimulate bone formation in vivo and in vitro. J.Clin.Invest 2003 Jun;111(11):1771-82.

[115] Giuliani N, Morandi F, Tagliaferri S, Lazzaretti M, Bonomini S, Crugnola M, Mancini C, Martella E, Ferrari L, Tabilio A, et al. The proteasome inhibitor bortezomib affects osteoblast differentiation in vitro and in vivo in multiple myeloma patients. Blood 2007 Jul 1;110(1):334-8.

[116] Oyajobi BO, Garrett IR, Gupta A, Flores A, Esparza J, Munoz S, Zhao M, Mundy GR. Stimulation of new bone formation by the proteasome inhibitor, bortezomib: implications for myeloma bone disease. Br.J.Haematol. 2007 Nov;139(3):434-8.

[117] Pennisi A, Li X, Ling W, Khan S, Zangari M, Yaccoby S. The proteasome inhibitor, bortezomib suppresses primary myeloma and stimulates bone formation in myelomatous and nonmyelomatous bones in vivo. Am.J.Hematol. 2009 Jan;84(1):6-14.

[118] Lund T, Soe K, Abildgaard N, Garnero P, Pedersen PT, Ormstrup T, Delaisse JM, Plesner T. First-line treatment with bortezomib rapidly stimulates both osteoblast activity and bone matrix deposition in patients with multiple myeloma, and stimulates

osteoblast proliferation and differentiation in vitro. Eur.J.Haematol. 2010 Oct;85(4): 290-9.

[119] Zangari M, Esseltine D, Lee CK, Barlogie B, Elice F, Burns MJ, Kang SH, Yaccoby S, Najarian K, Richardson P, et al. Response to bortezomib is associated to osteoblastic activation in patients with multiple myeloma. Br.J.Haematol. 2005 Oct;131(1):71-3.

[120] Heider U, Kaiser M, Muller C, Jakob C, Zavrski I, Schulz CO, Fleissner C, Hecht M, Sezer O. Bortezomib increases osteoblast activity in myeloma patients irrespective of response to treatment. Eur.J.Haematol. 2006 Sep;77(3):233-8.

[121] Delforge M, Terpos E, Richardson PG, Shpilberg O, Khuageva NK, Schlag R, Dimopoulos MA, Kropff M, Spicka I, Petrucci MT, et al. Fewer bone disease events, improvement in bone remodeling, and evidence of bone healing with bortezomib plus melphalan-prednisone vs. melphalan-prednisone in the phase III VISTA trial in multiple myeloma. Eur.J.Haematol. 2011 May;86(5):372-84.

[122] http://www.ema.europa.eu/ema/. 2012 Aug 31.

[123] Anderson G, Gries M, Kurihara N, Honjo T, Anderson J, Donnenberg V, Donnenberg A, Ghobrial I, Mapara MY, Stirling D, et al. Thalidomide derivative CC-4047 inhibits osteoclast formation by down-regulation of PU.1. Blood 2006 Apr 15;107(8):3098-105.

[124] Breitkreutz I, Raab MS, Vallet S, Hideshima T, Raje N, Mitsiades C, Chauhan D, Okawa Y, Munshi NC, Richardson PG, et al. Lenalidomide inhibits osteoclastogenesis, survival factors and bone-remodeling markers in multiple myeloma. Leukemia 2008 Oct;22(10):1925-32.

[125] Terpos E, Mihou D, Szydlo R, Tsimirika K, Karkantaris C, Politou M, Voskaridou E, Rahemtulla A, Dimopoulos MA, Zervas K. The combination of intermediate doses of thalidomide with dexamethasone is an effective treatment for patients with refractory/relapsed multiple myeloma and normalizes abnormal bone remodeling, through the reduction of sRANKL/osteoprotegerin ratio. Leukemia 2005 Nov;19(11):1969-76.

[126] Terpos E, Dimopoulos MA, Sezer O. The effect of novel anti-myeloma agents on bone metabolism of patients with multiple myeloma. Leukemia 2007 Sep;21(9): 1875-84.

Chapter 12

Rare Manifestations of Multiple Myeloma

Artur Jurczyszyn

Additional information is available at the end of the chapter

http://dx.doi.org/10.5772/53385

1. Introduction

Multiple myeloma (MM) or plasma cell myeloma, is a haematological disease representing 1-2% of all cancers and about 15% of haematological *malignancies*. The classic form of MM is characterized by generalized neoplastic changes in the bones accompanied by kidney damage, impaired haematopoiesis and susceptibility to infections. In laboratory tests, MM manifests itself by the presence of monoclonal protein, called paraprotein, in serum or urine. This results from the fact that pathological plasma cells produce a complete immunoglobulin (Ig), usually IgG or IgA, or only the kappa or lambda light chains. Solitary myeloma (osseous or extraosseous), non-secretory myeloma and secretory myeloma are rarer forms of MM. Sometimes, however, the clinical picture of MM is quite different from the classic manifestation described in the textbooks. This can cause diagnostic difficulties, thereby delaying treatment.

The atypical clinical and laboratory manifestations and paraneoplastic syndromes concomitant with a diagnosis of MM and described below, as are those that appear in the course of the disease, especially in progression. Although they do not represent a significant percentage of cases, knowledge of the rare clinical and laboratory variants of MM may assist in making a differential diagnosis in cases of doubt.

In addition to their low incidence, rare manifestations of MM share the lack of valid relevant scientific knowledge, which leads to difficulties in making firm therapeutic guidelines. In fact, most of the information on these conditions derives from case reports and/or small series studies, making it rather difficult to develop any uniform treatment approaches. As a result, several of rare manifestations of MM can well be controlled with standard regimens used for classic MM, like for example non-secretory myeloma. However the satisfactory strategies to control some of those conditions, such as plasma cell leukemia, are still unsatisfactory. These issues are best illustrated in the present work in the chapter discussing POEMS syndrome.

Furthermore, rare manifestations of MM are heterogonous also in their underlying cellular and/or molecular mechanisms. These can be either a plasma-cell clone (non-secretory myeloma), paraprotein or cytokines (some of the paraneoplastic disorders). Moreover, paraprotein may exhibit autoantibody activity or aggregate into insoluble depositions. This relates to some other uncommon conditions, including various types of amyloidosis and cryoglobulinemia. In amyloidosis, misfolding of proteins occurs. Otherwise soluble, misfolded protein molecules tend to aggregate as extracellular amyloid fibrils, leading to the damage of the various tissues and organs. In cryoglobulinemia, paraproteins present in circulating blood can become insoluble in a certain temperature, resulting in a wide spectrum of clinical symptoms depending on paraprotein properties (Merlini, Stone 2006).

Below, rare manifestations of MM are described in details. Their relative prevalence/incidence is given in Table 1. Table 2 provides short summary of the diagnostic and clinical characteristics of the rare manifestations of MM, except for POEMS syndrome described in more details in Table 3.

Rare manifestation of MM		**Percentage of all MM cases**
Non-secretory myeloma		1-5%
Myeloma IgD, IgM and IgE		
	IgD	2%
	IgM	0.2-0.5%
	IgE	Very rare
Plasma cell leukemia		0.5-3.0%
POEMS syndrome		Very rare
Rare paraneoplastic syndromes accompanying myeloma		Extremely rare
Family myeloma		Extremely rare

Supporting references can be found in corresponding sections of the main text.

Table 1. Rare manifestations of multiple myeloma (MM) and their prevalence/incidence.

http://dx.doi.org/10.5772/53385

Rare manifestation of MM	Major diagnostic criteria
Non-secretory myeloma	Bone marrow cytology and immunohistochemistry: the infiltration of clonal plasma cells. The clinical picture: classic osteolytic lesions and a decrease in the level of normal (non-clonal) immunoglobulins.
Myeloma IgD	Diagnosis: problematic because routine test does not detect the monoclonal protein peak in 60% of patients, and when it is detected, the concentration is usually smaller than 20 g/l. An overproduction of light chains (usually lambda) is observed in 90-96% of patients. The clinical picture: a variant of the light chain disease. Usually affects younger patients, the disease course is more aggressive and often accompanied by amyloidosis and extramedullary infiltrations. Lymphadenopathy, renal failure and hypercalcemia are common. Myopathy and carpal tunnel syndrome can be present.
Myeloma IgM	Diagnosis: the presence of IgM monoclonal protein in serum; it is necessary to differentiate with Waldenström's macroglobulinemia. The clinical picture: the clonal proliferation of plasma cells in bone marrow aspiration and the presence of hypercalcemia, renal failure and osteolytic foci.
Myeloma IgE	Frequent presence of plasma cells in peripheral blood, osteoblastic lesions, hepatosplenomegaly and amyloidosis.
Plasma cell leukemia	Diagnosis: at least 20% plasma cells in a peripheral blood smear and/or the absolute number of plasma cells in the peripheral blood exceeding 2 g/l with a concomitant monoclonal gammopathy. The clinical picture: extraosseous infiltrations, often with the involvement of the central nervous system, and accompanied by organomegaly and lymphadenopathy.
Rare paraneoplastic syndromes accompanying myeloma	Sweet's syndrome: granolocytosis, fever and painful erythematous skin changes caused by skin granulocytic infiltrations that subside following treatment with corticosteroids. Bullous epidermal separation or pemphigus: subepidermal bubbles and secondary ulcers.
Family myeloma	The exact genetic cause remains unknown but autosomal inheritance with low gene penetrance is most probable. An annual immunoelectrophoresis of the urine and serum protein least two cases of MM in first or second-degree relatives are present.

Supporting references can be found in corresponding sections of the main text. Detailed diagnostic criteria of POEMS syndrome can be found in Table 3.

Table 2. Major diagnostic procedures and criteria of rare manifestations of multiple myeloma (MM).

Disease	Definitionof the disease	References
POEMS syndrome	All four criteria must be met: 1. The presence of the monoclonal protein (in serum and/or in urine), especially the light chain type λ. 2. Peripheral polyneuropathy. 3. The presence of at least one "great" criterion: • osteosclerotic changes in the skeletal system • Castleman's disease • high levels of vascular endothelial growth factor. 4. The presence of at least one "small" criterion: • the enlargement of the internal organs (liver, spleen, lymph nodes) • pleural effusion, ascites, oedema • abnormal secretion of the endocrine glands (adrenal glands, thyroid, parathyroid, pancreas, gonads, with the exception of diabetes or hypothyroidism) •skin lesions (hyperpigmentation, hypertrichosis, peripheral cyanosis, abnormal structure of the nails) • optic disc oedema, • thrombocythaemia, polycythemia.	Kyle et al. 2009 Dispenzieri et al. 2003 Dispenzieri et al. 2007 Rajkumar et al. 2011

Table 3. The criteria for diagnosis of POEMS syndrome.

2. Non-secretory myeloma

Non-secretory myeloma is one of the least frequent forms of MM. The classic diagnostic methods of immunoelectrophoresis and immunofixation do not detect any monoclonal protein in either urine or serum. These patients are usually referred to a haematologist as part of a diagnosis for anaemia or bone changes. It is estimated that this form represents 1-5% of all MM cases [Kyle et al. 2003, Blade, Kyle 1999]. The diagnosis is based on a bone marrow examination (cytology and immunohistochemistry). This will confirm the infiltration of clonal plasma cells, although immunohistochemical tests do not confirm the existence of light kappa or lambda chains in 15% of patients with non-secretory myeloma. The clinical picture reveals classic osteolytic lesions and a decrease in the level of normal (non-clonal) immunoglobulins [Kyle et al. 2003, Blade, Kyle 1999] in 92% of patients. Although classic diagnostic tests do not indicate the presence of monoclonal protein, the ratio of free light chains in serum (FLCr) is abnormal in more than 2/3 of patients. This test is recommended for these patients to evaluate the effectiveness of the therapy [Durie 2006, Dispenzieri 2009]. A more detailed analysis of the immunofixation test, together with the results of the test for free light chains, allows the presence of monoclonal protein in serum to be ascertained. The proportion of patients with "true" non-secretory myeloma is consequently found to be much smaller than 2%. Repeated bone marrow smear tests are the only way to assess the activity of the disease [Durie 2006] in these patients. Cytogenetic abnormalities in patients with non-secretory myeloma do not differ from those observed in the secretory form [Blade, Kyle 1999]. Both the prognosis and the therapeutic recommendations are the same for patients with non-secretory myeloma and the classic form of the disease, i.e. secretory myeloma. Some studies, however, indicate that the prognosis for patients with non-secretory myeloma treated using autologous transplantation is better than for the patients suffering from the classic form of the disease [Terpos et al. 2003].

3. Myeloma IgD, IgM and IgE

The monoclonal production of immunoglobulin IgD A is a rare laboratory manifestation of MM, observed in approximately 2% of patients with MM. Diagnostic problems arise from the fact that the routine test does not detect the monoclonal protein peak in 60% of patients, and when it is detected, the concentration is usually smaller than 20 g/l. An overproduction of light chains (usually lambda) is observed in 90-96% of patients. This makes the clinical picture a variant of the light chain disease [Blade, Kyle 1999, Kuliszkiewicz-Janus et al. 2005, Shimamoto, 1991, Blades et al. 1994, Jancelewicz et al. 1975]. The clinical picture is also slightly different, although this usually affects younger patients – the disease course is more aggressive and often accompanied by amyloidosis and extramedullary infiltrations. Lymphadenopathy is observed in 10% of patients [Shimamoto, 1991, Blades et al. 1994]. Renal failure is observed in 33% of cases at the moment of diagnosis and hypercalcemia in 20% [Homan et al. 1990]. The disease is often accompanied by neurological symptoms such as myopathy and carpal tunnel syndrome, which is probably associated with the coexistence of amyloidosis. IgD myeloma is often associated with connective tissue diseases. This can hinder diagnosis due to the resulting low concentration of monoclonal protein. Previous analyses suggest that the mean survival time of patients with IgD MM is 13.7-21 months. This is shorter than for the classic IgG and IgA MM [Blade et al. 1994, Jancelewicz et al. 1975]. More recent analyses, however, indicate that 30% of patients with IgD myeloma live more than 3 years and 20% more than 5 years [Blade et al. 1994]. Shimamoto regards the presence of the lambda chain and leukocytes in excess of 7 g/l as adverse factors responsible for the shorter progression-free time in patients with IgD MM. Depending on the number of prognostic factors, patients are classified into three prognostic groups: 0, 1 and 2 [Shimamoto et al. 1991]. Based on a retrospective analysis of 36 patients undergoing ablative chemotherapy, the probability of 3-year survival and progression-free time were 69% and 38% respectively [Sharma et al. 2010]. Some authors indicate that the use of myeloablative chemotherapy reduces the differences between IgD MM and the classic forms of the disease [Sharma et al. 2010, Maisnar et al. 2008], but this remains a matter for discussion [Morris et al. 2010].

MM IgM is even less frequent (0.2-0.5% of patients with MM) [Reece et al. 2010, MacLennan 1992, Avet-Loiseau et al. 2003]. Although the presence of IgM monoclonal protein in serum is one of the clinical features common to the disease and Waldenström's macroglobulinemia (WM), the overall clinical picture is different. The differing prognoses and therapeutic recommendations make a correct diagnosis all the more important. The clonal proliferation of plasma cells usually observed in bone marrow aspiration, together with other characteristic clinical features of multiple myeloma such as hypercalcemia, renal failure and osteolytic foci, support a diagnosis of IgM MM much more frequently than a diagnosis of WM. These differential diagnostics may not be easy. Cytogenetic tests are helpful in these situations. Recent study results indicate that the presence of translocation t(11;14) associated with deregulation of cyclin D1 is specific for MM, but not for WM [Avet-Loiseau et al. 2003]. Another differentiating feature is that 6q deletion istypical of WM [Schop et al. 2006]. Some authors, however, indicate the limited sensitivity of cytogenetic testing in diagnosing MM IgM and therefore seek other differential diagnostic tests [Schuster et al. 2010]. One would be an increased expression of interleukin-1b (IL-1b). This substance is responsible for the increased production of interleukin 6 (IL-6) reported in patients with MM [Donovan et al. 2002]. The treatment of patients with IgM MM does not differ substantially from the treatment of patients with the classic form of MM. Some studies however, indicate a significantly worse prognosis compared with the classic forms, i.e. a much shorter survival time and progression-free time in patients with the rare form of MM [Morris et al. 2010]. Mean survival time is 30 months and myeloablative chemotherapy does not alter this prognosis [Reece et al. 2010, Schuster et al. 2010].

IgE myeloma is very rarely detected. Several cases of this variant have been described [Invernizzi et al. 1991, Hagihara et al. 2010, Chiu et al. 2010]. It manifests itself by the frequent presence of plasma cells in peripheral blood, osteoblastic lesions, hepatosplenomegaly and amyloidosis. The clinical course of this form of MM is usually aggressive and patients have a shorter survival time than those with the classic forms (16 months on average). This may be a result of a delayed diagnosis [Macro et al. 1999].

4. Plasma cell leukaemia

Plasma cell leukaemia is one of the most aggressive forms of MM. It is defined according to the Kyle criteria. Diagnosis is predicated on there being at least 20% plasma cells in a peripheral blood smear and/or the absolute number of plasma cells in the peripheral blood exceeding 2 G/l with a concomitant monoclonal gammopathy [Sher et al. 2010, Jimenez-Zepeda]. It should be noted that the presence of plasma cells in peripheral blood is symptomatic of several infectious diseases, e.g. septic shock, parvovirus B19 infection, infectious mononucleosis, and Dengue fever. These diseases, however, are not accompanied by the presence of monoclonal protein and the plasmacytosis abates with the other symptoms [Gawoski, Ooi 2003, Bai et al. 2006].

Plasma cell leukaemia is rare. It is estimated to constitute 0.5-3% of MM [Han et al. 2008]. Two forms of the disease should be distinguished: a primary form identified in the initial diagnosis; and a secondary form symptomatic of pre-existing classic MM. The primary form was more frequent than the secondary in previous analyses, but the number of patients with the primary and secondary forms is now similar [Sher et al.]. Complex cytogenetic abnormalities are found in 70% of cases of plasma cell leukaemia. These usually include hypodiploidia and structural abnormalities of chromosomes 1, 13 and 14 that are similar in both forms of the disease [Fonseca et al. 2004, Chang et al. 2009, Colovic et al. 2008]. Plasma cell leukaemia is the most aggressive clinical form of MM. Patients usually manifest extraosseous infiltrations, often with the involvement of the central nervous system, and accompanied by *organomegaly* and lymphadenopathy. The aggressiveness of the disease is also demonstrated by the significantly increased activity of serum lactate dehydrogenase, high levels of β2-microglobulin (in 65% of patients > 6 mg/l) and low serum albumin levels.

The prognosis remains poor, especially in the secondary form, where it is a consequence of the progression of the disease and increasing *chemoresistance*. Moreover, resistance very quickly develops in patients with primary leukaemia, despite their initial response to treatment. The average survival time is 8 months for patients with the primary form and 2 months for those with the secondary form [Garcia-Sanz et al. 1999, Tiedemann et al. 2008]. Because of the low incidence of the disease, there are no randomized controlled trials and thus no therapeutic recommendations. Traditional schemes for treatment of MM are usually ineffective. Even though prolongation of survival time was reported in patients after myeloablative chemotherapy assisted by autotransplantation, this treatment was less effective than it was in patients with the classic form of the disease. Allotransplantation is an alternative, especially in the primary disease, which often affects younger people. Due to the limited number of patients and lack of randomized studies, the effects of this treatment are difficult to assess, but previous reports indicate moderate effectiveness and high mortality (the mean survival time is 3 months) [Yeh et al. 1999].

New drugs, such as proteasome inhibitors and immunomodulatory drugs, are promising, although the effectiveness of this treatment remains unsatisfactory. As thalidomide is of limited efficacy and seems to have no significant effect on prolonging survival time in patients with plasma cell leukaemia (reported mean survival time is 3 months) [Petrucci et al. 2007], other authors have been presenting more promising data (survival time up to 14 months) [Johnston, Abdalla 2002]. The use of lenalidomide has enabled a response to be obtained in individual patients, as with resistance to other schemes, but this usually lasts 4-5 months [Musto et al. 2008, Benson and Smith 2007]. The results of bortezomib treatment are slightly more promising. This therapy, especially the combination therapy (VDT-PACE), enables a response to be obtained in more than 90% of patients, including those in whom the disease is initially chemoresistant. Mean survival time is 7-12 months [Albarracin, Fonseca 2011, Musto et al. 2007], although survival times of up to 20 months have also been reported [Sher et al. 2010, Ali et al. 2007]. Bortezomib appears to be able to overcome the adverse effects of cytogenetic abnormalities [Katodritou et al. 2009] – as it does with classic MM – and should therefore be considered a first-line treatment in patients with plasma cell leukaemia.

5. POEMS syndrome

The syndrome was first described in 1956 and was originally named the Crow–Fucasi syndrome. Since 1980, it has been known by the acronym POEMS, derived from the symptoms polyneuropathy, enlarged internal organs (organomegaly), endocrine disorders, monoclonal protein and skin changes.

The pathogenesis of POEMS syndrome is complex and not fully understood. The starting point must be the mutation of the plasma cells producing the light chains (usually λ) as this is what causes its clonal expansion. Karyotype tests of plasma cells usually reveal aneuploidy [Rose et al. 1997] and del13 [Bryce et al. 2007]. Whether a neoplastic clone produces its characteristic symptoms through the direct action of monoclonal protein on some target molecules and the secretion of various cytokines from neoplastic cells, or whether it happens in an indirect manner, is not precisely known. It is believed that high levels of pro-angiogenic and pro-inflammatory cytokines, especially IL-1β, TNF-α, IL-6 and a concentration of vascular endothelial growth factor (VEGF) are essential to the development of the clinical symptoms of POEMS syndrome [Gherardi et al. 1996, Hitoshi et al. 1994].

VEGF is considered to be the most important cytokine responsible for the development of POEMS syndrome. This is the cytokine that reacts with endothelial cells and causes the rapid and reversible increase in vascular filtration essential to angiogenesis and osteogenesis [Endo et al. 2002, Soubrier et al. 1997]. The increased production of VEGF is also a result of high concentrations of IL-1 and IL-6 [Soubrier et al. 1997]. VEGF 165 isoform is most commonly diagnosed. The concentration of VEGF correlates with the progression of the disease, but does not depend on the concentration of monoclonal protein [Watanabe et al. 1998].

POEMS syndrome is very rare. The incidence in Japan is 3 cases per million people per year [Arimura et al. 2007], and this is estimated to be even less in Western Europe and the United States of America. The peak incidence of POEMS syndrome occurs during the fifth and the sixth decades of life [Dispenzieri et al. 2007]. POEMS syndrome is a chronic disease and some patients live more than 10 years. Dispenzieri et al. have found that the mean survival time of patients with POEMS is 13.8 years [Dispenzieri et al. 2003]. In turn, Gherardi et al. have found that 7 out of 15 patients with POEMS syndrome live 5 years or more, including one case of 25 years [Gherardi et al. 1991].

The criteria for diagnosing POEMS syndrome are summarized in Table 3.

The characteristic symptoms of POEMS syndrome should have a temporal relationship. The most important symptom, i.e. the one that enables POEMS to be differentiated from other plasma cell dyscrasias, is the ascertainment of single or multiple osteosclerotic changes. A conclusive diagnosis of POEMS syndrome is unlikely in the absence of bone changes. Skin changes, most commonly hypertrichosis and hyperpigmentation, may occur in POEMS patients. Enlarged mammary glands and testicular atrophy may occur in men. Peripheral blood count abnormalities, especially thrombocythemia and polyglobulia, are frequently detected by morphological examinations.

The concentrations of serum monoclonal protein and the level of Bence-Jones protein in urine are lower than in patients with MM. Renal failure, high calcium plasma concentration, and pathological bone fractures are rarely observed. The percentage of plasma cells is usually less than 5% in bone marrow examinations. High concentrations of IL-1β, TNF-α, IL-6 and VEGF in serum are typical of POEMS [Soubrier et al. 1997].

Polyneuropathy is the predominant clinical symptom (100% of patients with POEMS syndrome) [Kelly Jr. et al. 1983]. Initially, sensory disturbances occur mainly in the lower limbs.

Gait disorders may appear later. This process is progressive and movement is difficult in 50% of patients. This can eventually cause disability. Bone pain and pathologic fractures are rare. Other symptoms include progressive weight loss and muscle atrophy.

About 1/3 of patients develop ascites and fluid in the pleural cavities [Dispenzieri et al. 2007]. In 50% of patients, the liver, and less frequently the spleen and the lymph nodes, is enlarged. A histopathological examination of the enlarged lymph node often indicates angiofollicular lymph node hyperplasia (Castleman's disease) [Dispenzieri et al. 2003, Nakanishi et al. 1984]. Some patients may develop venous and arterial thrombosis [Kang et al. 2003]. Impaired secretion of endocrine glands, most commonly hypogonadism, hypothyroidism, glucose metabolism and adrenal insufficiency, is diagnosed in about 84% of patients. Most patients have impaired secretion in four or more endocrine glands. This may be accompanied by failure of the gonads, thyroid, pancreas and adrenal glands.

Because the predominant symptom is polyneuropathy, patients with POEMS syndrome are initially referred to neurologists - usually with suspected Guillain-Barré syndrome or chronic inflammatory demyelinating polyradiculoneuropathy.

Once the monoclonal protein accompanying the polyneuropathy has been detected, a differential diagnosis should include AL, monoclonal gammopathy and MM.

The concentration of VEGF is one of the most sensitive tests to differentiate POEMS syndrome from the other diseases mentioned above. The plasma of patients with POEMS syndrome has a high VEGF concentration. VEGF concentration in patients with the other diseases mentioned above is low [Gherardi et al. 1996, Watanabe et al. 1998].

The rare incidence of POEMS syndrome and the lack of definitive knowledge as to its causes mean that there are no standards of treatment. For the same reason, there are no randomized clinical trial results to evaluate the effectiveness of any given method of treatment. Methods of treating POEMS syndrome patients have mainly been devised from clinical reports, case reports and retrospective observations (usually at a single centre), and the experience gained from treating other plasma cells *dyscrasias*.

Radiotherapy is the treatment of choice for POEMS syndrome patients with isolated bone lesions. If there are numerous bone changes and these coexist with other symptoms typical of POEMS syndrome, it is recommended that patients be treated similarly to those with MM. In older patients, the treatment is based on alkylating drugs, while the therapy for younger patients includes high-dose chemotherapy-assisted auto-SCT [Dispenzieri et al. 2003].

The final confirmation of the hypothesis that VEGF is the major cytokine responsible for the development of POEMS syndrome, will have a significant impact on changing the way that POEMS patients are treated; the way which will be predominantly focused on VEGF..Neither intravenous immunoglobulins nor plasmapheresis treatments benefit patients with POEMS syndrome [Dispenzieri et al. 2007]. The concomitant treatment with plasmapheresis and corticosteroids was found to be more effective [Ku et al. 1995]. Melphalan is the drug that has been used to treat *dyscrasias* the longest. The results of retrospective studies, in which melphalan was mainly used in combination with prednisone (the treatment duration was 12-24 months), indicate that a response to the treatment was obtained in 40% of patients [Dispenzieri et al. 2003]. Cyclophosphamide allows for remission of the disease in a limited number of patients. This treatment may be used in young patients who are candidates for auto-SCT.

The results of high-dose chemotherapy-assisted auto-SCT are promising [Sanada et al. 2006], as a response is obtained in over 90% of patients (Table 4). Transplant related mortality is determined to be approximately 7%. This is higher than in MM patients treated with auto-SCT and lower than in AL patients treated with auto-SCT [Gertz et al. 2002]. High dose chemotherapy assisted auto-SCT reduces the symptoms of polyneuropathy. When combined with radiotherapy, this reduction can last months or even years [Ganti et al. 2005]. The clinical response to the treatment correlates more closely to the VEGF concentration than to the monoclonal protein level [Nakano et al. 2001]. A *complete* haematological remission is not required to obtain a clinical improvement. The effectiveness of the most common ways of treating patients with POEMS syndrome is shown in Table 4.

Treatment	Response to the treatment	References
Corticosteroids	≥15%	Dispenzieri et al. 2003 Nakanishi et al. 1984 Orefice et al. 1994
Treatment with alkylating drugs	≥40%	Dispenzieri et al. 2003 Reitan et al. 1980
Radiation therapy	≥50%	Dispenzieri et al. 2003 Iwashita et al. 1977 Reitan et al. 1980
Auto-SCT	≥90%	Sanada et al. 2006 Ganti et al. 2005 Jaccard et al. 2002

Auto-SCT (*auto-stem cells transplantation*) – autologous transplantation of the stem cells obtained from peripheral blood.

Table 4. The effectiveness of the most commonly used treatments in patients with POEMS syndrome.

Apart from the methods of treating POEMS syndrome mentioned above, there are few reports on the effectiveness of therapy combined with bevacizumab and thalidomide in patients diagnosed with a relapse of POEMS syndrome after auto-SCT. The combination of cyclophosphamide, dexamethasone and bevacizumab is another example of a modern combination therapy, described by Samaras et al., to treat POEMS syndrome relapse after auto-PBSCT [Badros et al. 2005, Straume et al. 2006]. There are also case reports describing the treatment of patients with POEMS syndrome using lenalidomide [Dispenzieri et al. 2007]. Recently, Szturz et al. [2012] reported on the successful application of lenalidomide in Castleman disease, a condition that can accompany POEMS syndrome. Other drugs used to treat POEMS syndrome patients include interferon α [Coto et al. 1991], tamoxifen, trans retinoic acid, thalidomide, ticlopidine, argatroban and strontium (^{89}Sr) [Dispenzieri et al. 2007]. The effectiveness of these drugs is limited and further clinical trials are required.

Lenalidomide seems to be one of the most promising immunomodulatory drugs to treat POEMS syndrome, but further clinical studies are required [Dispenzieri et al. 2007].

High dose chemotherapy assisted auto-SCT remains the best therapeutic method, although it also has the highest mortality rate.

6. Rare paraneoplastic syndromes accompanying myeloma

Sweet's syndrome is one of the paraneoplastic syndromes that may accompany MM. This is a group of symptoms including granolocytosis, fever and painful erythematous skin changes caused by skin *granulocytic* infiltrations that subside following treatment with corticosteroids [Paydas et al. 1993]. These changes are also found in the mouth, the joints and the internal organs. Sweet's syndrome is extremely rare (0.25% of patients with MM) and is most likely caused by an increased sensitivity to the growth factor. This can be explained by an increased production of interleukin 6 (IL-6) [Bayer-Garner, Cottler-Fox, Smoller 2003].

Bullous epidermal separation (epidermolisis bullosa) may also coexist with MM. This is associated with the production of IgG antibodies against the *non-collagenous* domain of type VII collagen. This leads to the formation of subepidermal bubbles and secondary ulcers [Radfar 2006]. Pemphigus has a similar clinical picture. This is a rare complication observed in MM patients and is usually associated with IgA MM. This disease develops extremely rarely and is sometimes also associated with gammopathy of undetermined significance. It has been suggested that treatment should include bortezomib [Adam et al. 2010]. There are many skin symptoms associated with monoclonal gammopathy: leukocytoclastic vasculitis, pyoderma gangrenosum and Schnitzler syndrome. These, however, are rare and discussing them is beyond the scope of this chapter [Harati et al. 2005].

7. Family myeloma

The cause of MM remains unknown [Lynch et al. 2008, Alexander et al. 2007, Morgan, Davies, Lineta 2002]. It seems that the hereditary cause is negligible, although family cases of this cancer have been observed. It has also been described in connection with gammopathy of undetermined significance [Lynch et al. 2008]. Large population studies also indicate that MM, prostate cancer and malignant melanoma run in families, as do central nervous system neoplasms, although the results of some studies do not confirm this [Eriksson, Hallberg 1992, Camp, Werner, Cannon-Albright, 2008]. The risk of familial MM is small. It is estimated that the probability of first-degree relatives developing MM is 3.2 per 1000 cases and women are usually affected. Autosomal inheritance with low gene *penetrance* is believed to be responsible for the onset of the disease. The risk of familial gammopathy of undetermined significance is slightly higher, although still small. Had there been at least two cases of MM in first or second-degree relatives, an annual immunoelectrophoresis of the urine and serum protein in people 40 years and over would be recommended. If MM had occurred in anyone under 40 years old, the test would be recommended to relatives 35 years and over [Gerkes et al. 2007].

The described forms of MM are extremely rare. They are an important diagnostic problem because of their atypical clinical manifestation. The course of the disease is usually aggressive and the prognosis is serious. It is therefore essential that it be quickly and accurately diagnosed. The lack of prospective studies of large groups of patients is an additional problem. This makes these atypical clinical forms a therapeutic as well as a diagnostic challenge.

Author details

Artur Jurczyszyn

Department of Haematology University Hospital, Cracow, Poland

References

[1] Adam Z. et al. IgA pemphigus associated with monoclonal gammopathy completely resolved after achievement of complete remission of multiple myeloma with bortezomib, cyclophosphamide and dexamethasone regimen. Wien Klin Wochenschr 2010; 122: 311–314.

[2] Albarracin F., Fonseca R. *Plasma cell leukemia.* Blood Rev 2011 Feb 2.

[3] Alexander D.D. et al. *Multiple myeloma: a review of the epidemiologic literature.* Int J Cancer 2007; 120 (suppl. 12): 40–61.

[4] Ali R. et al. Efficacy of bortezomib in combination chemotherapy on secondary plasma cell leukemia. Leuk Lymphoma 2007; 48: 1426–1428.

[5] Arimura K., Hashiguchi T. *Crow-Fukase syndrome: clinical features, pathogenesis and treatment in Japan*. W: Yamamura T., Kira J., Tabira T. (red.) *Current topics in neuroimmunology*. Bologna 2007: 241–245.

[6] Avet-Loiseau H. et al. Translocation t(11;14)(q13;q32) is the hallmark of IgM, IgE, and nonsecretory multiple myeloma variants. Blood 2003; 101: 1570–1571.

[7] Bai L.Y. et al. Acalculous cholecystitis mimicking plasma cell leukemia. Ann Hematol 2006; 85: 487–488.

[8] Badros A., Porter N., Zimrin A. *Bevacizumab therapy for POEMS syndrome.* Blood 2005; 106: 1135.

[9] Bayer-Garner I.B., Cottler-Fox M., Smoller B.R. *Sweet syndrome in multiple myeloma: a series of six cases.* J Cutan Pathol 2003; 30: 261–264.

[10] Benson D.M. Jr., Smith M.K. *Effectiveness of lenalidomide (Revlimid) for the treatment of plasma cell leukemia.* Leuk Lymphoma 2007; 48: 1423–1425.

[11] Blade J., Kyle R.A. *Nonsecretory myeloma, immunoglobulin D myeloma, and plasma cell leukemia.* Hematol Oncol Clin North Am 1999; 13: 1259–1272.

[12] Blade J., Lust J.A., Kyle R.A. *Immunoglobulin D multiple myeloma: presenting features, response to therapy, and survival in a series of 53 cases.* J Clin Oncol 1994; 12: 2398–1404.

[13] Bryce A.H., Ketterling R.P., Gertz M.A. et al. *Cytogenetic analysis using multiple myeloma targets in POEMS syndrome. Proceedings of American Society of Oncology Meeting.* Chicago 2007.

[14] Camp N.J., Werner T.L., Cannon-Albright L.A. *Familial myeloma.* N Engl J Med 2008; 359: 1734–1735; author reply 1735.

[15] Chang H. et al. Genetic aberrations including chromosome 1 abnormalities and clinical features of plasma cell leukemia. Leuk Res 2009; 33: 259–262.

[16] Chiu W. et al. IgE-type multiple myeloma with the late development of IgA2 kappa and plasma cell leukaemia. Pathology 2010; 42: 82–84.

[17] Colovic M. et al. Thirty patients with primary plasma cell leukemia: a single center experience. Med Oncol 2008; 25: 154–160.

[18] Coto V., Auletta M., Oliviero U. et al. *POEMS syndrome: an Italian case with diagnostic and therapeutic implications.* Ann Ital Med Interna 1991; 6: 416–419.

[19] Dispenzieri A., Kyle R.A., Lacy M.Q. et al. *POEMS syndrome: definitions and long-term outcome.* Blood 2003; 101: 2496–2506.

[20] Dispenzieri A., Klein C.J., Mauermann M.L. *Lenalidomide therapy in a patient with POEMS syndrome.* Blood 2007; 110: 1075–1076.

[21] Donovan K.A. et al. IL-1beta expression in IgM monoclonal gammopathy and its relationship to multiple myeloma. Leukemia 2002; 16: 382–385.

[22] Durie B.G. et al. International uniform response criteria for multiple myeloma. Leukemia 2006; 20: 1467–1473.

[23] Endo I., Mitsui T., Nishino M. et al. *Diurnal fluctuation of edema synchronized with plasma VEGF concentration in a patient with POEMS syndrome.* Intern Med 2002; 41: 1196–1198.

[24] Eriksson M., Hallberg B. *Familial occurrence of hematologic malignancies and other diseases in multiple myeloma: a case-control study.* Cancer Causes Control 1992; 3: 63–67.

[25] Fonseca R. et al. Genetics and cytogenetics of multiple myeloma: a workshop report. Cancer Res 2004; 64: 1546–1558.

[26] Garcia-Sanz R. et al. Primary plasma cell leukemia: clinical, immunophenotypic, DNA ploidy, and cytogenetic characteristics. Blood 1999; 93: 1032–1037.

[27] Ganti A.K., Pipinos I., Culcea E. et al. *Successful hematopoietic stem-cell transplantation inmulticentric Castleman disease complicated by POEMS syndrome.* Am J Hematol 2005; 79: 206–210.

[28] Gawoski J.M., Ooi W.W. *Dengue fever mimicking plasma cell leukemia.* Arch Pathol Lab Med 2003; 127: 1026–1027.

[29] Gerkes E.H. et al. Familial multiple myeloma: report on two families and discussion of screening options. Hered Cancer Clin Pract 2007; 5: 72–78.

[30] Gertz M.A., Lacy M.Q., Dispenzieri A. et al. *Stem cell transplantation for the management of primary systemic amyloidosis.* Am J Med 2002; 113: 549–555.

[31] Gherardi R.K., Belec L., Soubrier M. et al. *Overproduction of proinflammatory cytokines imbalanced by their antagonists in POEMS syndrome.* Blood 1996; 87: 1458–1465.

[32] Gherardi R.K., Malapert D., Degos J.D. *Castleman disease – POEMS syndrome overlap* [letter; comment]. Ann. Intern Med 1991; 114: 520–521.

[33] Hagihara M. et al. An unusual case of IgE-multiple myeloma presenting with systemic amyloidosis 2 years after cervical plasmacytoma resection. Int J Hematol 2010; 92: 381–385.

[34] Han X. et al. Lymphoma survival patterns by WHO subtype in the United States, 1973–2003. Cancer Causes Control, 2008; 19: 841–858.

[35] Harati A. et al. Skin disorders in association with monoclonal gammopathies. Eur J Med Res 2005; 10: 93–104.

[36] Hitoshi S., Suzuki K., Sakuta M. *Elevated serum interleukin-6 in POEMS syndrome reflects the activity of the disease.* Intern Med 1994; 33: 25–33.

[37] Homan, H. et al. IgD multiple myeloma with renal involvement: case report. Jpn J Med 1990; 29: 212–215.

[38] Invernizzi F. et al. *A new case of IgE myeloma.* Acta Haematol 1991; 85: 41–44.

[39] Iwashita H., Ohnishi A., Asada M. et al. *Polyneuropathy, skin hyperpigmentation, edema, and hypertrichosis in localized osteosclerotic myeloma.* Neurology 1977; 27: 675–681.

[40] Jaccard A., Royer B., Bordessoule D. et al. *High-dose therapy and autologous blood stem cell transplantation in POEMS syndrome.* Blood 2002; 99: 3057–3059.

[41] Jancelewicz Z. et al. *IgD multiple myeloma. Review of 133 cases.* Arch Intern Med 1975; 135: 87–93.

[42] Jimenez-Zepeda V.H., Dominguez V.J. *Plasma cell leukemia: a rare condition.* Ann Hematol 2006; 85: 263–267.

[43] Johnston R.E., Abdalla S.H. *Thalidomide in low doses is effective for the treatment of resistant or relapsed multiple myeloma and for plasma cell leukaemia.* Leuk Lymphoma 2002; 43: 351–354.

[44] Kang K., Chu K., Kim D.E. et al. *POEMS syndrome associated with ischemic stroke.* Arch Neurol 2003; 60: 745–749.

[45] Katodritou E. et al. Extramedullary (EMP) relapse in unusual locations in multiple myeloma: Is there an association with precedent thalidomide administration and a correlation of special biological features with treatment and outcome? Leuk Res 2009; 33: 1137–1140.

[46] Kelly J.J. Jr., Kyle R.A., Miles J.M., Dyck P.J. *Osteosclerotic myeloma and peripheral neuropathy.* Neurology 1983; 33: 202–210.

[47] Kuliszkiewicz-Janus M. et al. Immunoglobulin D myeloma – problems with diagnosing and staging (own experience and literature review). Leuk Lymphoma 2005; 46: 1029–1037.

[48] Kyle R.A. et al. Review of 1027 patients with newly diagnosed multiple myeloma. Mayo Clin Proc 2003; 78: 21–33.

[49] Kyle R.A., Rajkumar S.V. *Criteria for diagnosis, staging, risk stratification and response assessment of multiple myeloma.* Leukemia 2009; 23: 3–9.

[50] Lynch H.T. et al. *Familial myeloma.* N Engl J Med 2008; 359: 152–157.

[51] MacLennan I.C. *In which cells does neoplastic transformation occur in myelomatosis?* Curr Top Microbiol Immunol 1992; 182: 209–214.

[52] Macro M. et al. *IgE multiple myeloma.* Leuk Lymphoma 1999; 32: 597–603.

[53] Maisnar V. et al. High-dose chemotherapy followed by autologous stem cell transplantation changes prognosis of IgD multiple myeloma. Bone Marrow Transplant 2008; 41: 51–54.

[54] Merlini G., Stine M.J. *Dangerous small B-cell clones.* Blood 2006; 108: 2520–2530.

[55] Morris C. et al. Efficacy and outcome of autologous transplantation in rare myelomas. Haematologica 2010; 95: 2126–2133.

[56] Musto P. et al. Efficacy and safety of bortezomib in patients with plasma cell leukemia. Cancer 2007; 109: 2285–2290.

[57] Musto P. et al. Salvage therapy with lenalidomide and dexamethasone in relapsed primary plasma cell leukemia. Leuk Res 2008; 32: 1637–1638.

[58] Nakanishi T., Sobue I., Toyokura Y. et al. *The Crow-Fukase syndrome: a study of 102 cases in Japan.* Neurology 1984; 34: 712–720.

[59] Nakano A., Mitsui T., Endo I. et al. *Solitary plasmacytoma with VEGF overproduction: report of a patient with polyneuropathy*. Neurology 2001; 56: 818–819.

[60] Orefice G., Morra V.B., De Michele G. et al. *POEMS syndrome: clinical, pathological and immunological study of a case*. Neurol Res 1994; 16: 477–480.

[61] Paydas S. et al. *Sweet's syndrome associated with G-CSF*. Br J Haematol 1993; 85: 191–192.

[62] Petrucci M.T. et al. Thalidomide does not modify the prognosis of plasma cell leukemia patients: experience of a single center. Leuk Lymphoma 2007; 48: 180–182.

[63] Rajkumar S.V. *Multiple myeloma: 2011 update on diagnosis, risk-stratification, and management*. Am J Hematol 2011; 86: 57–65.

[64] Radfar L. et al. Paraneoplastic epidermolysis bullosa acquisita associated with multiple myeloma. Spec Care Dentist 2006; 26: 159–163.

[65] Reece D.E. et al. Outcome of patients with IgD and IgM multiple myeloma undergoing autologous hematopoietic stem cell transplantation: a retrospective CIBMTR Study. Clin Lymphoma Myeloma Leuk 2010; 10: 458–463.

[66] Reitan J.B., Pape E., Fossa S.D. et al. *Osteosclerotic myeloma with polyneuropathy*. Acta Med Scand 1980; 208: 137–144.

[67] Rose C., Zandecki M., Copin M.C. et al. *POEMS syndrome: report on six patients with unusual clinical signs, elevated levels of cytokines, macrophage involvement and chromosomal aberrations of bone marrow plasma cells*. Leukemia 1997; 11: 1318–1323.

[68] Sanada S., Ookawara S., Karube H. et al. *Marked recovery of severe renal lesions in POEMS syndrome with high-dose melphalan therapy supported by autologous blood stem cell transplantation*. Am J Kidney Dis 2006; 47: 672–679.

[69] Schop R.F. et al. 6q deletion discriminates Waldenstrom macroglobulinemia from IgM monoclonal gammopathy of undetermined significance. Cancer Genet Cytogenet 2006; 169: 150–153.

[70] Schuster S.R. et al. IgM multiple myeloma: disease definition, prognosis, and differentiation from Waldenstrom's macroglobulinemia. Am J Hematol 2010; 85: 853–855.

[71] Sharma M. et al. The outcome of IgD myeloma after autologous hematopoietic stem cell transplantation is similar to other Ig subtypes. Am J Hematol 2010; 85: 502–504.

[72] Sher T. et al. Plasma cell leukaemia and other aggressive plasma cell malignancies. Br J Haematol 2010; 150: 418–427.

[73] Shimamoto Y., Anami Y., Yamaguchi M. *A new risk grouping for IgD myeloma based on analysis of 165 Japanese patients*. Eur J Haematol 1991; 47: 262–267.

[74] Singh D., Kumar L. *Myelomatous ascites in multiple myeloma*. Leuk Lymphoma 2005; 46: 631–632.

[75] Soubrier M., Dubost J.J., Serre A.F. et al. *Growth factors in POEMS syndrome: evidence for a marked increase in circulating vascular endothelial growth factor*. Arthritis Rheum 1997; 40: 786–787.

[76] Straume O., Bergheim J., Ernst P. *Bevacizumab therapy for POEMS syndrome*. Blood 2006; 107: 4973–4974.

[77] Szturz P. et al. *Lenalidomide: a new treatment option for Castleman disease*. Leuk Lymphoma 2012; 53: 2089–2091.

[78] Terpos E. et al. Plasmacytoma relapses in the absence of systemic progression post-high-dose therapy for multiple myeloma. Eur J Haematol 2005; 75: 376–383.

[79] Tiedemann R.E. et al. *Genetic aberrations and survival in plasma cell leukemia.* Leukemia 2008; 22: 1044–1052.

[80] Watanabe O., Maruyama I., Arimura K. et al. *Overproduction of vascular endothelial growth factor/vascular permeability factor is causative in Crow-Fukase (POEMS) syndrome*. Muscle Nerve 1998; 21: 1390–1397.

[81] Yeh K.H. et al. Long-term disease-free survival after autologous bone marrow transplantation in a primary plasma cell leukaemia: detection of minimal residual disease in the transplant marrow by third-complementarity-determining region-specific probes. Br J Haematol 1995; 89: 914–916.

Chapter 13

Pain and Multiple Myeloma

Emine Ozyuvaci, Onat Akyol and Tolga Sitilci

Additional information is available at the end of the chapter

http://dx.doi.org/10.5772/55528

1. Introduction

Multiple myeloma is a plasma cell malignancy characterized with clonal expansion of malignant plasma cells within the bone marrow and followed by osteolytic bone disease. It accounts for approximately 1% of all malignant diseases and represents about 10% of hematologic malignancies. Data from cloning and gene-sequencing studies strongly imply that the malignant clone in MM arises from a late cell in B-cell development. Investigation of a patient with suspected myeloma should include the screening tests. Electrophoresis of serum and concentrated urine should be performed, followed by immunofixation to confirm and type any M-protein present.

The common clinical presentations are fatigue and bone pain with or without associated fractures or infection. Mechanical impacts like intraosseous tumor pressure, microfractures, periost irritation, muscle spasm, nerve entrapment and compression of nerves by the collapsed vertebrae are reasons of severe myeloma pain.

Radiographic skeletal survey and bone marrow aspiration and biopsy are performed for diagnosis. Angtuaco EJ et al reported a radiologic review and explained that MR imaging bone marrow surveys in patients with MM demonstrate the broad spectrum of involvement, the results of treatment, the areas of potential complications, and the sites of focal disease for safe bone biopsies [1].

Pain characteristics clinically can be summarised as, pain is worse in supine position, especially at night or awakens from sleep, band like distribution around body, not relieved with rest and nonsteroidal anti-inflammatory drugs (NSAIDS), associated symptoms like fever, weight loss and progressive neurologic deficite in lower extremities. Somatic, visceral and neuropathic components can be easily involved in myeloma pain [2].

Chronic pain is extremely prevalent among patients with cancer. According to studies cancer pain can be relieved in more than 70% of patients using a simple opioid- based regimen.

Whether there is a relatively lesser degree of opioid responsiveness in chronic cancer pain, then adjuvant analgesics are neccessary. Adjuvant analgesics describe the drug with a primary indication other than pain, but with analgesic properties in some painful conditions, they are usually coadministered with analgesics (acetaminophen, NSAIDS, opioids) when treating cancer pain. Common causes of chronic pain in cancer patients as multiple myeloma patients are releated to peripheral neuropathy due to chemotheraphy, radiotheraphy and tumor invasion, chronic postsurgical incisional pain, phantom pain, musculoskeletal pain, visceral pain from viscera or tumor.

The pain is one of the most common symptoms at diagnosis experienced by myeloma patients and it may also be an indicator of a subsequent relapse. Up to 67% of patients report pain at diagnosis, although this may have been present for several months before [3]. At diagnosis, pain may be due to the disease process itself (predominantly from destructive bone disease, but occasionally from plasmacytomas directly affecting neural tissues), or it may signify a co-morbidity (e.g. degenerative arthritis or osteoporosis).

Later in the course of the disease, pain often arises as a sideeffect of therapies, e.g. thalidomide or bortezomib neuropathy. Particularly in older patients, it is important to always consider co-morbidities, such as arthritis or osteoporosis, mimicking bony malignant pain; diabetes or carpal tunnel syndrome mimicking peripheral neuropathy (PN); and postherpetic neuralgia as a common cause of persistent pain.

Assessment of pain, should start with taking a history but may involve imaging by X ray, bone scan, CT or MRI. Myeloma patients should be evaluated for the presence and severity of pain regularly. Pain severity can be assessed by visual analogue scales (VAS), numerical rated scales (NRS) or verbal rated scales (VRS) [4]. To diagnose the presence of neuropathic pain, the Leeds assessment of neuropathic symptoms and signs scale (LANSS) can be used [5].

The pain is usually in constant and dull at first but, as the disease progresses, it becomes more severe until it is agonizing and constant. Severity of pain may be particularly devastating and can negatively affect the quality of patient life and their functional status. This should be managed using a multi-modal, mechanism-based approach including evidence-based pharmacological therapies alongside non-drug methods such as radiotherapy, bisphosphonates, and where appropriate, interventional and psychological techniques.

The critical importance of pain management as part of routine cancer care has been forcefully advanced by WHO, international and national professional organisations, and governmental agencies.

American Pain Society Quality of Care Task Force reviewed recommendations for faciliating improvements in the quality of cancer pain management.

- Recognize and treat pain promptly (emphasis on comprehensive assessment and importance of preventive and prompt treatment based on evidence for neuroplasticity)
- Involve patients and families in pain management plan (emphasis on customization of care and participation of patient in treatment plan)

- Improve treatment patterns (eliminate inappropriate practices, provide multimodal therapy)
- Reassess and adjust pain management plan as needed (respond not only to pain intensity but to functional status and side effects)
- Monitor processes and outcomes of pain management (new standardized indicators and comments about forthcoming national performance indicators)

According to the European Society of Medical Oncology (ESMO) clinical practice guidelines with WHO ladder, general approach to management of cancer pain is,

STEP I: Mild pain (NRS: 1–4) is treated with non-opioid analgesics such as acetaminophen/ paracetamol or a NSAID

Paracetamol is a useful analgesic in cancer-related pain and other chronic pains and should be prescribed at a dose of up to 1 gram qid (p.o. or i.v. in patients who cannot take oral medication, e.g. because of vomiting or mucositis).

NSAIDS should be avoided apart from very short term use (eg 3-5 days) with acute severe pain, eg bone fracture. They should not be used in the presence of renal impairment, and used with extreme caution in myeloma patients in view of the risk of precipitating renal compromise

For patients with mild pain (<5/10), normal release tramadol is a reasonable choice of analgesic agent. Tramadol has 1/5th the potency of oral morphine and the starting dose is 50mg 6 hourly prn or qid. Codeine can also be used but it is a pro-drug of morphine, and 10-15% of the population is unable to convert it into active morphine, leaving them with unacceptable toxicity [6].

STEP II: Traditionally, patients with moderate pain (NRS: 5–7) have been treated with a combination product containing acetaminophen plus a weak immediate-release opioid

For patients with mild to moderate pain or whose pain is not adequately controlled by paracetamol or a NSAID given regularly by mouth, the addition of a step II opioid (eg, codeine or tramadol; table 1) given orally might achieve good pain relief without troublesome adverse effects. Alternatively, low doses of a step III opioid (eg, morphine or oxycodone; table 1) may be used instead of codeine or tramadol.

STEP III: In severe pain (NRS: 8–10), morphine, oxycodone, and hydromorphone can use and the data show no important differences between morphine, oxycodone, and hydromorphone given by the oral route. Morphine is most commonly used. Oral administration is the preferred route. If given parenterally, the equivalent dose is one-third of the oral medication. The buccal, sublingual and nebulized routes of administration of morphine are not recommended because at the present time there is no evidence of clinical advantage over the conventional routes.

Patients with chronic moderate (5-7/10) or severe pain (>7/10) can be started on tramadol as above, but will usually need to go onto more potent opioids rapidly if they do not respond. Hydromorphone or oxycodone, in both immediate-release and modified-release formulations for oral administration are effective alternatives to oral morphine. Oxycodone is twice the

Oral opioid	Characteristics and comments
Codeine	Step II drug only: use alone or in combination with paracetamol; daily doses ≥360 mg not recommended
Tramadol	Step II drug only: use alone or in combination with paracetamol; daily doses ≥400 mg not recommended
Hydrocodone	Step II drug only: used as a substitute for codeine in some countries
Oxycodone	Step II opioid when used at low doses (eg, ≤20 mg per day) alone or in combination with paracetamol
Morphine	Step II opioid when used at low doses (eg, ≤30 mg per day)
Hydromorphone	Step II opioid when used at low doses (eg, ≤4 mg per day)

Table 1. Step II opioids

potency of morphine and is associated with less drowsiness and hallucinations. For rapid onset, the normal release preparation can be used 4-6 hourly or qid, but most patients eventually prefer the convenience of the bd sustained release forms [7].

Methadone is a valid alternative but may be more complicated to use because of marked interindividual differences in its plasma half-life and duration of action. Methadone use should be initiated by physicians with experience and expertise in its use. Strong opioids may be combined with ongoing use of a nonopioid analgesic (step I). Patients presenting with severe pain that needs urgent relief should be treated with parenteral opioids, usually administered by the subcutaneous (s.c.) or intravenous (i.v.) route. Intramuscular injections are painful and have no pharmacokinetic advantage.

Patches can be used to deliver either fentanyl or buprenorphine, both of which are very potent opioids. Fentanyl causes significantly less nausea, sedation and constipation compared to morphine [8]. When given the choice of fentanyl patches or oral morphine for chronic pain, patients prefer the patches [9]. They are usually the treatment of choice for patients who are unable to swallow, patients with poor tolerance to morphine and patients with poor compliance. Earlier worries regarding an inferior equipotency ratio of buprenorphine to oral morphine or of a ceiling effect and partial antagonistic effects of buprenorphine as compared with fentanyl have not been substantiated by newer publications [10]. Buprenorphine often initially causes nausea but this can be covered by the use of an anti-emetic such as metoclopramide and is otherwise well tolerated.

Immediate-release and slow-release oral formulations of morphine, oxycodone, and hydromorphone can be used for dose titration. The titration schedules for both types of formulation should be supplemented with oral immediate-release opioids given as needed. When using normal release oral medication, the dose can be titrated up daily by 30-50% until pain is controlled or unacceptable side effects occur. With sustained release oral medication it is advisable to wait 2-3 days between dose increments. With patches, doses should not normally be increased at less than 3 days intervals.

With all sustained release analgesics, it is essential to offer the patient a normal release 'rescue medication' for breakthrough pain. This is particularly important when breakthrough pain occurs quickly and predictably. It is important to distinguish this kind of 'incident pain' from pain arising from end of dose failure with sustained release medications, or spontaneous pains associated with neuropathy or opioid-induced hyperalgesia [11]. The 'breakthrough dose' is usually equivalent to +10% - 15% of the total daily dose. If more than four 'breakthrough doses' per day are necessary, the baseline opioid treatment with a slow-release formulation has to be adapted. Normal release oxycodone or morphine can be used, at 1/6th of the current 24 hour total opioid dose. However, often the absorption of these oral drugs can be too slow for breakthrough pain.. Opioids with a rapid onset and short duration are preferred for breakthrough doses. Fentanyl has a high bioavailability via the transmucosal route, which has led to the development of fast-acting (but short-lived) fentanyl formulations. These include fentanyl lozenges (Actiq ®); buccal tablets (Effentora®); or sublingual tablets [12]. Nasal sprays will also soon be available. Normally, a patient should not need to use more 2–3 of these relatively expensive fentanyl formulations per day for breakthrough pain; if more are being taken, either the background medication needs to be increased or the patient should be referred to a specialist. There is no place for pethidine in the treatment of pain in myeloma.

In addition, there is also worth noting that the recommendations for opioids for breakthrough of the EAPC. The pain exacerbations resulting from uncontrolled background pain should be treated with additional doses of immediate-release oral opioids, and that an appropriate titration of around-the-clock opioid therapy should always precede the recourse to potent rescue opioid analgesics. Breakthrough pain (eg, incident pain) can be effectively managed with oral, immediate-release opioids or with buccal or intranasal fentanyl preparations. In some cases the buccal or intranasal fentanyl preparations are preferable to immediate-release oral opioids because of more-rapid onset of action and shorter duration of effect. Additionally, immediate-release formulations of opioids with short half-lives should be used to treat pre-emptively predictable episodes of breakthrough pain in the 20–30 min preceding the provoking manoeuvre.

With all opioids, it is important to offer the patient a laxative and to keep checking for the development of constipation. Transdermal fentanyl and buprenorphine are associated with reduced incidence of constipation [13]. It is not necessary to routinely prescribe an anti-emetic with opioids, except for the first week when starting buprenorphine.

Respiratory depression is uncommon in patients treated chronically with opioids as long as dose increments are made carefully as outlined above. With the initiation of opioids, it is common to see a reduction in respiratory rate; however, this is usually balanced by changes in tidal volume so that minute ventilation initially remains steady. Care needs to be taken in patients with COPD or obstructive sleep apnoea, in whom the respiratory depression can occur even with low doses of opioids. True respiratory depression caused by opioids is diagnosed by a reduction in oxygen saturation ($SaO2 < 90\%$) or by arterial blood gases. If this occurs, naloxone can be given but care must be taken not to provoke a serious increase in pain. Advice on future opioid dosing should be sought from a specialist in pain or palliative medicine.

Recently a condition known as opioid-induced hyperalgesia has been consistently identified in animal studies and has also been demonstrated to occur in human studies. This condition is characterised by increasing reporting of pain in the presence of increasing opioid dosage. The pain can be localised to the original lesion but is often generalised to adjacent dermatomes. The skin in the affected area may show hyperalgesia (increased pain response on normal painful stimulus) or allodynia (pain felt even on light touch). The treatment involves reduction in the opioid dosage along with the introduction of an NMDA channel blocker such as ketamine or methadone [14].

Most opioids cause dose-related sedation; however, fentanyl and oxycodone are associated with reduced sedation compared to morphine [15]. Patients who experience intolerable sedation due to opioids (or other drugs, e.g. thalidomide) may be considered for a trial of a psychostimulant such as methylphenidate or modafanil; this should only be prescribed by a specialist in palliative medicine. In patients with opioid-related neurotoxic effects (delirium, hallucination, and myoclonus), dose reduction or opioid switching should be considered.

Patients receiving step III opioids who have side-effects and do not achieve adequate analgesia that are severe, unmanageable, or both, might benefit from switching to an alternative opioid.

When switching from one opioid drug to another, dose conversion ratios can be recommended with different levels of confidence (table 2). These conversion ratios are specific for patients in whom analgesia from the first opioid is satisfactory. Therefore, when the opioid is switched because of unsatisfactory analgesia, excessive side-effects, or both, clinical experience suggests that the starting dose should be lower than that calculated from published equianalgesic ratios. In all cases the dose needs to be titrated in accordance with clinical response.

For patients with continuing severe (>6/10) pain or those who are unable to tolerate analgesics because of adverse effects, help should be sought from a specialist service such as the palliative care team or chronic pain team.

Haematology teams should readily seek to share care of pain and other symptoms with local palliative and supportive care teams. Patients at home can be seen by community or hospice-based palliative care teams. Hospital chronic pain teams should be consulted for severe pain if palliative and supportive care teams are not available. Acute pain teams may be helpful if the patient has an acute severe pain, e.g. bone fracture causing immobilization, which may respond to interventional procedures, e.g. local nerve blockade or spinal delivery of opioids and local anaesthetic. Orthopaedic surgeons or interventional radiologists are able to perform cement vertebroplasty or kyphoplasty for uncontrolled pain arising from vertebral collapse. Psychologists can help with patients who have severe anxiety overlying pain and with other issues.

In many of multiple myeloma patients, musculoskeletal complications with enhanced bone destruction lead to pain with pathologic fractures, spinal cord compression and radiculopathy. Bone lesions result not only from the direct deposits of myeloma cells within the bone, but also from the release of soluble factors by both the tumor and the microenvironment, resulting in the stimulation of osteoclast activity and bone resorption. The inhibition of bone resorption and hypercalcaemia can be reduced by the use of bisphosphonates. This class of drugs

http://dx.doi.org/10.5772/55528

RELATIVE ANALGESIC RATIO	STRENGTH OF THE RECOMMENDATION FOR USE	
Oral morphine to oral oxycodone	1.5 : 1	Strong
Oral oxycodone to oral hydromorphone	4 : 1	Strong
Oral morphine to oral hydromorphone	5 : 1	Weak
Oral morphine to TD buprenorphine (*)	75 : 1	Weak
Oral morphine to TD fentanyl (**)	100 : 1	Strong

(*) Example: 60 mg oral morphine to 35 μg/h TD buprenorphine (equivalent to 0.8 mg per 24 h).

(**) Example: 60 mg oral morphine to 25 μg/h TD fentanyl (equivalent to 0.6 mg per 24 h).

TD=transdermal.

Table 2. Relative analgesic dose ratios

potentiate the effects of analgesics in improving myeloma bone pain with reducing bone releated events, but not mortality.

Management of spinal pain is often conservative, in the absence of instability/neurological compromise, orthopaedic, neurosurgical or interventional radiological advice should be sought in cases of persistent/refractory pain. Vertebroplasty and kyphoplasty are alternative options for controlling pain associated with vertebral collapse. Vertebroplasty and kyphoplasty are both vertebral body augmentation techniques of percutaneous injection of bone cement to the vertebral bodies. They are best performed soon after the vertebra collapses and may be ineffective if many months have elapsed. Both techniques carry the small risk of cement leakage leading to pulmonary embolism and neural compromise. It is therefore important that there is access to a spinal surgery service when these procedures are performed.

Vertebroplasty involves the percutaneous injection, under general anaesthetic and i.v. sedation and using radiological imaging, of polymethacrylate bone cement or equivalent biomaterial into the vertebral body. Several vertebrae can be treated simultaneously. The injection allows local pain relief and bone strengthening but will not restore vertebral height. No randomized studies on the use of vertebroplasty in myeloma have been published. However, a recent review of 67 cases demonstrated improvements in pain (89%), mobility (70%) and use of opioid analgesia (65%) [16].

Kyphoplasty involves the percutaneous insertion of a small, inflatable balloon into the vertebral body; when inflated it produces a potential space. The balloon is then removed and bone cement is injected to fill the cavity. Although more time consuming than vertebroplasty the complication rates appear lower with similar potential benefits of both pain relief and improved function to vertebroplasty but with reduced risk of cement leak. There is also the potential to restore vertebral height but this only occurs in a minority of patients. At the present time, the documented use of kyphoplasty in myeloma is limited to case reports and small case series although outcomes in myeloma do appear comparable to those in osteoporosis [17, 18].

Many patients with myeloma have subclinical or even clinical peripheral neuropathy (PN) at diagnosis, often due to co-morbidities. These patients are at risk of worsening PN when exposed to potentially neurotoxic drug treatments, such as thalidomide and bortezomib. The cause of PN in myeloma patients is multifactorial and when patients are assessed, it is important to grade the degree of neuropathy using a recognized scale, such as the National Cancer Institute (NCI), Common Toxicity Criteria [19], LANSS [20] or the Total Neuropathy Score [21].

PN in myeloma patients can be subdivided as follows:

- Disease- or M protein-associated peripheral neuropathy
- Peripheral neuropathy related to co-morbidities
- Chemotherapy-induced peripheral neuropathy

Disease- or M protein-associated peripheral neuropathy: Spinal cord or nerve root compression is a common neurological complication of myeloma due to compression by plasmacytoma, lytic or extramedullary disease and requires appropriate imaging and specific treatment including a specialist opinion as to the need for surgical intervention or radiotherapy.

The reported prevalence of sensory PN may depend on the study cohort, the methods of detection and the criteria used, with a recent study reporting rates of pretreatment sensory PN in up to 20% of patients, and neuropathic abnormalities in as many as 54%. [22].

The cause of the neuropathy in many cases of myeloma is not clear and may be multifactorial, and studies have also varied in relation to rates of small or large fibre or mixed PN. In those cases where amyloidosis and toxicity due to chemotherapy are not the cause, the M protein itself or other consequences of the underlying disease may play a part. Clinically, a symmetrical, distal sensory/motor neuropathy inducing paraesthesiae and numbness in the hands and feet is seen.

POEMS (Polyneuropathy, Organomegaly, Endocrinopathy, M-protein and Skin abnormalities) syndrome and AL amyloidosis are more specialized situations, PN is a significant clinical feature in 85–100% of patients affected by POEMS syndrome [23]. It is a consequence of axonal degeneration and demyelination, typically distal, symmetrical and initially sensory, but as the condition progresses, a disabling symmetrical weakness may develop.

PN affects 17% of patients with AL amyloidosis at diagnosis. The PN is typically axonal and characteristically painful, distal and symmetrical and often associated with an autonomic neuropathy. Cryoglobulinaemia is another recognized source of PN.

Peripheral neuropathy related to co-morbidities: Conditions such as diabetes mellitus, carpal tunnel and other nerve compression syndromes, including chronic inflammatory demyelinating polyradiculoneuropathy, chronic renal failure and vitamin B12 deficiency, should be actively sought and appropriately managed, with specialist input as needed.

Chemotherapy-induced peripheral neuropathy: Chemotherapy-induced peripheral neuropathy (CIPN), also known as treatment-emergent peripheral neuropathy, is a major aspect of myeloma management. CIPN has been a long recognized complication of vinca alkaloid and platinum-based treatments and may be significantly dose limiting, but these drugs are no longer in regular use in myeloma. There is emerging evidence for the incidence and natural history of PN due to novel therapies, including thalidomide-induced PN (TiPN) and bortezomib-induced PN (BiPN), which may be considered as distinct clinical entities.

TiPN may arise after prolonged administration of thalidomide, is mostly mild to moderate in severity and appears to be a cumulative effect [24]. Initial symptoms include sensory changes, such as paraesthesia and hyperaesthesia, motor symptoms and autonomic dysfunction. Later effects include loss of vibration and joint position sense, which may lead to ataxia and progressive gait disturbance. Nerve conduction studies do not reliably predict the onset of significant TiPN and do not necessarily correlate with the clinical findings. Reduction or temporary discontinuation of the drug usually leads to a clinical improvement in the symptoms whereas continuation of dose intense treatment in the face of neuropathy may cause permanent neurological damage. Mileshkin et al and other investigators have recommended that thalidomide therapy should not exceed 6 months as the risk of TiPN is unacceptably high [25].

BiPN is characterized by neuropathic pain and a lengthdependent distal sensory neuropathy with suppression of reflexes. Motor neuropathy may follow and infrequently results in mild to severe distal weakness in the lower limbs. There may also be a significant autonomic component, which manifests as dizziness, hypotension, diarrhoea or constipation and/or extreme fatigue. It is thought to occur at a certain threshold (within five cycles but rarely beyond) of treatment and may be more likely to occur within the setting of renal impairment, in keeping with other therapy related toxicities in this setting. Electrophysiological testing reveals a mainly distal sensorimotor axonal loss, with secondary demyelination. The symptoms of BiPN improve or completely resolve in the majority of patients after a median of 3 months following discontinuation of the drug, but in a proportion of cases, symptoms have taken up to 2 years to improve [26]. Apart from a graded dose reduction or withdrawal [27], the only treatment for BiPN is symptomatic relief. No effective prophylactic treatment is available and any use of nutritional supplements should be restricted to low doses to avoid harm from excessive doses of pyridoxine. In particular, caution should be exercized with supplements containing ascorbic acid, which may inhibit the anti-myeloma effect of bortezomib [28].

An accurate neurological history should be taken from all patients prior to commencement of neurotoxic agents and regularly during the course of therapy. Patients should be reviewed in person at the start of each cycle to ensure that emergent symptoms are detected and acted upon. Dose-reductions may be needed within a treatment cycle if symptoms are progressive, so as to avoid the irreversible neurological damage that may result from waiting until the next cycle to make a change.

Initial investigations should be tailored according to the history and examination. Vitamin B12 deficiency should be screened for periodically. Metabolic and autoimmune causes should also be considered. If there are prominent features of small fibre neuropathy, then AL amyloidosis should be excluded by tissue biopsy or serum amyloid P scan; any further investigations, such as electrophysiological studies or cerebrospinal fluid protein estimation, should be directed by a neurologist.

The management of PN should include symptom control along with treatment of any potentially reversible causes. Identification and correction of Vitamin B12 deficiency is important and optimal management of co-morbid causes, such as diabetes mellitus or alcohol excess, may also improve tolerance of neurotoxic drugs. An awareness of the spectrum of symptoms that herald CIPN is crucial. Such symptoms need to be carefully sought at each meeting with the patient.

Careful monitoring of patients receiving bortezomib and prompt dose and schedule modifications are essential. Temporary interruptions in therapy may also be beneficial, before resuming on a new schedule/dose. Recent data from front line protocols incorporating bortezomib suggest that a weekly regimen is as effective and associated with less neuropathy than twice-weekly regimens [29]. Although, the twice weekly regimens of subcutaneous bortezomib offers non-inferior efficacy to standard intravenous administration, with an improved safety profile for peripheral neuropathy in patients with relapsed multiple myeloma [30]. Continuation of dose intense treatment in the face of neuropathy may cause permanent neurological damage. Measurement of lying and standing blood pressures weekly in patients receiving bortezomib may detect autonomic neuropathy before it becomes a debilitating problem for the patient. The administration of intravenous normal saline prior to each dose of bortezomib may improve tolerance of the drug.

Neuropathic pain is often poorly responsive to standard analgesic regimes. There has been very little research specifically in the management of painful CIPN, and that has mostly been in solid tumours [31]. Opioids can be effective but if used alone in high dose are associated withsignificant adverse effects [32]. A multimodal approach using opioids together with other pain modulating drugs is now recommended [33]. Thus a calcium channel blocker should be added early (e.g. gabapentin or pregabalin); it may be necessary to add a sodium channel blocking agent, e.g. oxcarbazepine (carbamazepine should be avoided because of drug interactions); or an SNRI, e.g. amitryptiline or duloxetine.

Several studies have shown that adding gabapentin to an opioid in patients with cancer-related neuropathic pain can give improved analgesia with reduced adverse effects compared to using either agent alone [34]. The response to gabapentin correlated with the severity of the underlying neurotoxicity. Approximately 25% of patients receiving gabapentin experienced mild somnolence, but none discontinued it. Note that gabapentin may be associated with myelosuppression and so should be avoided around the time of stem cell transplant.

The haematologist who is not familiar with these agents should seek advice from the local chronic pain or palliative care service. For patients with continuing severe pain in spite of initiating these drugs or those who are unable to tolerate analgesics because of adverse effects, specialist help is essential. They will advise on dose modifications and can also initiate specialist options, such as ketamine, methadone or spinal analgesia.

http://dx.doi.org/10.5772/55528

In addition, topical treatments may be of benefit. Capsaicin cream 0.075% acts on peripheral nerve TRPV1 heat and pain receptors; menthol acts on TRPM8 receptors for cold and may both be helpful in patients with „cold" or „hot" dysaesthesia respectively [35]. Emollients, such as cocoa butter, may help some patients but the physiological mechanism is unclear. In other forms of superficial neuropathic pains (e.g. post-herpetic neuralgia or scar pain), the sodium channel blocker lidocaine can be used topically as a 5% plaster, applied to the affected area for 12 hours and then left off for 12 hours. Some patients obtain relief within a few days but the peak effect is reached with 2-4 weeks [36].

Complementary therapy can be defined as therapies that are used alongside, or integrated with, conventional health care. These differ from alternative therapies, which are designed to be used in place of conventional therapy. However, a clear definition of what constitutes complementary and alternative medicine has not yet been elucidated, and therefore discretion must be exercised when interpreting guidance pertaining to these therapies.

Complementary therapy has a role in the management of multiple myeloma when used as adjunct to conventional medicine. It improves patients' perceived quality of life and ability to cope with the effects of the disease. The development of an evidence-base to support complementary therapy use in myeloma is in the early stages of development.

Patients with myeloma may express preference for complementary therapy and place value in the role they have to play within the context of their cancer care plan – for the management of both the psycho-social and physiological effects associated with myeloma. Patients may value complementary therapy and the sense of control gained when they are used as part of their cancer treatment plan. Consequently, patient choice should be informed and respected by healthcare professionals in order to ensure the best overall treatment and care plan for myeloma is delivered.

There is a dearth of scientific evidence to support the effectiveness of complementary therapy in the management of myeloma; however, some studies have shown that complementary therapy can help patients with myeloma to: manage their symptoms, live with altered body image, promote relaxation, alleviate anxiety, reduce chemotherapy side-effects, improve sleep pattern, reduce stress and tension, reduce psychological distress/provide emotional support and improve well-being. Importantly, cancer patients using complementary therapy also perceive an improved quality of life.

Some complementary therapies, such as acupuncture, have been submitted to more rigorous evaluation and are acknowledged for their effective use in cancer treatment for the management of chemotherapy-associated nausea and vomiting. However, no convincing scientific-evidence has emerged to date that shows complementary therapy slows cancer progression [37].

The types of complementary therapies and frequency with which they are used by myeloma patients vary considerably. Among the most common therapies are homoeopathy, touch therapies such as aromatherapy, massage and reflexology, healing and energy therapies such as reiki, spiritual healing and therapeutic touch, hypnosis and hypnotherapy, acupuncture, herbal medicines and dietary interventions [38].

Author details

Emine Ozyuvaci, Onat Akyol and Tolga Sitilci

Istanbul Education and Research Hospital, Department of Anaesthesiology and Pain Management Center, Istanbul, Turkey

References

[1] Angtuaco EJ, Fassas A, Walker R, Sethi R, Barlogie B. (2004) Multiple Myeloma: Clinical Review and Diagnostic Imaging. *Radiology*, 231, 11-23.

[2] Kyle RA: Multiple myeloma: Review of 869 cases. *Mayo Clin Proc* 50:29-40, 1975

[3] Kariyawasan, C.C., Hughes, D.A., Jayatillake, M.M. & Mehta, A.B. (2007) Multiple myeloma: causes and consequences of delay in diagnosis. *Quarterly Journal of Medicine*, 100, 635–664.

[4] Shi, H.Y., Mau, L.W., Chang, J.K., Wang, J.W. & Chiu, H.C. (2009) Responsiveness of the Harris Hip Score and the SF-36: five years after total hip arthroplasty. *Quality of Life Research,* 18, 1053-1060.

[5] Bennett, M.I., Attal, N., Backonja, M.M., Baron, R., Bouhassira, D., Freynhagen, R., Scholz, J., Tölle, T.R., Wittchen, H.U. & Jensen, T.S. (2007) Using screening tools to identify neuropathic pain. *Pain,* 127, 199-203.

[6] Lötsch, J. & Geisslinger, G. (2006) Current evidence for a genetic modulation of the response to analgesics. *Pain,* 121, 1-5.

[7] Mucci-LoRusso, P., Berman, B.S., Silberstein, P.T., Citron, M.L., Bressler, L., Weinstein, S.M., Kaiko, R.F., Buckley, B.J. & Reder, R.F. (1998) Controlled-release oxycodone compared with controlled-release morphine in the treatment of cancer pain: a randomized, double-blind, parallel-group study. *European Journal of Pain,* 2, 239-249

[8] Clark, A.J., Ahmedzai, S.H., Allan, L.G., Camacho, F., Horbay, G.L., Richarz, U. & Simpson, K. (2004) Efficacy and safety of transdermal fentanyl and sustained-release oral morphine in patients with cancer and chronic non-cancer pain. *Current Medical Research and Opinion,* 20, 1419-1428.

[9] Ahmedzai, S. & Brooks, D. (1997) Transdermal fentanyl versus sustained-release oral morphine in cancer pain: preference, efficacy, and quality of life. The TTS-Fentanyl Comparative Trial Group. *Journal of Pain and Symptom Management,* 13, 254-261.

[10] Niscola P., Arcuri E., Giovannini M., Scaramucci L., Romani C., Palombi F., Trape`G., Morabito F. (2004) Pain syndromes in haematological malignancies: an overview. *The Hematology Journal* 5, 293–303

[11] Davies, A.N., Dickman, A., Reid, C., Stevens, A.M. & Zeppetella, G. (2009) Science Committee of the Association for Palliative Medicine of Great Britain and Ireland. The management of cancer-related breakthrough pain: recommendations of a task group of the Science Committee of the Association for Palliative Medicine of Great Britain and Ireland. *European Journal of Pain,* 13, 331-338.

[12] Lennernäs, B., Frank-Lissbrant, I., Lennernäs, H., Kälkner, K.M., Derrick, R. & Howell, J. (2010) Sublingual administration of fentanyl to cancer patients is an effective treatment for breakthrough pain: results from a randomized phase II study. *Palliative Medicine,* 24, 286-293.

[13] Clark, A.J., Ahmedzai, S.H., Allan, L.G., Camacho, F., Horbay, G.L., Richarz, U. & Simpson, K. (2004) Efficacy and safety of transdermal fentanyl and sustained-release oral morphine in patients with cancer and chronic non-cancer pain. *Current Medical Research and Opinion,* 20, 1419-1428.

[14] Ballantyne, J.C. & Mao, J. (2003) Opioid therapy for chronic pain. *New England Journal of Medicine,* 349, 1943-1953.

[15] Reid, C.M., Martin, R.M., Sterne, J.A., Davies, A.N. & Hanks, G.W. (2006) Oxycodone for cancer-related pain: meta-analysis of randomized controlled trials. *Archives of Internal Medicine,* 166, 837-843.

[16] McDonald, R.J., Trout, A.T., Gray, L.A., Dispenzieri, A., Thielen, K.R. & Kallmes, D.F. (2008) Vertebroplasty in multiple myeloma: outcomes in a large patient series. *American Journal of Neuroradiology,* 29, 642–648.

[17] Masala, S., Fiori, R., Massari, F., Cantonetti, M., Postorino, M. & Simonetti, G. (2004) Percutaneous kyphoplasty: indications and technique in the treatment of vertebral fractures from myeloma. *Tumori,* 90, 22–26.

[18] Lane, J.M., Hong, R., Koob, J., Kiechle, T., Niesvizky, R., Pearse, R., Siegel, D. & Poynton, A.R. (2004) Kyphoplasty enhances function and structural alignment in multiple myeloma. *Clinical Orthopaedics and Related Research,* 426, 49–53.

[19] Trotti, A., Colevas, A.D., Setser, A., Rusch, V., Jaques, D., Budach, V., Langer, C., Murphy, B., Cumberlin, R., Coleman, C.N. & Rubin, P. (2003) CTCAE v3.0: development of a comprehensive grading system for the adverse effects of cancer treatment. *Seminars in Radiation Oncology,* 13, 176-181.

[20] Bennett, M. (2001) The LANSS Pain Scale: the Leeds assessment of neuropathic symptoms and signs. *Pain,* 92, 147–157.

[21] Cavaletti, G., Frigeni, B., Lanzani, F., Piatti, M., Rota, S., Briani, C., Zara, G., Plasmati, R., Pastorelli, F., Caraceni, A., Pace, A., Manicone, M., Lissoni, A., Colombo, N., Bianchi, G. & Zanna, C. (2007) The Total Neuropathy Score as an assessment tool for grading the course of chemotherapy-induced peripheral neurotoxicity: comparison

with the National Cancer Institute - Common Toxicity Scale. *Journal of the Peripheral Nervous System*, 12, 210–215.

[22] Richardson, P.G., Xie, W., Mitsiades, C., Chanan- Khan, A.A., Lonial, S., Hassoun, H., Avigan, D.E., Oaklander, A.L., Kuter, D.J., Wen, P.Y., Kesari, S., Briemberg, H.R., Schlossman, R.L., Munshi, N.C., Heffner, L.T., Doss, D., Esseltine, D.L., Weller, E., Anderson, K.C. & Amato, A.A. (2009) Single-agent bortezomib in previously untreated multiple myeloma: efficacy, characterization of peripheral neuropathy, and molecular correlations with response and neuropathy. *Journal of Clinical Oncology, 27*, 3518–3525.

[23] Dispenzieri, A. & Gertz, M.A. (2004) Treatment of POEMS syndrome. *Current Treatment Options in Oncology*, 5, 249–257.

[24] Cavaletti, G., Beronio, A., Reni, L., Ghiglione, E., Schenone, A., Briani, C., Zara, G., Cocito, D., Isoardo, G., Ciaramitaro, P., Plasmati, R., Pastorelli, F., Frigo, M., Piatti, M. & Carpo, M. (2004) Thalidomide sensory neurotoxicity: a clinical and neurophysiologic study. *Neurology*, 62, 2291–2293.

[25] Mileshkin, L., Stark, R., Day, B., Seymour, J.F., Zeldis, J.B. & Prince, H.M. (2006) Development of neuropathy in patients with myeloma treated with thalidomide: patterns of occurrence and the role of electrophysiologic monitoring. *Journal of Clinical Oncology*, 24, 4507–4514.

[26] El-Cheikh, J., Stoppa, A.M., Bouabdallah, R., de Lavallade, H., Coso, D., de Collela, J.M., Auran-Schleinitz, T., Gastaut, J.A., Blaise, D. & Mohty, M. (2008) Features and risk factors of peripheral neuropathy during treatment with bortezomib for advanced multiple myeloma. *Clinical Lymphoma & Myeloma*, 8, 146–152.

[27] Richardson, P.G., Briemberg, H., Jagannath, S., Wen, P.Y., Barlogie, B., Berenson, J., Singhal, S., Siegel, D.S., Irwin, D., Schuster, M., Srkalovic, G., Alexanian, R., Rajkumar, S.V., Limentani, S., Alsina, M., Orlowski, R.Z., Najarian, K., Esseltine, D., Anderson, K.C. & Amato, A.A. (2006) Frequency, characteristics, and reversibility of peripheral neuropathy during treatment of advanced multiple myeloma with bortezomib. *Journal of Clinical Oncology*, 24, 3113–3120.

[28] Perrone, G., Hideshima, T., Ikeda, H., Okawa, Y., Calabrese, E., Gorgun, G., Santo, L., Cirstea, D., Raje, N., Chauhan, D., Baccarani, M., Cavo, M. & Anderson, K.C. (2009) Ascorbic acid inhibits antitumor activity of bortezomib in vivo. *Leukemia*, 23, 1679–1686.

[29] Bringhen, S., Larocca, A., Rossi, D., Cavalli, M., Genuardi, M., Ria, R., Gentili, S., Patriarca, F., Nozzoli, C., Levi, A., Guglielmelli, T., Benevolo, G., Callea, V., Rizzo, V., Cangialosi, C., Musto, P., De Rosa, L., Liberati, A.M., Grasso, M., Falcone, A.P., Evangelista, A., Cavo, M., Gaidano, G., Boccadoro, M. & Palumbo, A. (2010) Efficacy and safety of once weekly bortezomib in multiple myeloma patients. *Blood*, 116, 4745–4753.

[30] Moreau, P., Pylypenko, H., Grosicki, S., Karamanesht, I., Leleu, X., Grishunina, M., Rekhtman, G., Masliak, Z., Robak, T., Shubina, A., Arnulf, B., Kropff, M., Cavet, J., Esseltinc, DL., Feng, H., Girgis, S., van de Velde, H., Deraedt, W., Harousseau, JL. (2011) Subcutaneous versus intravenous administration of bortezomib in patients with relapsed multiple myeloma: a randomised, phase 3, non-inferiority study. *Lancet*, 12, 431-440

[31] Tsavaris, N., Kopterides, P., Kosmas, C., Efthymiou, A., Skopelitis, H., Dimitrakopoulos, A., Pagouni, E., Pikazis, D., Zis, P.V. & Koufos, C. (2008) Gabapentin monotherapy for the treatment of chemotherapy-induced neuropathic pain: a pilot study. *Pain Medicine*, 9, 1209–1216.

[32] Rowbotham, M.C., Twilling, L., Davies, P.S., Reisner, L., Taylor, K. & Mohr, D. (2003) Oral opioid therapy for chronic peripheral and central neuropathic pain. *New England Journal of Medicine*, 348, 1223–1232.

[33] Raphael, J., Hester, J., Ahmedzai, S., Barrie, J., Farqhuar-Smith, P., Williams, J., Urch, C., Bennett, M.I., Robb, K., Simpson, B., Pittler, M., Wider, B., Ewer-Smith, C., Decourcy, J., Young, A., Liossi, C., McCullough, R., Rajapakse, D., Johnson, M., Duarte, R. & Sparkes, E. (2010) Cancer Pain: Part 2: Physical, Interventional and Complimentary Therapies; Management in the Community; Acute, Treatment-Related and Complex Cancer Pain: A Perspective from the British Pain Society Endorsed by the UK Association of Palliative Medicine and the Royal College of General Practitioners. *Pain Medicine*, 11, 872–896.

[34] Ho, T.W., Backonja, M., Ma, J., Leibensperger, H., Froman, S. & Polydefkis, M. (2009) Efficient assessment of neuropathic pain drugs in patients with small fiber sensory neuropathies. *Pain*, 141, 19–24.

[35] Vriens J, Nilius B, Vennekens R (2008) Herbal compounds and toxins modulating TRP channels. *Curr Neuropharmacol*. 6:79-96.

[36] Binder A, Bruxelle J, Rogers P, Hans G, Bösl I, Baron R (2009). Topical 5% lidocaine (lignocaine) medicated plaster treatment for post-herpetic neuralgia: results of a double-blind, placebo-controlled, multinational efficacy and safety trial. *Clin Drug Investig*. 29:393-408.

[37] Leukemia and Lymphoma Society. (2006) Integrative medicine and complementary and alternative therapies as part of blood cancer care. HYPERLINK "http://www.leukemia-lymphoma.org/attachments/" http://www.leukemia-lymphoma.org/attachments/ National/br_1150734030.pdf.

[38] Molassiotis, A., Margulies, A., Fernandez-Ortega, P., Pud, D., Panteli, V., Bruyns, I., Scott, J.A., Gudmundsdottir, G., Browall, M., Madsen, E., Ozden, G., Magri, M., Selvekerova, S., Platin, N., Kearney, N. & Patiraki, E. (2005) Complementary and alternative medicine use in patients with haematological malignancies in Europe. *Complementary Therapies in Clinical Practice*. 11, 105–110.

Chapter 14

Quality of Life Issues of Patients with Multiple Myeloma

Klára Gadó and Gyula Domján

Additional information is available at the end of the chapter

http://dx.doi.org/10.5772/55625

1. Introduction

The great advance in the field of anti-myeloma therapy in the last few decades has resulted in a huge improvement of overall and disease-free survival. Nevertheless, multiple myeloma (MM) is still an incurable disease.

There are two issues emerging. On one hand, the patient lives together with the illness for a long time, and on the other hand, the thought of incurable illness hangs over their head like the sword of Damocles for a longer time. Quality of life (QoL) issues are coming into focus because of the longer survival times.

Problems related to the disease such as pain, fatigue, bone fracture-induced inconveniences, complications such as infections, neuropathy, thrombosis, osteonecrosis of the jaw, mucositis, as well as invasive interventions emphasize the importance of supportive care.

The social and economic environment of the patients, their participation in the world of labor, financial resources, changes in their family and in their circle of friends all have a great impact on the QoL of patients.

The stigmata of chronic illness and malignancy also contribute to the development of depression thus influencing quality of life. At the last stage of life it is a very hard task for the patient to face dying.

At the same time, family members are also in a troublesome situation. To accept the incurable illness of a beloved member of the family is a great psychical burden. Beside these, the increase of physical burden may cause insoluble task for the folks and this may generate sense of guilt.

Nowadays, the measuring of QoL is in a class by itself. QoL has become a prognostic factor. Several studies have demonstrated that better quality of life goes hand in hand with better prognosis. This is also the case with multiple myeloma.

Results of examinations of QoL may help us to provide professional and effective support to the patient and their family through a holistic approach. Multidisciplinary co-operation is essential.

2. Main features of Multiple Myeloma

Multiple myeloma is the second most common hematological cancer and represents 10% of all hematological malignancies and 1 % of all cancers. The annual incidence of the disease in the US is 4 in 100,000. Approximately 100,000 new cases of MM are diagnosed each year worldwide [1]. MM accounts for 1% of all cancer-related deaths (approximately 72,000 deaths annually). The vast majority of the patients diagnosed with MM are 70-80 years old. MM is characterized by unregulated plasma cell proliferation in the bone marrow. These malignant plasma cells produce and secrete abnormal immunoglobulin (Ig) or immunoglobulin fragments. The monoclonal lg in the sera can cause hyperviscosity and this is one of the major symptoms of the disease. Clinical features and typical laboratory findings of MM include fatigue, bone pain, osteolythic bone lesions, pathologic bone fracture, anemia, hypercalcaemia, renal insufficiency, elevation of monoclonal Ig in the sera and/or in the urine and elevated erythrocyte sedimentation rate. The etiology of MM is unknown but aside from several environmental factors that are suspected, more and more cytogenetic alterations involved with the oncogenic process are detected [2,3].

3. The aims of MM treatment

Despite the huge advance in the field of MM treatment, the disease has still remained incurable.

The main goal of treatment is the prolongation of survival. By the 1980's to 1990's, the survival of untreated patients had increased from mere months to 3-5 years. The introduction of intensive treatment, such as high-dose chemotherapy with autologous stem cell transplantation (ASCT), further prolonged the overall survival. Novel agents, including immunomodulatory drugs, such as thalidomide and lenalidomide, and the proteosome inhibitor bortezomib have dramatically changed the results in the past decade. Besides overall survival, disease-free survival has also been prolonged and the life expectancies of refractory and relapsed patients are also largely improved [4].

The only curative treatment option is allogeneic stem cell transplantation due to antitumor immunity mediated by donor lymphocytes. However, morbidity and mortality related to graft-versus-host disease remain a challenge and regarding the average age of MM patients it remains an option for only a minority of patients.

Depending on stage of the disease, median survival varies between 5-10 years for patients with ISS stage I disease undergoing stem-cell transplant and/or receiving novel anti-myeloma regimens [5]. However, outcomes have typically been poor for patients with high-risk disease and despite recent therapeutic advances the outlook for such patients remains unfavorable [6].

4. Consequences of MM being a disease of the elderly

The incidence of multiple myeloma (MM) increases with age and with the aging of the population, the number of adults with MM is expected to double in the next 20 years. Intensification of anti-myeloma therapy has resulted in a huge prolongation of survival data but this data mainly refers to younger patients who are eligible for these treatment modalities.

Older patients are ineligible for high-dose therapy because it causes an unacceptably high mortality rate in that patient population. Several co-morbidities of this setting or poor performance status prevent the success of intensive treatment.

On the other hand the significance of supportive measures for these patients has become a greater value. Besides the extended duration of survival, to improve the quality of survival by alleviating symptoms and achieving disease control while minimizing the adverse effects of the treatment has become a major goal [7].

Factors affecting prognosis include burden of disease, type of cytogenetic abnormality present, patient related factors (such as age and performance status) and treatment response factors.

Asymptomatic myeloma (smoldering myeloma) does not require any treatment, only observation (watch and wait) is needed.

The choice of first-line treatment depends on a combination of factors.

For patients under 70 and with good performance status, the treatment of choice is high-dose chemotherapy with ASCT.

The majority of patients are transplantation-ineligible because of poor performance status or co-morbidities. These patients are therefore offered a less intensive single-agent or combination chemotherapy. Typically, combination therapies include chemotherapy with an alkylating agent and corticosteroids. More recent treatment options may also include combination therapies that incorporate drugs such as thalidomide, bortezomib and lenalidomide [8].

Regarding the maintenance therapy, if complete remission (CR) has been reached there is no need for maintenance therapy with thalidomide or lenalidomide because there is no significant difference in OS. In the case of lenalidomide, a significantly increased risk of secondary malignancies was reported [9]. Maintenance is advised for patients who have not reached CR. In these cases, one of the new drugs (thalidomide, lenalidomide or bortezomib) is the drug of choice [10].

However, in line with all these improvements in the field of chemotherapy, some new questions have emerged. The patient has gained a longer life, but is this life good enough? Is it worth the sea of difficulties during the treatment period and even afterward? To answer these questions, QoL measurements can offer valuable meaning.

5. Definition of quality of life and importance of QoL measuring

QoL can be defined in many ways. As a general term it is used to indicate the well-being of people and societies. A person's environment, physical and mental health, education, recreation, social well-being, freedom, human rights and happiness are also significant factors.

The World Health Organization (WHO) defines QoL as individuals' perception of their position in life in the context of the culture and value systems in which they live and in relation to their goals, expectations, standards, and concerns [11].

As illness and its treatment affect the psychological, social, and economic well-being, as well as the biological integrity of individuals, any definition should be all encompassing while allowing individual components to be delineated. This allows the impact of different disease states or interventions on overall or specific aspects of QoL to be determined.

QoL is measured in a variety of contexts. Aside from healthcare, it is also used in international development and political science. This results in diverse definitions being given to the term. Factors that are considered are both qualitative and quantitative. Many local, national and international organizations conduct surveys and psychological tests to determine an individual or society's life quality for different purposes.

A major rule for physicians is the principle of "nil nocere". While making an effort to reach better and better disease control for cancer patients, we often neglect the repercussions of the patient in regards to "being ill", to the consequences of the treatment, and to the disease per se. The main purpose for all clinicians is therefore to improve the quality of the patient's life and to avoid iatrogenic harm. It is not enough to make implicit, subjective judgments about QoL when treating a patient. Making explicit, objective assessments about QoL using validated tools and instruments is needed. Formal assessment of QoL is now a mandatory requirement in most clinical trials.

6. Health-Related Quality of Life (HRQoL)

WHO defines health as "A state of complete physical, mental, and social well-being not merely the absence of disease." The measurement of health and the effects of health care must include not only an indication of changes in the frequency and severity of diseases but also an estimation of well being and this can be assessed by measuring the improvement in the QoL related to health care [11].

HRQoL can be defined as self-perceived aspects of wellbeing that are related to or affected by the presence of a disease or treatment [12]. A multidimensional HRQoL instrument was defined as any quality of life instrument assessing two or more of the three core domains described by the World Health Association: physical, social, and psychological wellbeing [13]. As a multidimensional construct, it includes perceptions, both positive and negative, of several dimensions such as physical, emotional, social and cognitive functioning. It also includes the negative aspects of somatization disorder and symptoms caused by a disease and/or its treatment [14]. Studies undertaken in different settings or in different countries might display slight divergences as HRQoL is also modulated by cultural and care patterns.

Over the past 20 years there has been a growing interest in the inclusion of HRQoL measures to assess the effects of a condition and/or its therapies on a person's health. In response to this interest, methods to assess health status and HRQoL have proliferated. There are now a number of valid and reliable instruments available for use in research investigations, which are the culmination of years of research with various populations, and reflect the target populations' perceptions of their health status and HRQoL [15].

HRQoL-measurement instruments validated for use in cancer patients have two basic categories. Questionnaires specifically designed for the disease explore the repercussions of the most typical symptoms and side-effects and are appropriate for comparing different treatment modalities or changes in patients. The general instruments are applicable to any population and are better suited to studies that seek to ascertain the disease's repercussion on HRQoL, taking the general population as reference [16]. Among the former, the most used in Europe for MM patients are the European Organization for Research and Treatment of Cancer Core Cancer Quality Life Questionnaire (EORTC QLQ-C30) and its MM-specific module (EORTC-QLQ-MY24/MY20). Among the latter, the Medical Outcomes Survey Short-Form General Health Survey (SF-36) is the most widely used.

There are also symptom-specific instruments, assessing the patient's reflections directly concerning pain, fatigue, neuropathy and nausea.

For example, the Functional Assessment of Chronic Illness Therapy (FACIT) system which is an established, comprehensive set of health-related quality-of-life measures includes a 27-item general measure, the Functional Assessment of Cancer Therapy (FACT-G), which can be combined with disease or treatment-specific subscales. The FACT-G captures four domains of health-related quality of life: physical, social, emotional and functional well-being. The supplemental subscales measure additional concerns of a specific disease or treatment. For example, the multiple myeloma subscale (FACT-MM) includes MM-relevant items There are also symptom-specific measures, such as FACT-An for patients with anemia or fatigue, FACT-Bone Pain: for patients with bone pain and treatment-specific measures assessing the QoL changing due to treatment such as FACT&GOG-Ntx: for patients with neurotoxicity [17].

7. Importance of quality of life issues

In the case of MM, disease severity and type of treatment (high-dose chemotherapy and ASCT, the use of novel agents such as bortezomib, thalidomide or lenalidomide) have a clear influence on the patient's subjective perception of the disease. Their effects on HRQoL are also modulated by personality traits, personal resources and the availability and perception of social and family support.

Clinical applications of HRQoL tools may include prognostication, monitoring response to treatment, prioritizing problems or facilitating communication. The use of HRQoL instruments in clinical practice has also been shown to independently improve HRQoL in general oncology patients [18]. Some authors who have demonstrated reduced HRQoL in myeloma have concluded that HRQoL assessment should become a normal part of clinical care [19, 20].

Besides the typical primary parameters of clinical trials for measuring the treatment effect, such as tumor volume and time to progression, recognition of HRQoL is also an important endpoint in clinical research. In circumstances when the studied treatment modality results only a modest improvement in respect to primary parameters, with little benefit for the patient but with a significant side-effect profile, it may be a helpful outcome to detect the declination of HRQoL compared to the control. Clinical trials incorporating QoL assessments can provide more information and help clarify the relative harms and benefits of palliative chemotherapy and aid patient decisions when survival gains are small.

Delineation of side-effect profile by means of HRQoL assessment can assist in determining the types of supportive interventions that may be needed to ameliorate the side-effects.

QoL can also represent an independent prognostic factor. It is known that patients with a good QoL at the beginning of treatment manage better than those with a worse baseline value and there is a growing amount of evidences that QoL can be used as an effective prognostic indicator in respect to several kinds of malignancies [21].

QoL data can be a useful predictor of patient response to treatment and can affect decision-making about therapeutic options. This data allows patients to make informed and individualized decisions on the most appropriate treatment and any required supportive interventions.

HRQoL may be applied by the healthcare system to allocate resources by economic reality. As demand is always larger than resources, the optimal allocation of the financial means has great economic importance.

8. Myeloma-specific HRQoL aspects

MM is a chronic, incurable disease that is associated with reduced quality of life. MM patients have to face the problems of living with a chronic illness longer as a result of prolonged survival. However, they are also faced with the difficulties related to a malignant disease. Disease symptoms, concerns with certain therapeutic modalities and also the QoL changes due to organ transplantation emerge. Generation of pathologic bone fracture, bone pain, fatigue because of anemia and malignant disease itself, neurological symptoms due to hypercalcaemia have a profound impact on the QoL of MM patients.

Chronic renal failure develops in one third of MM patients. Chronic dialysis treatment implicates several life style changes.

Most anti-myeloma therapies involve intravenous injections or infusions. Regular laboratory check-ups require repeated blood sample collections that require multiple encounters with needles. Taking bone marrow for diagnosis and several times afterward for control examinations is very painful unless it is performed in narcosis.

ASCT has considerable effects on QoL. High-dose chemotherapy presents significant side effects and subsequently a reduction of QoL. This is due mainly to infections, mucositis, increased use of blood products and prolonged stays in the hospital.

Side-effects of several lines of treatments include polyneuropathy, deep vein thrombosis, loss of hair and constipation. Osteonecrosis of the jaw caused by bisphosphonates, though a rare event, results in severe deterioration of QoL.

Recurrent infections due to the patients' immunocompromised status, the disease itself and also due to the several lines of treatment used to control the disease also contribute to the worsening of QoL.

9. Questionnaires for evaluating MM

Osborne et al. systematically reviewed the different HRQOL instruments applied for evaluating myeloma patients in their recent study. Thirteen different HRQOL instruments were identified across 39 studies. Only one disease-specific instrument was identified (EORTC-QLQ-MY24/MY20). Other measures were general cancer tools (EORTC-QLQ-C30, FACT-An), treatment specific (EORTC-QLQ-HDC19, FACT-BMT), or generic [SF-36, SF-12, SEIQoL-DW, EQ-5D, 15D, life ingredient profile (LIP), Quality of Life Index (QLI)]. The SEIQoLDW was the only individualised instrument (with domains defined by respondents). No instrument was developed specifically for clinical use, or in palliative settings – although the search strategy was designed to identify these. [22].

No single instrument covered all issues identified as important by people with myeloma. The most comprehensive coverage was found in the EORTC-QLQ-MY24 (myeloma-specific module, used in conjunction with core cancer questionnaire EORTC-QLQ-C30), the FACT-BMT and the QLI.

However, each tool has its strengths and the choice of tool will depend on the context in which it is used. To describe the incidence of side effects in a particular group, the EORTC tools may be more appropriate. However, in clinical practice, we may want a tool to focus more on the particular concerns of each patient (such as the SEIQoL-DW). These tools are time-consuming, require specialized training, are difficult to compare between studies and different interviewers and can be less feasible in certain groups such as those with chronic disease or the elderly.

Existing tools tend to be designed for use in research settings and their adaptation or the development of new tools specifically for use in clinical practice would be beneficial [22].

10. HRQoL studies in MM

Though HRQoL examinations are widely used especially in cancer patients and they are an integral component of clinical trials with new drugs, MM patients are relatively poorly studied in this respect. A PubMed search with terms of "multiple myeloma and quality of life or health-related quality of life" has resulted in only 51 items.

These studies targeted the comparison of HRQoL of MM patients in different countries [23], treated with different therapeutic schedules, receiving new drugs [24], underwent

ASCT or tandem ASCT [25], special issues of the elderly [26], the effect of anemia and fatigue and also the effect of personality on disease outcome [27]. Methodological aspects are also emphasized [20].

11. Disease-specific complaints and HRQoL of MM patients

Patients with MM experience a very high symptom burden and low HRQOL. In a study published in 2012, the Eindhoven Cancer Registry was used to select all patients diagnosed with MM from 1999 to 2010. Patients were asked at baseline and 1 year later. Patients with MM reported statistically significant and clinically relevant worse scores on all EORTC QLQ-C30 scales compared to the norm. Also, patients with MM reported a mean decrease (e.g., worsening) between baseline and 1-year follow-up scores for: QoL (74% of patients had a deteriorated score), fatigue (50%), nausea and vomiting (71%), pain (59%) and dyspnoea (66%). The most bothering symptoms during the past week were tingling hands/feet (32%), back pain (28%), bone aches/pain (26%), pain in arm/shoulder (19%) and feeling drowsy (18%). Also, 37% worried about their future health, 34% thought about their disease and 21% worried about dying [28].

12. QoL differences in transplant-ineligible myeloma patients treated with different drug combinations

The phase 3 VISTA study (ClinicalTrials.gov NCT00111319) in transplant-ineligible myeloma patients demonstrated superior efficacy with bortezomib-melphalan-prednisone (VMP; nine 6-wk cycles) vs. melphalan-prednisone (MP) but also increased toxicity. HRQoL was evaluated using the EORTC-QLQ-C30 questionnaire. Results demonstrated clinically meaningful, transitory HRQoL decrements with VMP and relatively lower HRQoL vs. MP during early treatment cycles, associated with the expected additional toxicities. However, HRQoL is not compromised in the long term, recovering by the end-of-treatment visit to be comparable vs. MP. Analyses by bortezomib dose intensity indicated better HRQoL in patients receiving lower dose intensity [29].

13. HRQoL assessment in MM patients undergoing autologous stem cell transplantation

HRQoL assessment in this patient setting is important as patients and even clinicians are reluctant to choose this modality for fear of declination of QoL. However, it is not the best choice for every patient. HRQoL studies may contribute to the appropriate patient selection.

In a population-based study, the Nordic Myeloma Study Group found a survival advantage for high-dose therapy and ASCT compared to conventional chemotherapy in MM patients who were less than 60 years of age. HRQoL was integrated into the trial, using the EORTC QLQ-C30 questionnaire. Of the 274 patients receiving intensive therapy, 221 (81%) were compared to 113 (94%) of 120 patients receiving conventional melphalan-prednisone treatment. Prior to treatment, there were no statistically significant differences in any HRQoL score between the two groups. One month after the start of induction chemotherapy, the patients on intensive treatment had lower scores that gradually improved and at 12 and 24 months, the HRQoL was similar to that of the control patients. At 36 months, there was a trend toward less fatigue, pain, nausea, and appetite loss in the intensive-treatment group. Despite the moderate HRQoL reduction associated with the early intensive chemotherapy phase, the 18 months of prolonged survival seem to be associated with a good HRQoL [30].

QOL results of an Australian study on MM patients who underwent dose-reduced tandem ASCT were published in 2011. Patients younger than 60 years old received conditioning with melphalan 140 mg/m^2 and patients who were Older than or equal to 60 years old received 100 mg/m^2. EORTC QLQ-C30 and the QLQ-MY24 questionnaires were conducted after each ASCT and thereafter every 3 months for 24 months. Mean global health measure improved from 3.44 before transplant to 4.50 (1being very poor and 7 being excellent) at the second and subsequent follow-up visits and the mean global QoL score improved from 3.61 to 4.71. Pain symptoms were reduced and physical functioning improved throughout the period of post-transplant follow-up. The study showed that dose-reduced tandem ASCT was well tolerated with low toxicity although there was a transient reduction in QoL during both transplants. Post-transplant follow-up showed significant improvement in overall HRQoL that reflects positively on the overall disease-outcome [31].

In a University of Arkansas study, the decreases in functioning after transplantation were less pronounced than anticipated. At stem cell collection, physical deficits were common, with most patients scoring 1 standard deviation below population norms for physical well-being (70.2%) and functional well-being (57.5%), and many reporting at least moderate fatigue (94.7%) and pain (39.4%). Clinically meaningful levels of anxiety (39.4%), depression (40.4%) and cancer-related distress (37.0%) were evident in a notable proportion of patients. After transplantation, there was a worsening of transplant-related concerns, depression and life-satisfaction. However, pain improved and social functioning was well preserved. Older patients were not more compromised than younger ones. In multivariate analyses, they reported better overall QoL and less depression than before transplantation [32].

14. QoL assessment of elderly MM patients

Thalidomide with melphalan and prednisone (MPT) was defined as standard treatment in elderly patients with MM. In a randomized trial (HOVON49), a prospective HRQoL study was initiated in order to assess the impact of thalidomide on QoL. Patients aged 65 years and older with newly diagnosed MM were randomized to receive melphalan plus prednisone (MP) or MPT, followed by thalidomide maintenance in the MPT arm. 284 patients were included (MP, n=149; MPT n=135). HRQoL was assessed with the QLQ-

C30 and the myeloma-specific module (QLQ-MY24) at baseline and at predetermined intervals during treatment. The QLQ-C30 subscales physical function and constipation showed an improvement during induction in favour of the MP arm. During thalidomide maintenance, the scores for the QLQ-MY24 paraesthesia became significantly higher in the MPT arm. The QLQ-C30 subscales pain, insomnia and appetite loss and the QLQ-MY24 item sick scored marginally better during thalidomide maintenance. The overall QoL-scale QLQ-C30-HRQoL showed a significant time trend towards more favorable mean values during protocol treatment without differences between MP and MPT. For the QLQ-C30 subscales emotional function and future perspectives, difference in favour of the MPT arm from the start of treatment was observed with no significant 'time × arm' interaction, indicating a persistent better patient perspective with MPT treatment. The study concluded that the higher frequency of toxicity associated with MPT does not translate into a negative effect on HRQoL and that MPT holds a better patient perspective [33].

Quality-of-life assessment may be an independent and valuable addition to the known prognostic factors in multiple myeloma. In a randomized trial (NMSG 4/90), patients treated with melphalan/prednisone were compared to a melphalan/prednisone + interferon alpha-2b treated patient group in 486 newly diagnosed multiple myeloma. Univariate analysis showed a highly significant association with survival from the start of therapy for physical functioning as well as role and cognitive functioning, global quality of life, fatigue and pain. In multivariate analysis, physical functioning and W.H.O. performance status were independent prognostic factors when analysed in a Cox regression model with the somatic variables beta-2 microglobulin, skeletal disease and age. The best prediction for survival from the start of therapy was obtained by combining the beta-2 microglobulin and physical functioning scores in a variable consisting of three risk factor levels with an estimated median survival of 17, 29 and 49 months, respectively [34].

15. Assessment of the correlation of psychological well-being and QoL in MM

A cross-sectional survey was conducted aiming to identify the nature and range of needs, as well as levels of quality of life (QoL), of both patients living with myeloma and their partners. Patients and their partners were recruited from 4 hospitals in the United Kingdom at a mean post-diagnosis time of 5 years. A total of 132 patients and 93 of their partners participated. One-quarter of the patients and one-third of the partners reported unmet supportive care needs. About 27.4% of patients reported signs of anxiety and 25.2% reported signs of depression. Almost half the partners (48.8%) reported signs of anxiety and 13.6% exhibited signs of depression. Anxious/depressed patients had more than double the unmet needs than non-anxious/depressed patients ($P<0.05$). QoL was moderate, with key areas of impairment being physical, emotional, social and cognitive functioning. Patients complained of several symptoms, including tiredness (40.7%), pain (35.9%), insomnia (32.3%), peripheral neuropathies (28.3%) and memory problems (22.3%). About 40.8% were worried about their health in the future [35].

http://dx.doi.org/10.5772/55625

16. Conclusion

Investigation of QoL has become increasingly important in economically developed countries. HRQoL assessment is becoming a current and integral part of clinical studies with new drugs. Measuring of QoL is becoming more and more important for decision making in the field of health policy.

MM is a currently incurable disease, but survival can be significantly prolonged by the administration of new therapeutic modalities. The mean age at the time of diagnosis is over 60, so it is especially important to choose the least harmful treatment for the patient so the best quality of life can be achieved. Results of QoL examinations can help us find the most appropriate treatment for our patients.

Abbreviations

ASCT: autologous stem cell transplantation; **EORTC:** European Organization for Research and Treatment of Cancer; **HRQoL:** health-related quality of life; **Ig:** immunoglobulin; **MM:** multiple myeloma; **QoL:** quality of life; **WHO:** World Health Organization

Author details

Klára Gadó* and Gyula Domján

*Address all correspondence to: gadok@freemail.hu

Semmelweis University, Faculty of Medicine, 1st Department of Internal Medicine, Budapest, Hungary

References

[1] Ferlay, J, Shin, H. R, Bray, F, Forman, D, Mathers, C, & Parkin, D. M. Estimates of worldwide burden of cancer in (2008). GLOBOCAN 2008. Int J Cancer. 2010;, 127, 2893-917.

[2] Raab, M. S, Podar, K, Breitkreutz, I, Richardson, P. G, & Anderson, K. C. Multiple myeloma. Lancet. (2009). , 374(9686), 324-39.

[3] Sirohi, B, & Powles, R. Epidemiology and outcomes research for MGUS, myeloma and amyloidosis. Eur J Cancer. (2006). , 42, 1671-83.

[4] Cherry, B. M, Korde, N, Kwok, M, Roschewski, M, & Landgren, O. Evolving therapeutic paradigms for multiple myeloma: back to the future. Leuk Lymphoma. (2012). doi:10.3109/10428194.2012.717277)

[5] Greipp, P. R. San Miguel J, Durie BG, et al. International staging system for multiple myeloma. J Clin Oncol. (2005). , 23, 3412-20.

[6] Attal, M, Harousseau, J. L, Stoppa, A. M, Sotto, J. J, et al. A prospective randomized trial of Autologous Bone Marrow Transplantation and chemotherapy in Multiple Myeloma. N Engl J Med. (1996). , 335, 91-97.

[7] Wildes, T. M, Vij, R, Petersdorf, S. H, Medeiros, B. C, & Hurria, A. New Treatment Approaches for Older Adults with Multiple Myeloma. J Geriatr Oncol. (2012). Epub 2012 Feb 28., 3(3), 279-290.

[8] Kyle, R. A, & Rajkumar, S. V. Criteria for diagnosis, staging, risk stratification and response assessment of multiple myeloma. Leukemia. (2009). , 23, 3-9.

[9] Attal, M, & Olivier, P. Cances Lauwers V, et al. Maintenance treatment with lenalidomide after transplantation for myeloma. Analysis of secondary malignancies within the IFM trial. Haematologica (2011). suppl 1):s23., 2005-02.

[10] Richardson, P. G, Laubach, J. P, Schlossman, R. L, Ghobrial, I. M, Mitsiades, C. S, Rosenblatt, J, Mahindra, A, Raje, N, Munshi, N, & Anderson, K. C. The Medical Research Council Myeloma IX trial: the impact on treatment paradigms. Eur J Haematol. (2012). , 88(1), 1-7.

[11] Kuyken, W, Orley, J, Hudelson, P, & Sartorius, N. Quality of life assessment across cultures. Int. J. Mental Hlth, 23, 5. (WHOQOL): position paper from the World Health Organization. Soc. Sci. Med., (1994).

[12] Ebrahim, S. Clinical and Public-Health Perspectives and Applications of Health-Related Quality-Of-Life Measurement. Soc Sci Med. (1995). doi:O., 41, 1383-1394.

[13] WHOQOL-GroupThe World Health Organization quality of life assessment (WHOQOL): Position paper from the World Health Organization. Soc Sci Med. (1995). , 41(10), 1403-9.

[14] Osoba, D. Lessons Learned from Measuring Health-Related Quality-Of-Life in Oncology. J Clin Oncol. (1994). , 12, 608-616.

[15] Naughton, M. J, & Shumaker, S. A. The case for domains of function in quality of life assessment. Qual Life Res. (2003). Suppl , 1, 73-80.

[16] Ferrans, C. E. In: Outcomes Assessment in Cancer. Measures, Methods, and Applications. 1. Lipscomb J, Gotay CC, Snyder C, editor. Cambridge: Cambridge University Press; (2005). Definitions and conceptual models of quality of life; , 14-30.

[17] Webster, K, Cella, D, & Yost, K. The Functional Assessment of Chronic Illness Therapy (FACIT) measurement system: properties, application, and interpretation. Health Qual Life Outcomes. (2003). , 1, 79-86.

[18] Velikova, G, Booth, L, Smith, A. B, Brown, P. M, Lynch, P, Brown, J. M, et al. Measuring Quality of Life in Routine Oncology Practice Improves Communication and Patient Well-Being: A Randomized Controlled Trial. J Clin Oncol. (2004). , 22(4), 714-24.

[19] Sherman, A. C, Simonton, S, Latif, U, Plante, T. G, & Anaissie, E. J. Changes in quality-of-life and psychosocial adjustment among multiple myeloma patients treated with high-dose melphalan and autologous stem cell transplantation. Biol Blood Marrow Transplant. (2009). , 15(1), 12-20.

[20] Osborne, T. R, Ramsenthaler, C, Siegert, R. J, Edmonds, P. M, Schey, S. A, & Higginson, I. J. What issues matter most to people with multiple myeloma and how well are we measuring them? A systematic review of quality of life tools. Eur J Haematol. (2012). Sep 18. doi:ejh.12012.

[21] Fallowfield, L. Quality of life: a new perspective for cancer patients. Nat Rev Cancer. (2002). , 2(11), 873-9.

[22] Osborne, T. R, et al. What issues matter most to people with multiple myeloma and how well are we measuring them? A systematic review of quality of life tools. Eur J Haematol. (2012). Sep 18. doi:ejh.12012.

[23] Kontodimopoulos, N, Samartzis, A, Papadopoulos, A. A, & Niakas, D. Reliability and Validity of the Greek QLQ-C30 and QLQ-MY20 for Measuring Quality of Life in Patients with Multiple Myeloma. ScientificWorldJournal. (2012).

[24] Alegre, A, Oriol-rocafiguera, A, Garcia-larana, J, Mateos, M. V, Sureda, A, Martinez-chamorro, C, Cibeira, M. T, Aguado, B, Knight, R, & Rosettani, B. Efficacy, safety and quality-of-life associated with lenalidomide plus dexamethasone for the treatment of relapsed or refractory multiple myeloma: the Spanish experience. Leuk Lymphoma. (2012). Epub 2012 Mar 1., 53(9), 1714-21.

[25] Naumann-winter, F, Greb, A, Borchmann, P, Bohlius, J, Engert, A, & Schnell, R. First-line tandem high-dose chemotherapy and autologous stem cell transplantation versus single high-dose chemotherapy and autologous stem cell transplantation in multiple myeloma, a systematic review of controlled studies. Cochrane Database Syst Rev. (2012). Oct 17;10:CD004626. doi:CD004626.pub3.

[26] Verelst, S. G, & Termorshuizen, F. Uyl-de Groot CA, Schaafsma MR, Ammerlaan AH, Wittebol S, Sinnige HA, Zweegman S, van Marwijk Kooy M, van der Griend R, Lokhorst HM, Sonneveld P, Wijermans PW; Dutch-Belgium Hemato-Oncology Cooperative Group (HOVON). Effect of thalidomide with melphalan and prednisone on health-related quality of life (HRQoL) in elderly patients with newly diagnosed multiple myeloma: a prospective analysis in a randomized trial. Ann Hematol. (2011). Epub 2011 Apr 7., 90(12), 1427-39.

[27] Strasser-weippl, K, & Ludwig, H. Psychosocial QOL is an independent predictor of overall survival in newly diagnosed patients with multiple myeloma. Eur J Haematol. (2008). Epub 2008 Jul 11, 81(5), 374-9.

[28] Mols, F, Oerlemans, S, Vos, A. H, Koster, A, Verelst, S, & Sonneveld, P. van de Poll-Franse LV. Health-related quality of life and disease-specific complaints among multiple myeloma patients up to 10 yr after diagnosis: results from a population-based study using the PROFILES registry. Eur J Haematol. (2012). doi:j. 1600-0609.2012.01831.x. Epub 2012 Aug 1, 89(4), 311-9.

[29] Delforge, M, & Dhawan, R. Robinson D Jr, Meunier J, Regnault A, Esseltine DL, Cakana A, van de Velde H, Richardson PG, San Miguel JF. Health-related quality of life in elderly, newly diagnosed multiple myeloma patients treated with VMP vs. MP: results from the VISTA trial. Eur J Haematol. (2012). doi:j.1600-0609.2012.01788.x. Epub 2012 May 7., 89(1), 16-27.

[30] Gulbrandsen, N, Wisløff, F, Brinch, L, Carlson, K, Dahl, I. M, Gimsing, P, Hippe, E, Hjorth, M, Knudsen, L. M, Lamvik, J, Lenhoff, S, Løfvenberg, E, Nesthus, I, Nielsen, J. L, & Turesson, I. Westin J; Nordic Myeloma Study Group. Health-related quality of life in multiple myeloma patients receiving high-dose chemotherapy with autologous blood stem-cell support. Med Oncol. (2001)., 18(1), 65-77.

[31] Khalafallah, A, Mcdonnell, K, Dawar, H. U, et al. Quality of life assessment in multiple myeloma patients undergoing dose-reduced tandem autologous stem cell transplantation. Mediterr J Hematol Infect Dis. (2011). e2011057. Epub 2011 Nov 28.

[32] Sherman, A. C, Simonton, S, Latif, U, Plante, T. G, & Anaissie, E. J. Changes in quality-of-life and psychosocial adjustment among multiple myeloma patients treated with high-dose melphalan and autologous stem cell transplantation. Biol Blood Marrow Transplant. (2009)., 15(1), 12-20.

[33] Verelst, S. G, & Termorshuizen, F. Uyl-de Groot CA, Schaafsma MR, Ammerlaan AH, Wittebol S, Sinnige HA, Zweegman S, van Marwijk Kooy M, van der Griend R, Lokhorst HM, Sonneveld P, Wijermans PW; Dutch-Belgium Hemato-Oncology Cooperative Group (HOVON). Effect of thalidomide with melphalan and prednisone on health-related quality of life (HRQoL) in elderly patients with newly diagnosed multiple myeloma: a prospective analysis in a randomized trial. Ann Hematol. (2011). Epub 2011 Apr 7., 90(12), 1427-39.

[34] Wisløff, F, & Hjorth, M. Health-related quality of life assessed before and during chemotherapy predicts for survival in multiple myeloma. Nordic Myeloma Study Group. Br J Haematol. (1997)., 97(1), 29-37.

[35] Molassiotis, A, Wilson, B, Blair, S, Howe, T, & Cavet, J. Unmet supportive care needs, psychological well-being and quality of life in patients living with multiple myeloma and their partners. Psychooncology. (2011)., 20(1), 88-97.

Chapter 15

Multiple Myeloma in Horses, Dogs and Cats: A Comparative Review Focused on Clinical Signs and Pathogenesis

A. Muñoz, C. Riber, K. Satué, P. Trigo,
M. Gómez-Díez and F.M. Castejón

Additional information is available at the end of the chapter

http://dx.doi.org/10.5772/54311

1. Introduction

Multiple myeloma (MM) or plasma cell myeloma is a neoplastic proliferation of plasma cells that primarily involves the bone marrow but may originate from extramedullary sites [1-4]. Although it is uncommon in veterinary medicine, it has been reported in several species, including cats, dogs and, horses [1,3,5-10]. The frequency of MM in cats is slightly <1% of all malignant neoplasms. Canine MMs account for only 0.3% of all malignancies in dogs. MMs account approximately 2% of all hematopoietic neoplasms in both dogs and cats [4]. Most of the reports in the literature are limited to 1 to 16 case studies [4,11-16]. However, in a recent report regarding the incidence of bone disorders diagnosed in dogs, MM was the second most frequently diagnosed neoplastic condition in canine bone marrow [17].

Similarly, MM is an extremely rare disorder in horses. Ten cases, nine from the literature and a new case, were described by Edwards et al. [1] and only six additional cases have been described lastly [3,6-8,18]. Because of the uncommonly diagnosis of equine MM, the prevalence of this neoplasm is unknown in the horse.

2. Data of the patients with multiple myeloma

MM is generally a disease of older animals, although some reports exist in young animals. In dogs, the average age of diagnosis is between 8 and 12 year-old [9-10,15,19-25].There is a report of MM in a younger dog, 4-year-old [26]. There is no apparent gender predisposition in dogs. Further, the largest retrospective study to date (60 dogs) included 30 males and 30 females [27].

The mean age of diagnosis in cats ranges between 12.5 and 14 years, and most of the cats with MM are older than 7 year-old [28,29,4,30,31,32,33,9]. According to the literature, the youngest cat with MM was 1.5 year-old [31]. A myeloma-related disorder has been described for a 19-month-old cat [34]. Males accounted for about 55-56%. The age and gender in dogs and cats with MM are similar to those described in human patients. In a large retrospective study of 1027 people, the average age of diagnosis was 66 years and 59% were men [35].

MM is also a neoplasm of elderly horses, with mean age of 11 years at the moment of the diagnosis [1]. Horses with this condition have ranged in age from three months to 25 years. The youngest animals were a 1.6-year-old Quarter Horse mare [36] and a 3 month-old Quarter Horse colt [37]. Although it was suggested initially that it could be more common in Quarter Horses [1], there are too few reports in equids for statistical interpretation of this data. Both male (geldings and stallions) and female horses are represented equally.

3. Current knowledge of the etiology and predisposing factors of MM in companion animals

Factors associated with the development of MM in companion animals have not been identified. In human patients, exposure to high doses of ionizing radiation has been linked to MM development according to some studies [38-40]. In relation to x-rays, the results of many cohort studies in human beings have been inconsistent, in some cases suggesting that frequent exposure has a negligible effect and in other that it is a significant risk [41-43]. In one report of equine MM, one horse was used regularly for teaching radiology and Pusterla et al. [3] suggested that it might exists an association between exposure to x-rays and neoplastic transformation.

Genetic and hereditary factors may also play a role in MM development [44-45]. Recurrent infections or antigen stimulation have been proposed as predisposing factors, although epidemiological studies have not been confirmed this association [46]. Infections with several virus diseases in human patients appear related to an elevated MM risk, although some data do not support a potentially causal relationship between these infections and MM [46-50]. In cats, a link between MM and virus such as feline leukemia virus (FeLV) and feline immunodeficiency virus (FIV) has not been identified, but a diagnosis of the disease among sibling suggests a familiar association [29]. The role of oncogenes, tumor-suppresor genes, cytokines, and their interaction with the bone marrow environment in the etiopathogenesis of the MM are currently being investigated in animal models. Overexpression of cell cycle regulators, such as cyslin D1 and disregulation of receptor tyrosine kinase have been implicated in the pathogenesis of plasma cell tumors and MM [51]. Progression of B cell lymphoma to MM and of solitary plasma cell tumors to MM in dogs and cats have been reported [52-53].

http://dx.doi.org/10.5772/54311

4. Clinical signs

The infiltration of various organ systems by neoplastic cells, the production of cytokines by the tumor or the bone marrow microenvironment, and the high circulating level of a single type of immunoglobulin lead to a wide array of clinical manifestations. Therefore, the clinical signs of MM vary with the level of plasma cell proliferation, the location and spread of the neoplastic plasma cells, and the nature and extent of the proteinuria [3,4,9-10,15,33,54]. The clinical signs are generally non-specific and include lethargy, renal failure, hemostatic abnormalities, anorexia, diarrhea and vomiting in small animals and weight loss, anorexia, fever, increased susceptibility to infections and limb edema in horses [1,3,8,11,36].

4.1. Increased susceptibility to infections

MM patients are usually immunocompromised and thus highly susceptible to infections [55]. MM associated immunodeficiency is likely a multifaceted phenomenon secondary to decreased concentration of polyclonal immunoglobulin [56], suppression of macrophage-related factors influencing the normal B cell differentiation to plasma cells [57] in response to antigenic stimulation [58], decreased T helper cell function, increased rate of γ-globulin catabolism, neoplastic infiltration of bone marrow resulting in leukopenia [59], dysfunctional and/or decreased numbers of neutrophils, and defective complement activation [3-4].

In cats with MM, the most common infectious processes include periodontitis, chronic recurrent upper respiratory infections and terminal bacteriemia [4]. In horses with MM, the most common system affected by infectious disease is the lung, with several cases of severe pneumonia [1,3,37,60].

4.2. Bone pain and skeletal lesions

Bone pain is considered one of the most common presenting complaints in human patients [61-62]. Skeletal abnormalities are commonly recognized in small animals, but uncommon in horses with MM [1,3,63]. Horses frequently had bone lesions, therefore, bone pain might manifest more as a gait abnormality and therefore, it could be misdiagnosed.

The percentage of cats with MM and radiographically-evident skeletal lesions was 58.3% [2,4,13,63-66], similar to the 50-60% occurrence reported for dogs [27,64]. Skeletal lesions can be either solitary (well-circumscribed with areas of osteolysis or punched-out lytic areas) or multiple (generalized osteopenias) [4,27]. Rarely, pathologic fractures are seen. Skeletal lesions are typically identified in bones involved in active hematopoiesis (e.g. ribs, vertebrae, pelvis, and proximal and distal aspects of long bones). Other causes of focal osteolysis are rare in companion animals, but include carcinomas [67], giant cell tumors of bone [68], benign aneurismal bone cysts [69-71] and bone lesions secondary to tumor invasion [70,72-73]. Generalized osteopenias have also been diagnosed radiographically [4]. Demineralization of bone in humans is detected through measurement of bone mineral density, a technique not used routinely in veterinary medicine. Generalized osteopenias is not specific for MM, and may also be seen with nutritional, renal and metabolic disorders [74-77].

4.3. Bleeding disorders

Bleeding is a prominent feature of MM in human beings [78-82]. Clinically, hemorrhages occur in approximately one-third of dogs and one fourth of cats with MM [4,27,29]. In horses, the most common clinical manifestation is epistaxis [1,3,6].

The pathogenesis of bleeding diathesis is likely multifactorial. The M-component may interfere with normal coagulation and lead to hemostatic defects by various mechanism that include inhibition of platelet aggregation and release of platelet factor, adsorption of minor clotting factors, induction of abnormal fibrin polymerization and functional decrease in calcium. In instances where myelophthisis is present due to profound bone marrow infiltration, thrombocytopenia may develop and contribute to hemorrhagic events [24].

4.4. Hyperviscosity syndrome

The hyperviscosity syndrome (HVS) in characterized by clinico-pathologic abnormalities that occur secondarily to increased serum viscosity, which is associated with the M-component. HVS is most commonly associated with immunoglobulin-M macroglobulinemia due to the high molecular weight of IgM [85]. However, it also can occur in presence of IgA, and rarely with IgG [27]. HVS leads to bleeding diathesis, neurological signs (such as seizures, depression, coma), congestive heart failure, renal failure and ophthalmic abnormalities, including tortuous and dilated retinal vessels, retinal hemorrhages and retinal detachment, sludging of blood within small vessels and impaired delivery of nutrients and oxygen to tissues [84].

Approximately 20% of dogs with MM develop this syndrome and it has been reported in cats [4,13,19,23,54,85]. There is a report that measured serum viscosity in a horse with MM [86]. The horse had a serum concentration of globulin of 9.6 g/dl (reference range 3.5-4.5 g/dl) and a relative serum viscosity of 7 (reference range 1.4-1.7). In horses, edema is a common clinical signs in MM [1,3]. The genesis of limb edema is unknown, although blood hyperviscosity may be contributory. Increased vascular permeability has been proposed as a cause of edema accompanying osteosclerosis myeloma in human beings [87].

4.5. Renal disease

Renal disease occurs in approximately 22-50% of dogs and about 30% of cats with MM [4,27]. The pathogenesis of renal disease is commonly multifactorial and several mechanisms have been implicated in human patients [88-89]. In the majority of the cases, renal impairment is caused by the accumulation and precipitation of light chains, which forms casts in the distal tubules, resulting in renal obstructions. In addition, myeloma light chains are also directly toxic on proximal renal tubules, further adding to renal dysfunction [89-90]. Circulating monoclonal light chains are relatively freely filtered through the glomerulus, reaching the proximal tubule, where they are catabolized. Free light chains are endocytosed by proximal tubule cells, through a receptor-mediated process, by binding to the tandem scavenger receptor system cubilin/megalin. Then, they are endocytosed through the clathrin-dependent endosomal/lysosomal pathways and degraded within lysosomes [91-94]. In

MM, excess light chain production overcomes the capacity of the tubular cells to catabolize the free light chains that appear in the tubular fluid of distal nephron segments. Therefore, they form tubular casts with Tamm-Horsfall protein (uromodulin), a glycoprotein-synthesized by the cells in the medullary thick ascending limb of the loop of Henle with affinity for monoclonal light chains. Light chains interact through their complementary determining region with a specific binding site on the Tamm-Horsfall protein and form aggregates and casts that subsequently lead to the tubular obstruction of the distal tubule and the thick ascending loop of Henle [95-97]. Tubular obstruction increases intraluminal pressure, reduces glomerular filtration rate and reduces interstitial blood flow, thus further compromising the renal function [90]). The rates of cast formation increase when light chains increase, although there is considerable diversity among the nephrotoxicity of light chains. The variable region of the light chain determines nephrotoxicity of the specific light chain by determining the affinity with Tomm-Horsfall protein [98-99]. It has been indicated that Tamm-Horsfall protein interacts with the hypervariable regions of the light chains. This region contains the amino acids that give diversity, and allow for interactions with several proteins to promote antigen binding by immunoglobulins [100-101]. In addition, the variable region of the light chain determines the specific type of renal damage. Both lambda and kappa light chains are nephrotoxic, but lambda light chains are more frequently involved in the formation of amyloid than kappa [102]. The relationship between the type of light chain and the severity and type of renal damage has not been investigated in animals yet.

In addition of casts formation, endocytosis of light chains by renal tubular cells induces proinflammatory cytokine production (interleukin-6 and 8, tumor necrosis factor-α). These proinflammatory cytokines promote infiltration by inflammatory cells that produce metalloproteinases and increase transforming growth factor-b production, resulting in matrix protein deposition and fibrosis and further compromising the ability of the nephron to restore function [103]. Light chains endocytosis might also cause tubular cell necrosis, leading to more severe renal dysfunction [104], but the exact mechanism has not been described. It has been hypothesized that the aggregation of light chains after endocytosis initiates a cascade leading to tubular cell death [105].

Other mechanisms that lead to renal insufficiency are tumor infiltration within the renal parenchyma, hypercalcemia, amyloidosis, decreased renal perfusion due to the HVS, dehydration, ascending urinary tract infections and Bence-Jones proteinuria [4, 27]. In human patients with MM, hypercalcemia is the second most common cause of renal failure. Hypercalcemia is also probably an important predisposing factor to renal dysfunction in animals with MM, since a tight relationship between renal failure and hypercalcemia has been described in many reports in veterinary medicine [106-108] Hypercalcemia interferes with renal function and impairs renal concentrating ability, causes vasoconstriction of renal vasculature and enhances diuresis.

4.6. Heart disease

Heart disease may occur in patients with MM as a consequence of HVS related to myocardial hypoxia and increased cardiac workload. In addition, amyloid deposition in the myocardium and anemia may exacerbate the severity of this condition [109]. Approximately 50% of the cats with MM in one study had idiopathic heart murmur [4]. Recently, three cases of cats evaluated for congestive heart failure with acute collapse, tachypnea, increased respiratory effort, and pulmonary crackles, have been reported secondarily to HVS [54].

4.7. Other clinical signs

Neurological manifestations often complicate the course of MM, but direct involvement of the central nervous system in rare in human patients, although there are some cases reported [110-113]. Similarly, neurological signs are uncommon manifestations of MM in animals. However, it is well recognized that MM may lead to abnormalities of the central nervous system either as a result of spinal cord compression by the neoplasm arising within a vertebra or due to pathological fracture of a vertebra weakened by tumor infiltration [114-115]. It could also be due to the HVS where sludging of blood within the vasculature results in central nervous system hypoxia [116]. Neurological signs associated with MM have been reported in horses [1,7], cats [31] and dogs [22,114]. Edwards et al. [1] described the cases of three horses with rear leg paresis and/or ataxia. Spinal cord compression by an extradural tumor mass was observed in one of the two horses in which the spinal canal was examined. McConkey et al. [7] observed a horse with hind ataxia progressing to paralysis, with dysphagia and ptyalism. These clinical signs were attributed to neoplastic involvement of the trigeminal nerve. Similarly, Appel et al. [31] presented the case of a cat with hind limb locomotor difficulties, signs of pain along the lumbar portion of the vertebral column, with altered motor function and moderate muscle atrophy. In this case, survey radiographs revealed osteolytic lesions in lumbar vertebras [31].

In MM patients, peripheral neuropathy has for a long time been considered as mainly secondary to the tumor, following a direct compression (radicular or medullar), light chain deposits (amyloidosis), cryoglobulinemia or an autoimmune mechanism [117-121]. A paraneoplastic polyneuropathy is seen in association with IgM monoclonal gammopathy associated with MM, Waldenstrom's macroglobulinemia, primary amyloidosis and lymphoma, as well as monoclonal gammopathy of undetermined significance. IgM-M proteins have autoantibody activity and have been shown to bind to myelin associated glycoprotein resulting in a demyelinating peripheral neuropathy [121]. However, increased levels of cytokines are thought to cause the paraneoplastic neuropathy rather than an immune-mediated mechanism [122-123]. Furthermore, with the use of new drugs, the iatrogenic neurotoxicity has become the leading cause of peripheral neuropathy in people [124-126]. The commonest nerve involvement appears to be in the form of sensory-motor axonal neuropathy followed by sensory-motor demyelinating neuropathy [117].

In companion animals, paraneoplastic neuropathies have been reported sporadically in malignant tumors, and include bronchogenic carcinoma, insulinoma, leiomyosarcoma, hemangiosarcoma, undifferentiated sarcoma, synovial sarcoma and adrenal adenocarcinoma [114,127-129]. Viviers and Dobson [22] described the case of a 12-year-old female German Shepherd dog that developed progressive hindlimb followed by forelimb ataxia with tetraplejia. Neurological examination suggested lower motor dysfunction. MM was diagnosed

http://dx.doi.org/10.5772/54311

by biochemical evaluation, radiography and bone marrow aspirate. An electromyogram revealed positive sharp waves and fibrillation potentials in the skeletal muscles of the limbs, suggesting a polyneuropathy. Motor function started to improve four weeks after commencing treatment. According to the authors, polyneuropathy in this dog appeared as a paraneoplastic syndrome secondary to MM [22].

Cutaneous involvement in MM has also been described in animals, although it seems to be unusual. Mayer et al. [24] described the case of an 8-year-old Rottweiler dog with more than 50 soft cutaneous and subcutaneous nodules, ranging from 0.5 to 2.5 cm in diameter, located primarily on the ventral aspects of the thorax and abdomen and the medial aspect of the thighs. Histopathological examination of excised subcutaneous modules revealed MM. More recently, Fukumoto et al. [16] presented the case of a 7-year-old male, mixed breed dog with more than 40 cutaneous nodules ranging from 0.5 to 1.0 cm in diameter, mainly on the abdomen and inguinal region. Cutaneous involvement has not been described in horses with MM.

5. Diagnosis aids of multiple myeloma in veterinary medicine

5.1. Hematology

Anemia is a prominent feature of MM, it is commonly associated with clinical progression in human patients and occurs in more than two thirds of all patients [130-132]. Similarly, approximately 30% of dogs and 75% of cats with MM have a normocytic normochromic non-regenerative anemia [4,10,26-27,32-33] and anemia is also invariably present in horses with MM.

The pathogenic mechanisms involved in the anemia are chronic inflammation, tumor hemorrhage and/or hemostatic abnormalities, myelophthisis, increased red blood cell destruction induced by the HVS, plasma expansion secondary to the osmotic effect of the paraproteins and red cell destruction by neoplastic cells [4,27,29]. In cats, erythrophagocytosis by neoplastic plasma cells [32], mast cells [133]), lymphocytes [134-135] and histocytes [136] has been observed. In the same way, there are several reports of phagocytic plasma cells in people with MM [137]. Although erythrophagocytic plasma cells in humans with MM are rare, neoplastic plasma cells have been observed with phagocytosed platelets and granulocytes [138]. The mechanism of hemophagocytosis in MM is unclear, as plasma cells have not phagocytic function under normal circumstances. Results of the direct antiglobulin test in humans are almost always negative, suggesting hemophagocytosis by neoplastic cells is not an autoimmune function [137]. It has been speculated that phagocytic plasma cells may arise as an expansion of a rare B-cell clone with innate phagocytic potential [137]. A single case of phagocytic plasma cells aberrantly expression CD15 (normally found on neutrophils and monocytes and involved in phagocytosis) has been reported in human beings [139].

Nevertheless, anemia of chronic disease appears to be of utmost importance in MM. Interleukin-1 and tumor necrosis factors are capable of suppressing erythropoiesis [130]. Anemia has broad implications in these patients. First, the low hemoglobin concentration and packed cell volume have been associated with poor quality of life in people, and affect daily activity. Second, anemia has an impact on the cardiovascular system. In fact, anemia has been shown to induce or aggravate hypoxia and ischemic complications. Third, anemia has been shown to be a poor prognostic factor in MM [140-142].

Data concerning white blood cell count (total and different subpopulations) are not consistent in animals with MM. It has been found lymphopenia [24,30,32], leukocytosis due to neutrophilia [4,8], neutropenia with lymphocytosis [31], leukopenia [1,25,37], leukocytosis with neutrophilia and lymphocytosis [31], neutropenia [16], neutrophenia with lymphopenia [18], pancytopenia [10] and absence of white blood cell abnormalities [3,6,22].

Thrombocytopenia is reported in approximately one third of all canine patients of MM [10,25,27]. It has also been described in cats [4,29] and horses [18,37]. However, there are many other reports of MM in veterinary medicine with patients that show normal number of platelets [3,6-8,16,22,24,31-32]. Thrombocytopenia that could promote bleeding disorders, is proposed to result from infiltration of bone marrow by malignant plasma cells, consumption of platelets as part of thrombohemorrhagic syndrome, such as disseminated intravascular coagulation, shortened platelet half-life or immune-mediated destruction, even though the latter 2 mechanisms have yet to be verified in veterinary medicine [10,27,30,64,142-143].

5.2. Blood clinical biochemistry

5.2.1. Serum protein concentrations and serum protein electrophoresis

Hyperproteinemia, specifically hypoalbuminemia and hyperglobulinemia is very common in MM, but not an invariable feature. Hypoalbuminemia has been described consistently in MM in dogs [9,15-16,22-24], cats [3,9,29,32] and horses [1,3,18]. However, in the three animal species, there are some reports that reported serum albumin concentrations within the reference range in animals [6-8,31].

The mechanisms of the hypoalbuminemia are unknown, but in human beings is primarily related to the extent of the proliferation of the MM and it is therefore of diagnostic and prognostic importance [144]. Several studies have suggested that low serum albumin concentrations correlate with increased serum concentrations of interleukin-6, a potent myeloma cell growth factor, reflecting disease severity and cell proliferation [145-146]. Interleukin-6 is a multifunctional, pro-inflammatory cytokine that stimulates B cell maturation and proliferation and overproduction has been demonstrated in a variety of B-cell malignancies [147].

The neoplastic plasma cells are responsible for an overproduction of a homogeneous or monoclonal immunoglobulin product, known as paraproteins o M-component. The paraproteins may be complete immunoglobulin, free light chains, light chains fragments or polymers, or partial immunoglobulins missing one or both chains [148]. The term monoclonal gammopathy is commonly used to define hyperglobulinemia characterized by an electrophoretic pattern with a sharply defined peak that is usually in the β- or γ- region and is narrower than the albumin peak [9,149]. When 2 narrow peaks with these features are recognized, the term biclonal gammopathy is often used. Monoclonal gammopathies are associated with production of a single clone of immunoglobulin owing to clonal expansion of neoplastic lymphoid cells, such as plasma cells in MM and B cells in lymphoma [9]. In contrast, a polyclonal gammopathy is characterized by a broader peak or multiple peaks in the γ- or β-γ regions. Polyclonal gammopathies are associated with chronic antigenic stimulation that occurs in chronic infections and other inflammatory conditions [148,150-152]. The term oligoclonal gammopathy refers to an electrophoretic pattern that is similar to a monoclonal one, but in which the globulin peak is slightly wider than the albumin peak [9,149]. Oligoclonal gammopathy may occasionally occur in animals with chronic inflammation or infectious disease [9].

Although monoclonal gammopathy is the laboratory landmark of MM, other conditions occasionally can induce a monoclonal gammopathy in animals, such as chronic inflammation (leishmaniosis, ehrlichiosis, chronic pioderma, feline infectious peritonitis) [149-150,153-155], amyloidosis [156-157], B-cell lymphoma [149], Waldenströms macroglobulinemia [158-159] and monoclonal gammopathy of undefined significance (MGUS) [160]. The inclusion criterion for MGUS are M-protein and <10% bone marrow plasmacytosis, with no evidence of lytic lesions, light chain proteinuria or other clinical, hematologic, and biochemical abnormalities [161-162]. MGUS occurs in 1-2% of people over the age of 50 and 3% of people over the age of 70 [162]. A significant proportion (25%) of these will evolve within 20 years into MM, primary amyloidosis, macroglobulinemia or another lymphoproliferative disease [162].

In dogs affected by MM, the incidence of IgA and IgG is comparable, whereas in cats and horses IgG is most commonly involved [1,3-4,27]. In fact, of the 25 published feline MM with immunoelectrophoresis results, 20 had IgG gammopathies, and 5 had IgA gammopathies [2,13-14,85]. Similarly, there are some reports of IgA gammopathies in horses with MM [3,8].

Biclonal gammopathy, with two M-components has been reported in humans [163-165], even though it was found to be very rare, occurring in about 1% of human beings with MM [166]. Biclonal gammopathies have been described in lymphoproliferative disorders in dogs and cats [2,9,19,23,167-168] including MM. The term biclonal is applied to the electrophoretic pattern and does not always correlate with true biclonal expansion because the biclonal electrophoretic may arise from a single clone of B-cells, usually mature plasma cells that produce one type of immunoglobulin with different dimerization patterns [9]. The biclonal pattern may also occur from production of two different classes of immunoglobulins, usually IgG and IgA, by two separate cell clones [23]. However, production of separate heavy chain isotypes by a single clone of neoplastic cells, may result from isotype switching, which occurs normally during B-cell maturation [9].

The prevalence of biclonal gammopathy in companion animals is unknown, but it could be higher than reported. In many clinical veterinary laboratories, serum protein electrophoresis is performed using cellulose acetate as the support medium. However, better separation of protein fractions may be obtained using agar cell electrophoresis or capillary zone electrophoresis. Facchini et al. [9] reported two cases (dog and cat) with gammopathies associated with MM that were interpreted as oligoclonal by standard cellulose acetate electrophoresis but were determined to be biclonal con capillary zone electrophoresis.

MMs in veterinary patients lacking hyperglobulinemia have also been described [10]. The authors propose that the lack of hyperglobulinemia resulted from either M-protein associated secondary hypogammaglobulinemia or the IgA nature of the M protein. Secondary hypogammaglobulinemia with an immunosuppressive phenomenon associated with MM is reported to occur in about 10% of human MM patients, and in a report, is most commonly seen in secretory immunoglobulin A- MM [169-172]. The mechanism underlying MM-associated hypogammaglobulinemia is unclear, but recent work suggest that appropriate B-cell maturation and immunoglobulin production are impaired by defects in CD4+, CD45R+, naïve T cells and increases in CD8+, CD11b1+ memory T cells [173-174]. The depression of normal immunoglobulin production associated with exuberant M protein production has been described anecdotally, but not specifically described in dogs with MM [64]. Seelig et al. [10] supported their hypothesis in the immunoglobulin quantification data, which indicate massive production of the immunoglobulin A M-protein and mild to moderate decreases in immunoglobulins G and M in a dog.

Cryoglobulinemia has also been described in human patients with MM [175-176]. Cryoglobulins are proteins, usually immunoglobulins that precipitate as serum is cooled to temperature less than body temperature and dissolve upon rewarming. They are most commonly evident as a white gelatinous material but may sometimes appear crystalline or flocculent [177] Cryoglobulinemia is rare in animals and are limited descriptions in dogs with MM [114,178], in a dog with Waldenström's macroglobulenia [179], in a cat [28], in a horse with lymphoma [180], and in several horses with glomerulonephritis [181-182]. In human patients, cryoglobulins are classified into 3 groups on the basis of their immunoglobulin composition. In type-1 cryoglobulinemia a single monoclonal immunoglobulin, usually IgM is present. This is most commonly associated with lymphoproliferative disorders such as MM, Waldenström's macroglobulinemia, lymphoma, and lymphocytic leukemia, but occasionally can develop in conjunction with immune-mediated diseases [177]. In type II cryoglobulinemia, a monoclonal immunoglobulin, usually IgM complexes with polyclonal IgG, whereas in type III cryoglobulinemia, polyclonal immunoglobulins, usually immunoglobulin M complex with polyclonal immunoglobulin G. Type II and III cryoglobulinemia and may develop secondary to infection, immune-mediated diseases or very rarely, lymphoproliferative disease. In some instances, an underlying disease is not found and the cryoglobulinemia is described as essential. Using this classification system, type-I and mixed cryoglobulinemia in dogs, horses and cats have been described. Two dogs with MM had type-I immunoglobulin A cryoglobulinemia [114,178] and the dog with Waldenström's macroglobulinemia had type-I immunoglobulin M cryoglobulinemia [179]. Another dog had an essential mixed immunoglobulin G-M cryoglobulinemia and cryofibrinogenemia [183], and although a thorough investigation for the underlying disease was not performed, the diagnosis was supported by resolution and lack of recurrence of clinical signs when the dog was maintained in a warm environment [183]. A cat had type I immunoglobulin G cryoglobulinemia in association with MM [28].

The typical clinical signs of cryoglobulinemia are purpura, cold intolerance, acrocyanosis and ulceration, necrosis and gangrene of the skin of the distal extremities [184]. However of the cases of cryoglobulinemia reported in the veterinary literature, only 1 dog [183] and 2 horses [180,182] had typical lesions. Necrosis of the pinnae occurred in the dog [183] and in 1 of the horses [180] and distal limb swelling and ulceration in other horse [182]. Similarly, <50% of human patients with cryoglobulinemia have typical clinical signs even in cold conditions [184]. The lesions develop as a result of precipitation of cryoglobulin in small-diameter blood vessels, which causes vascular occlusion and tissue ischemia. Subsequently, inflammation may develop at the site of precipitation secondary to complement fixation by immunoglobulin G [185]. Despite extensive investigation, the physical and chemical characteristics accounting for the temperature-dependent solubility of cryoglobulins have not been determined. Proposed mechanisms include altered amino acid or carbohydrate content of the cryoglobin, leading to abnormal interactions between water and the protein [185].

5.2.2. Serum urea and creatinine concentrations

Azotemia is present in half of MM human patients when first evaluated [78-79]. Similarly, many animals with MM show azotemia when presented [1,4,10,24,27,29], whereas there are other cases with serum urea and creatinine concentrations within the reference limits [3,6,22]. Probably these differences depend on the existence of renal kidney and on the degree of hydration.

5.2.3. Serum total and ionized calcium concentrations

Hypercalcemia has been reported in approximately 15-20% of dogs and 20-25% of cats affected by MM [4,29,65]. Similarly, hypercalcemia seems to be common in horses with MM [1,3,8], although there is a report of hypocalcemia in one horse with MM [18].

Hypercalcemia is a complication of uncontrolled osteolysis, influenced in part by osteoclast activation factor and in human patients has been associated with extensive osteolytic disease [86]. However, MM-associated hypercalcemia is not reported as frequently as bone lysis [4,27,35,64], perhaps because disease progression is usually slow, allowing for appropriate metabolic controls. Other mechanisms of hypercalcemia are the release of an osteoclast activating factor by either the bone marrow microenvironment or by neoplastic cells located in bone [186-190]. In humans, interleukin-1, interleukin-6, tumor necrosis factor and the receptor activator of the nuclear factor kappa B ligand (RANKL) all modulated osteoclast activity and may contribute to hypercalcemia [191]. Paratyroid hormone related peptide (PTH-rP) also may contribute to the pathogenesis of MM-related hypercalcemia. It seems that essentially every cell of the body makes PTHrP under normal conditions [192-193]. It has a broad range of physiological functions, including stimulation of bone resorption, vasorelaxation, and cell proliferation, regulation of placental calcium transport, organogenesis, parturition, lactation, and vascular smooth muscle proliferation and development of the skeletal system [193]. Despite its wide distribution of the body, PTHrP is normally present in minute amounts in the circulation [193-194] and high serum PTHrP concentrations have been found in conjunction only with pathologic conditions, principally malignancy [194-195]. PTHrP may be synthesized by normal cells activated by the presence of a malignancy or by neoplastic cells. There is a report of a horse with MM and high concentrations of PTHrP [8]). High levels of PTHrP have been also described in other neoplasms, such as thymoma [196], nasal carcinoma [197], squamous cell carcinomas [198], angiomyxoma [199], mammary carcinoma [200], lymphoma [201-203] adenocarcinoma of the apocrine gland of the anal sac [203] and malignant melanoma [204].

The measurement of ionized calcium is recommended to confirm hypercalcemia in these patients, because binding of calcium by the M protein will increase total calcium concentration, while ionized calcium will remain within normal limits [205]. Therefore, increased ionized calcium concentrations supports true hypercalcemia. There is a recent report that present a case of MM in a dog with increased total serum calcium concentration, but with serum ionized calcium concentrations within normal limits [25]. The authors suggested that the majority of the calcium was protein-bound to serum M proteins. In fact, serum calcium exists in two major fractions, free and protein bound. A small portion of calcium is bound to other small anions such as citrate, lactate, and phosphate. Because ionized calcium is the physiologically active species of blood calcium, it is ordinarily maintained within very narrow limits by rigidly controlled mechanisms [205-206]. Approximately half of normal total serum calcium is bound to negatively charged sites on albumin. Human MM has been reported to bind calcium on the Fab portion of the globulin molecules [148].

MM is frequently complicated by an increase in the concentration of ionized calcium, which if persistent leads to secondary nephrogenic diabetes insipidus and loss of the renal medullary concentration gradient causing polyuria and polydipsia [25].

5.2.4. Alterations in the coagulation profile

Approximately 50% of dogs affected by MM have abnormal prothrombin and partial thromboplastin times [149,207] and these abnormalities have also been found in horses [6,18,37,86] and cats [4,29]. However, other animals with MM had normal bleeding times [3,22].

Coagulation defects can result from paraproteins interference with clotting factors, protein coating of platelets leading to thrombocytopenia and binding of the Fab fragment of the M-protein to fibrin, preventing aggregation [116,208].

5.2.5. Alterations in serum sodium concentrations

Three horses with MM were hyponatremia [1]. The decreased concentrations could have resulted from displacement of the aqueous phase of plasma by the hyperglobulinemia. However, true hyponatremia in human beings with MM has been described. Suggested mechanism include displacement of sodium by cationic paraproteins, decreased plasma water secondary to unusual hydration characteristics of paraproteins, and syndrome of inappropriate antidiuretic hormone release [209-210]. Alterations in serum sodium concentrations do not appear to be common in small animals.

5.2.6. *Alterations in serum cholesterol concentrations*

Hypocholesterolemia has been noted in approximately 69% of affected cats in one study [4]. Similarly, hypocholesterolemia was found in a horse with MM [1]. The incidence in cats is higher than in human patients [211-212]. Serum cholesterol concentrations are thought to be correlated inversely with globulin concentrations [35,211]. It has been postulated that the hypocholesterolemia is the result of a down-regulation of cholesterol production by the liver to maintain oncotic pressure in the face of hyperglobulinemia [78]). The main causes of hypocholesterolemia in veterinary medicine include protein-losing enteropathies, severe malnutrition, hepatic insufficiency or hyperthyroidism [213-215].

5.3. Urinalysis

Proteinuria, detected by routine urinalysis is present in 90%of human patients with MM [216-221]. In the same way, proteinuria using dipsticks has been found in horses [1,3,6], dogs [10,22] and cats [4,28,30,32] with MM. However, dipsticks detect primarily albuminuria and therefore, the sulfosalicylic acid test (SSA) provides greater sensitivity for globulin detection but specificity is low due to the concomitant detection of albumin, globulin, Bence Jones proteins, proteases and polypeptides. False positive SSA results may occur with penicillin and its derivatives, tolbutamide or sulfisoxazole metabolites, or certain contrast media in the urine [222]. In people, false positive results for Bence Jones proteins detected by means of heat precipitation can occur due to excessive amount of polyclonal light chain proteins in patients affected by a variety of conditions, including connective tissue diseases, non-plasmacytic tumors and chronic renal failure [4,216,222]. Therefore, urine protein electrophoresis remains the preferred diagnostic modality to detect monoclonal proteinuria, even is not always used in veterinary medicine.

Bence Jones proteinuria has been estimated to occur in approximately 25-40% of dogs an approximately 65% of cats with MM [4,27,29]. Similarly, it has been determined in horses with MM [1,3].

5.4. Diagnostic ancillary aids

Survey radiographies and echographies are required for screening of skeletal lesions and identification of abdominal organ neoplasia respectively. Furthermore, a funduscopic examination should be carried out in patients suspicious of MM, mainly in small animals, in order to rule out ocular lesions associated with the HVS, such as retinal hemorrhages, retinal detachment, venous tortuosity, dilation, sacculation, and blindness.

As explained before, skeletal lesions vary from areas of osteopenias observed in early stages of the disease to lytic lesions typical of later stages. Biopsy and histopathology of a lytic lesion may sometimes be necessary for a definitive diagnosis. Survey radiographies are commonly performed now in small animals with MM, because increased clinician awareness of the lesions, better quality radiographs and increased knowledge about the disease. In horses with MM, survey radiographies are less used, probably because of the higher incidence of skeletal lesions of other origin (sport horses). Lung radiography is recommended in equine patients with MM in order to rule out pneumonia, one common finding in these cases [3,18]. In addition, hepatomegaly (58%), splenomegaly (25%), cardiomegaly (67%) and renomegaly (9%) have been detected in cats with MM [4,29].

The most common ultrasonographic abnormalities involved the spleen and the liver and to a lesser extent the kidneys [4]. In cats, the most consistent finding in MM is splenic enlargement and diffuse or nodular hypoechogenicity. The most consistent hepatic abnormality is diffuse hyperechogenicity and enlargement [4]. Bone marrow cytology should be done to confirm the diagnosis. A detailed description of the histopathological characteristics in bone marrow and in other organs after necropsy, consistent with MM is out of the scope of the present review.

5.5. Diagnostic criteria

Current published recommendations for determining a diagnosis in veterinary medicine indicate that the animal should have at least 2 of the following 4 criteria: 1) Bone marrow plasmacytosis with >20% plasma cells; 2) Monoclonal gammopathy based on serum protein electrophoresis; 3) Osteolysis and 4) Light chain (Bence-Jones) proteinuria (2). These criteria are unweighted for animal patients. In human patients, criteria are weighted as 'major' and 'minor' and accommodate lower plasma cell percentages (17). In people, confirmation of MM requires first that the patient be symptomatic (i.e. have bone pain) or have anemia, hypercalcemia, azotemia, hypoalbuminemia, or bone demineralization. The diagnostic criteria of MM are then applied. Major criteria include: 1) plasmacytoma(s) with biopsy; 2) marrow plasmatocytosis >30%; 3) M-protein with >3.5 g/dl immunoglobulin G or 2.0 g/dl immunoglobulin A and 4) κ or λ chain excretion on 24-h urine protein electrophoresis. The 4 minor criteria include: a) marrow plasmacytosis with 10-30% plasma cells; b) M-protein at values less than indicated above; c) lytic bone lesions and d) >50% normal serum immunoglobulin concentration. If the diagnosis includes major criteria, then any 2 of the 4 will suffice, or major criterion 1 plus minor criterion b, c, or d; or major criterion 3 plus minor criterion a or c. If the diagnosis is based on only minor criteria, then it must include the first and second criteria (a and b), plus 1 of the remaining 2 criteria (c or d). This system has been recently incorporated for the diagnosis in animals [4,10,24,31-32]. However, some modifications have been introduced. Plasma cell atypia has been included as a criterion when marrow plasmacytosis was between 10 and 20%. In humans, nuclear-cytoplasmic maturation asynchrony, nuclear immaturity, and pleomorphism are considered reliable markers for distinguishing neoplastic cells from reactive plasma cells [223]. In addition, reactive plasma cells usually do not exceed 5% of all nucleated cells in marrow and are well differentiated [223-224].

6. Treatment options in veterinary patients with mm

Treatment of MM with oral melphalan and glucocorticoids (prednisone or prednisolone) is the standard of therapy due to its dual ability to reduce the bulk of the tumor and the symptoms of the decrease [16,22-25,31-33,225]. Although complete eradication is only rarely achieved, chemotherapy is often effective in decreasing tumor burden, reducing serum immunoglobulin levels, promoting bone remodeling and providing symptomatic relief. Further, this treatment leads to improved quality and possible duration of life [27,225] and is also used in human patients with MM [226-230].

Melphalan is an alkylating agent whose oral absorption is unpredictable, requiring administration to be made preferable on the empty stomach. In dogs, melphalan is initially administered at 0.1 mg/kg PO once a day for 10 days and then 0.05 mg/kg PO every other day. In cats, they are administered at 0.5-2.0 mg/kg PO once a day. Melphalan is combined with glucocorticoids, prednisone [22,24-25,42] or less common, prednisolone [25,30-31]. Glucocorticoids have been shown to induce apoptosis in vitro via inhibition of Iκβ activation and decreased nuclear factor κB activity [231-232]. Prednisone in dogs with MM is generally administered at 1.0 mg/kg for the first 10 days of therapy and then, decreased to 0.5 mg/kg every other day [22,24-25,32,225]. This combination treatment is continued indefinitely, until relapse or myelosuppression.

Other alkylating drugs including cyclophosphamide, chlorambucil and 1(2-chloroethyl)-3-cyclohexyl-1-nitrosourea (CCNU) have also been used to treat MM in small animals [10,233]. The addition of cyclophosphamide to a prednisone- melphalan regimen may be beneficial to patients with severe clinical signs and/or hypercalcemia. Due to its platelet-sparing effect, cyclophosphamide may be used in place of melphalan in thrombocytopenic patients, although this drug can have severe suppressive effects on other bone marrow lineages [234-237]. Chorambucil, administered at 0.2 mg/kg PO once daily has been used successful for the treatment of immunoglobulin M macroglobulinemia in dogs [159].

Combination chemotherapy protocols incorporating vincristine, carmustine, melphalan, cyclophosphamide and prednisone or vincristine, melphalan, cyclophosphamide and prednisone have been used in human beings, but outcomes are essentially comparable to those of patients with melphalan and prednisone alone [238-241]. The administration of high dose dexamethasone in conjunction with vincristine and doxorubicin was investigated in humans with refractory MM and resulted in a response greater than 50%. Rapid tumor response, alleviation of bone pain, resolution of hypercalcemia and absence of damage to bone marrow stem cells were remarkable advantages to this treatment combination [239]. Anecdotally, in dogs, responses of a few months duration have been achieved with a combination of doxorubicin, vincristine and prednisone in lymphoma [242-243] and in MM [10].

The efficacy of inteferon for the treatment of MM is controversial [244-245]. While a response rate of approximately 20% was reported in humans with relapsed MM, the addition of interferon to standard chemotherapy approaches failed to provide a significant benefit to the overall survival time in a meta-analysis of 2286 patients [244]. However, there is other report that stated that even though most interferon benefits to MM patients are relatively small when viewed in the light of survival expectancies, they seem clinically relevant. Since median overall survival of conventionally treated MM patients ranges between 30 and 50 months, 3-7 months gains of life amount to a increase of 10-25% [244].

High-dose chemotherapy in association with autologous transplantations using bone marrow or blood-derived stem cells is now widely accepted for the treatment of hematological malignancies including MM. This approach yielded to complete remissions in refractory human patients, but mortality rate due to bone marrow suppression was high. Contamination of most bone marrow and blood stem cell samples with neoplastic cells within the autograph resulted in recurrence of disease, emphasizing the need of optimize purging techniques [246-250]. Autologous bone marrow transplant has also been added to chemotherapy in the treatment of some malignancies in companion animals, such as lymphoma and acute myeloid leukemia [251-253].

In human patients with MM, biphosphonates such as pamidronate, have been used to prevent or to delay the onset of bone lesions and associated bone pain [254-257]. Bisphosphonates have been administered in dogs with appendicular osteosarcoma [258-259] and with malignant histiocytosis [260], but they have not been used in veterinary patients with MM.

Treatment of patients affected by indolent MM with the anti-angiogenic agent thalidomide resulted in a 66% response rate and the drug appeared to have potential to delay the onset of clinical signs associated with the disease [261-262]. The efficacy of thalidomide for the treatment of refractory relapsed MM has also been confirmed [263-265]. Studies evaluating the possible efficacy of thalidomide for the treatment of MM in companion animals are lacking. Bortezomib, a proteasome inhibitor, induces apoptosis of MM cells and inhibits their binding to bone marrow stromal cells, which otherwise would trigger the transcription of interleukin-6 via an NFκB-dependent pathway. In different studies a 25% response rate was achieved in human beings with MM and an overall survival time of 16 months. Furthermore, addition of dexamethasone to the treatment regimen improved responses in 19% of treated patients [227-228,264,266].

Additional, some patients experience severe clinical signs secondary to hypercalcemia, renal dysfunction, HVS or pathologic fractures will require palliative therapy specifically directed to the clinical complications of the disease.

7. Prognosis of companion animals with multiple myeloma

Unfortunately, the prognosis of companion animals with MM is poor. The mean survival time in dogs treated with MM and treated with melphalan, cyclophosphamide and prednisone is 540 days after diagnosis [27]. In dogs, negative prognostic factors include extensive bone lesions, hypercalcemia and light chain proteinuria. Renal insufficiency and poor initial response to therapy also may be associated with decreased survival times [27]. In a study of 9 cats with MM, it was found that hypercalcemia, pathologic fractures, anemia, Bence-Jones proteinuria, azotemia, persistent elevations in serum protein concentrations at 8 weeks after treatment and little or no clinical improvement were poor prognostic indicators and reflected a more aggressive form of the disease [29]. Survival time for such cats did not exceed 14 days, with a median of 5 days. In contrast, normocalcemia, lack of azotemia, absence of pathologic fractures, no anemia, absence of Bence-Jones proteinuria and a normal serum protein 8 weeks after commencement of treatment reflected a less aggressive form with a median survival of 387 days (range between 120 and 720 days) [29].

In a study, a possible relationship between prognosis and immunoglobulin isotype was suggested in cats with MM [2], even though there are few detailed cases. Although immunoglobulin A appears to be less commonly produced than immunoglobulin G in cats, as described before, the published cases with immunoglobulin A paraproteins had visceral involvement and decreased survival time (ranging from a few days to 6 months) [12,65,267-268]. Either immunoglobulin has been associated with clinical signs of HVS, including cardiac insufficiency, retinal hemorrhages and neurological signs [85,268]. This phenomenon relates to the size of the paraproteins and the degree of hyperglobulinemia. Since immunoglobulin A may assume a dimeric or multimeric form, it may be more commonly associated with hyperviscosity than immunoglobulin G. HVS can contribute to decreased survival time in animals with MM [13,23,54,85].

The lifespan of horses diagnosed of MM usually does not exceed two years [1,3,6,8]. There is not any published case of equine MM that attempted chemotherapy and most horses are euthanized owing to the advance stage of the disease.

Author details

A. Muñoz[1], C. Riber[1], K. Satué[2], P. Trigo[3], M. Gómez-Díez[3] and F.M. Castejón[3]

*Address all correspondence to: pv1mujua@uco.es

1 Department of Animal Medicine and Surgery, School of Veterinary Medicine, University of Córdoba, Córdoba, Spain

2 Department of Animal Medicine and Surgery, School of Veterinary Medicine, Cardenal Herrera-CEU University, Valencia, Spain

3 Equine Sport Medicine Centre, School of Veterinary Medicine, University of Córdoba, Córdoba, Spain

References

[1] Edwards DE, Parker JW, Wilkinson JE, Helman RG. Plasma Cell Myeloma in the Horse. A Case Report and Literature Review. Journal of Veterinary Internal Medicine 1993; 7(3) 169-176.

[2] Bienzle D, Silverstein DC, Chaffin K. Multiple Myeloma in Cats: Variable Presentation and Different Immunoglobin Isotypes in Two Cats. Veterinary Pathology 2000;37(4) 364-369.

[3] Pusterla N, Stacy BA, Vernaw W, De Cock HEV, Magdesian KG. Immunoglobulin A Monoclonal Gammopathy in Two Horses with Multiple Myeloma. Veterinary Record 2004;155(1) 19-23.

[4] Patel RT, Caceres A, French AF, McManus M. Multiple Myeloma in 16 Cats: a Retrospective Study. Veterinary Clinical Pathology 2005;34(4)341-352.

[5] Thrall MA. Lymphoproliferative Disorders. Lymphocytic Leukemia and Plasma Cell Myeloma. Veterinary Clinics of North America: Small Animal Practice 1981;11 321-347.

[6] Geelen SN, Bernardina WE, Grinwis GC, Kalsbeek HC. Monoclonal Gammopathy in a Dutch Warmblood Mare. Veterinary Quarterly 1997;19(1) 29-32.

[7] McConkey S, Lopez A, Pringle J. Extramedullary Plasmacytoma in a Horse with Ptyalism and Dysphagia. Journal of Veterinary Diagnostic Investigation 2000;12(3) 282-284.

[8] Barton MH, Sharma P, LeRoy B, Howerth EW. Hypercalcemia and High Serum Parathyroid Hormone-Related Protein Concentration in a Horse with Multiple Myeloma. Journal of American Veterinary Medical Association 2004;225(3) 409-413.

[9] Facchini RV, Bertazzolo W, Zuliani D, Bonfanti U, Caldin M, Avalline G, Roccabianca P. Detection of Biclonal Gammopathy by Capillary Zone Electrophoresis in a Cat and a Dog with Plasma Cell Neoplasia. Veterinary Clinical Pathology 2010;39(4) 440-446.

[10] Seelig DM, Perry JA, Avery AC, Avery PR. Monoclonal Gammopathy without Hyperglobulinemia in 2 Dogs with IgA Secretory Neoplasms. Veterinary Clinical Pathology 2010;39(4) 447-453.

[11] Jacobs T. Multiple Myeloma in a Cat with Paraparesis. Feline Practice 1994;22(4) 28-32.

[12] McDonald WJ, Burton SA, Fuentealba IC. Plasma Cell Myeloma Producing an Immunoglobulin A Paraprotein in a Cat. Canadian Veterinary Journal 1994;35(3) 157.

[13] Weber NA, Tebeau CS. An Unusual presentation of Multiple Myeloma in Two Cats. Journal of American Animal Hospital Association 1998;34(6) 477-483.

[14] King AJ, Davies DR, Irin PJ. Feline Multiple Myeloma: Literature Review and Four Case Reports. Australian Veterinary Practice 2002;32 146-151.

[15] Zeugswetter F, Kleiter M, Wolfesberger B, Schwendenwen I, Miller I. Elevated Fructosamine Concentrations Caused by IgA Paraproteinemia in Two Dogs. Journal of Veterinary Science 2010;11(4) 359-361.

[16] Fukumoto S, Hanazono K, Kawasaki N, Hori Y, Higuchi S, Sasaki T, Temma K, Uchide T. Anaplastic Atypical Myeloma with Extensive Cutaneous Involvement in a Dog. Journal of Veterinary Medical Science 2012;74(1) 111-115.

[17] Weiss DJ. A Retrospective Study of the Incidence and the Classification of Bone Marrow Disorders in the Dog at a Veterinary Teaching Hospital (1996-2004). Journal of Veterinary Internal Medicine 2006;20(4) 955-961.

[18] Kim DY, Taylor HW, Eades SC, Cho DY. Systemic AL Amyloidosis Associated with Multiple Myeloma in a Horse. Veterinary Pathology 2005;42(1) 81-84.

[19] Kato H, Momoi Y, Omori K, Youn HY, Yamada T, Goto N, Ono K, Watari T, Tsujimoto H, Hasegawa A. Gammopathy with Two M-Components in a Dog with Ig-Type Multiple Myeloma. Veterinary Immunology and Immunopathology 1995;49(1-2) 161-168.

[20] Marks SL, Moore PF, Taylor DW, Munn RJ. Nonsecretory Multiple Myeloma in a Dog: Immunohistologic and Ultrastructural Observations. Journal of Veterinary Internal Medicine 1995;9(1) 50-54.

[21] Peterson EN, Meininger AC. Immunoglobulin A and Immunoglobulin G Biclonal Gammopathy in a Dog with Multiple Myeloma. Journal of American Animal Hospital Association 1997;33(1) 45-47.

[22] Villiers E, Dobson J. Multiple Myeloma with Associated Polyneuropathy in a German Shepherd Dog. Journal of Small Animal Practice 1998;39(5) 249-251.

[23] Ramaiah SK, Seguin MA, Carwile HE, Raskin RE. Biclonal Gammopathy Associated with Immunoglobulin A in a Dog with Multiple Myeloma. Veterinary Clinical Pathology 2002;31(2) 83-89.

[24] Mayer MN, Kerr ME, Grier CK, McDonald VS. Immunoglobulin A Multiple Myeloma with Cutaneous Involvement in a Dog. Canadian Veterinary Journal 2008;49(7) 694-702.

[25] Tripp CD, Bryan JN, Wills TB. Presumptive Increase in Protein-Bound Serum Calcium in a Dog with Multiple Myeloma. Veterinary Clinical Pathology 2009;38(1) 87-90.

[26] Lautzenhiser SJ, Walker MC, Goring RL. Unusual IgM-Secreting Multiple Myeloma in a Dog. Journal of American Veterinary Medical Association 2003;223(5),645-648.

[27] Matus RE, Leifer CE, MacEwen EG, Hurvitz AI. Prognostic Factors for Multiple Myeloma in the Dog. Journal of American Veterinary Medical Association 1986;188(11) 1288-1292.

[28] Hickford FM, Stokol T, Van Gessel YA, Randolph JF, Schermerhorn T. Monoclonal Immunoglobulin G Cryoglobulinemia and Multiple Myeloma in a Domestic Shorthair Cat. Journal of Veterinary Medical Science 2000;217(7) 1029-1033.

[29] Hanna F. Multiple Myelomas in Cats. Journal of Feline Medicine and Surgery 2005;7(5) 278-287.

[30] Yamada O, Tamura K, Yagihara H, Isotani M, Azakami M, Sawada S, Ono K, Washizu T, Bankobara M. Light-Chain Multiple Myeloma in a Cat. Journal of Veterinary Diagnostic Investigation 2007;19(4) 443-447.

[31] Appel SL, Moens NM, Abrams-Ogg A, Woods JP, Nykamp S, Bienzle D. Multiple Myeloma with Central Nervous System Involvement in a Cat. Journal of American Veterinary Medical Association 2008;233(5) 743-747.

[32] Webb J, Chary P, Morthrup N, Almy F. Erythrophagocytic Multiple Myeloma in a Cat. Veterinary Clinical Pathology 2008;37(3) 302-307.

[33] Takeuchi Y, Iizuko H, Kanemitsu H, Fujino Y, Nakashima K, Uchida K, Ohno K, Nakayama H, Tsugimoto H. Myeloma-Related Disorder with Leukaemic Progression in a Cat. Journal of Feline Medicine and Surgery 2010;12(12) 982-987.

[34] Williams DH, Goldschmidt MH. Hyperviscosity Syndrome with IgM Monoclonal Gammopathy and Hepatic Plasmacytoid Lymphosarcoma in a Cat. Journal of Small Animal Practice 1982;23(6) 311-323.

[35] Kyle RA, Gertz MA, Witzig TE. Review of 1027 Patients with Newly Diagnosed Multiple Myeloma. Mayo Clinic Proceedings 2003;78(1) 21-33.

[36] McAllister C, Quall C, Tyler R, Root CR. Multiple Myeloma in a Horse. Journal of American Veterinary Medical Association 1987;191(3) 337-339.

[37] Henry M, Prasse K, White S. Hemorrhagic Diathesis Caused by Multiple Myeloma in a Thee-Month-Old Foal. Journal of American Veterinary Medical Association 1989;194(3) 392-394.

[38] Wing S, Richarson D, Wolf S, Mihlan G, Crawford-Brown D, Wood J. A Case Control Study of Multiple Myeloma at Four Nuclear Facilities. Annual Epidemiology 2000;10(3) 144-153.

[39] Morgan GJ, Davies FE, Linet M. Myeloma Aetiology and Epidemiology. Biomedical Pharmacotherapy 2002;56(5) 223-234.

[40] Yiin JK, Anderson JL, Daniels RD, Seel EA, Fleming DA, Waters KM, Chen PH. A Nested Case-Control Study of Multiple Myeloma and Uranium Exposure among Workers at the Oak Ridge Gaseous Diffusion Plant. Radiation Research 2009;171(6) 637-645.

[41] Wang JX, Inskip JD, Boir JD, Li BX, Zhang JY, Fraumeni JF. Cancer Incidence among Medical Diagnostic X-ray Workers in China, 1950 to 1985. International Journal of Cancer 1990;45(5) 889-895.

[42] Boice JD, Morin NM, Glass AG, Friedman GD, Stovall M, Hoover RN, Fraumeni JF. Diagnostic X-ray procedures and Risk of Leukemia, Lymphoma and Multiple Myeloma. Journal of the American Medical Association 1991;265 1290-1294.

[43] Hatcher JL, Baris O, Olashan AF, Inskip PD, Savitz DA, Swanson GM, Pottern LM, Greenberg RS, Schwartz AG, Schoenberg JB, Brown LM. Cancer Diagnostic Radiation and the Risk of Multiple Myeloma (United States). Cancer Causes and Control 2001;12 755-761.

[44] Grass S, Preuss KD, Ahlgrimm F, Fadle N, Regitz E, Pfoehler C, Murawski N, Pfreundschuh M. Association of a Dominantly Inherited Hyperphosphorylated Paraprotein Target with Sporadic and Familiar Multiple Myeloma and Monoclonal Gammopathy of Undetermined Significance: a Case Control Study. Lancet Oncology 2009;10(10) 950-956.

[45] Greenberg AJ, Rajkumar SV, Vachon CM. Familiar Monoclonal Gammopathy of Undetermined Significance and Multiple Myeloma: Epidemiology, Risk Factors and Biological Characteristics. Blood 2012,119(23) 5359-5366.

[46] Becker N. Epidemiology of Multiple Myeloma. Recent Results in Cancer Research 2011;183(1) 25-35.

[47] Sjak-Shie NN, Vescio RA, Berenson JR. The Role of Human Herpesvirus-8 in the Pathogenesis of Multiple Myeloma. Hematology/Oncology Clinics of North America 1999;13(6) 1159-1167.

[48] Sadeghian MH, Katebi M, Ayatollali H, Keramati MR. Immunohistochemical Study Association between Human Herpesvirus 8 and Multiple Myeloma. International Journal of Hematology 2008;88(3) 283-286.

[49] Huang B, Li J, Zhou Z, Zheng D, Liu J, Chen M. High Prevalence of Hepatitis B Virus Infection in Multiple Myeloma. Leukemia and Lymphoma 2012;53(2) 270-274.

[50] Pinato DJ, Rossi D, Minh MT, Toniutto P, Boccato E, Minisini R, Gaidano G, Pirisi M. Hepatitis B Virus and Lymphomagenesis. Novel Insights into an Occult Relationship. Digestive and Liver Diseases 2012;44(3) 235-238.

[51] Cangul IT, Wunen M, Van Garderen E, Van den Ingh TS. Clinico-Pathological Aspects of Canine Cutaneous and Mucocutaneous Plasmacytomas. Journal of Veterinary Medicine A 2002;49(6),307-312.

[52] Burnett RC, Blake MK, Thompson LJ, Avery PR, Avery AC. Evolution of a B-cell Lymphoma to Multiple Myeloma after Chemotherapy. Journal of Veterinary Internal Medicine 2004;18(5) 768-771.

[53] Radhakrishnan A, Risbon RE, Patel RT, Ruiz B, Clifford CA. Progression of a Solitary Malignant Cutaneous Plasma Cell Tumor to Multiple Myeloma in a Cat. Veterinary Comparative Oncology 2004;2(1) 36-42.

[54] Boyle TG, Holowaychuk MK, Adams AK, Marks SL. Treatment of Three Cats with Hyperviscosity Syndrome and Congestive Heart Failure Using Plasmapheresis. Journal of American Animal Hospital Association 2001;47(1) 50-55.

[55] Paradisi F, Corti G, Cinelli R. Infectious in Multiple Myeloma. Infectious Diseases. Clinics of North America 2001;15(vii-viii) 373-384.

[56] Waldman TA, Broder S, Krakauer R, Durm M, Goldman c, Meade B. The Role of Suppresor Cells in the Pathogenesis of Common Variable Hypogammaglobulinemia

and the Immunodeficiency Associated with Myeloma. Federation Proceedings 1976;35(9) 2067-2072.

[57] Pilarski LM, Andrews FJ, Mant MJ, Ruether BA. Humoral Immune Deficiency in Multiple Myeloma Patients due to Compromised B Cell Function. Journal of Clinical Immunology 1986;6(6) 491-501.

[58] Dammacco F, Miglietta A, Bonomo L. Immune Functions in Patients with Multiple Myeloma (Delayed Cutaneous Reactivity and Lymphocytes Bearing Receptors for Sheep, Human and Mouse Erythrocytes). International Journal of Clinical and Laboratorial Research 1977;7 343-353.

[59] Jacobson DR, Zolla-Pazner S. Immunosuppresion and Infection in Multiple Myeloma. Seminars in Oncology 1986;13(3) 282-290.

[60] Schalm OW, Knight HD, Osburn BR. Idiopathic Gammopathy and Plasmacytosis in a Horse. California Veterinarian 1974;28 13-20.

[61] Drake MT. Bone Disease in Multiple Myeloma. Oncology (Williston Park) 2009;23(14) 28-32.

[62] Minter AR, Simpson H, Weiss BM, Landgren O. Bone Disease from Monoclonal Gammopathy of Undetermined Significance to Multiple Myeloma: Pathogenesis, Interventions and Future Opportunities. Seminars in Hematology 2011;48(1) 55-65.

[63] Drew RA, Greatorex JC. Vertebral Plasma Cell Myeloma Causing Posterior Paralysis in a Horse. Equine Veterinary Journal 1974;6(3) 131-134.

[64] MacEwen EG, Hurvitz AI. Diagnosis and Management of Monoclonal Gammopathies. Veterinary Clinics of North America 1977;7(1) 119-132.

[65] Sheafor SE, Gamblin RM, Couto CG. Hypercalcemia in Two Cats with Multiple Myeloma. Journal of American Animal Hospital Association 1982;18 79-82.

[66] Eastman CA. Plasma Cell Tumors in a Cat. Feline Practice 1990;24(1) 26-31.

[67] Rosol TJ, Tannehill-Gregg SH, LeRoy BE, Mandl S, Contag CH. Animal Models of Bone Metastasis. Cancer 2003;97(3) 748-757.

[68] McMannus PM, Wood AKW, Christiansen JS, Craig LE. Lytic Lesion in the Distal Humerus of a Dog. Veterinary Clinical Pathology 2001;30(3) 121-123.

[69] Biller DS, Johnson GC, Birchard SJ, Fingland RB. Aneurysmal Bone Cyst in a Rib of a Cat. Journal of American Veterinary Medical Association 1987;190(9) 1193-1195.

[70] Pernell RT, Dunstan RW, DeCamp CE. Aneurysmal Bone Cyst in a Six-Month-Old Dog. Journal of American Veterinary Medical Association 1992;201(12) 1897-1899.

[71] Miura N, Fujiki M, Miyoshi Y, Misumi K, Sakamoto H. Steroid Injection Therapy in a Feline Solitary Bone Cyst. Journal of Veterinary Medical Science 2003;65(4) 523-525.

[72] Shimada A, Yanagida M, Umemura T, Tsukamoto S, Suganuma T. Aneurysmal Bone Cyst in a Dog. Journal of Veterinary Medical Science 1996;58(10) 1037-1038.

[73] Simon D, Gruber AD, Hewicker-Trautwern M, Nolte I. Pathological Femoral Fracture due to a Rhabdomyosarcoma in a Cat. Journal of Small Animal Practice 2000;41(12) 566-570.

[74] Norrdin RW, Moffat KS, Thrall MA, Gasper PW. Characterization of Osteopenia in Feline Mucopolysaccharidosis VI and Evaluation of Bone Marrow Transplantation Therapy. Bone 1993;14 361-367.

[75] Henik RA, Forrest LJ, Friedman AL. Ricketts Caused by Excessive Renal Phosphate Loss and Apparent Abnormal Vitamin D Metabolism in a Cat. Journal of American Veterinary Medical Association 1999;215(11) 1620-1621.

[76] Tomsa K, Glauss T, Hauser B. Nutritional Secondary Hyperparathyroidism in Six Cats. Journal of Small Animal Practice 1999;40(11) 533-539.

[77] Schwarz T, Stork CK, Mellor D, Sullivan M. Osteopenia and other Radiographic Signs in Canine Hyperadrenocorticismo. Journal of Small Animal Practice 2000;41(11) 491-495.

[78] Kyle RA. Multiple Myeloma: Review of 869 Cases. Mayo Clinic Proceedings 1975;50(1) 29-40.

[79] Kapadia SB. Multiple Myeloma: A Clinicopathologic Study of 62 Consecutively Autopsied Cases. Seminar in Oncology 1986;13 282-290.

[80] Saif MW, Allegra CJ, Greenberg B. Bleeding Diathesis in Multiple Myeloma. Journal of Hemotherapy and Stem Cell Research 2001;10(5) 657-660.

[81] Castelli R, Ferrari B, Cortelezzi A, Guariglia A. Thromboembolic Complications in Malignant Haematological Disorders. Current Vascular Pharmacology 2010;8(4) 482-494.

[82] Coppola A, Tufano A, Di Capua M, Franchini M. Bleeding and Thrombosis in Multiple Myeloma and Related Plasma Cell Disorders. Seminars in Thrombosis and Hemostasis 2011;37(8) 929-945.

[83] Gentilini F, Calzolan C, Buonacucina A, Di Tommaso H, Militerno G, Famigli P, Bergamini P. Different Biological Behaviour of Waldenström Macroglobulinemia in Two Dogs. Veterinary Comparative Oncology 2005;3(2) 87-97.

[84] Hendrix DV, Gelatt KN, Smith PJ, Brooks DE, Whittaker CJ, Chmielewski NT. Ophtalmic Disease as the Presenting Complaint in Five Dogs with Multiple Myeloma. Journal of American Animal Hospital Association 1998;34(2) 121-128.

[85] Forrester SD, Greco DS, Relford RL. Serum Hyperviscosity Syndrome Associated with Multiple Myeloma in Two Cats. Journal of American Veterinary Medical Association 1992;200(1) 79-82.

[86] Jacobs RM, Kociba GJ, Ruoff WW. Monoclonal Gammopathy in a Horse with Defective Hemostasis. Veterinary Pathology 1983;20 643-647.

[87] Silberstein LE, Duggan D, Berkman EM. Therapeutic Trial of Plasma Exchange in Osteosclerotic Myeloma Associated with the POEMS Syndrome. Journal of Clinical Apheresis 1985;2(3) 253-257.

[88] Knudsen LM, Hjorth M. Hippe E. Renal Failure in Multiple Myeloma: Reversibility and Impact on the Prognosis. European Journal of Haematology 2000;65(3) 175-181.

[89] Clark AD, Shetty A, Soutar R. Renal Failure and Multiple Myeloma: Pathogenesis and Treatment of Renal Failure and Management of Underlying Myeloma. Blood Reviews 2002;13(2) 119-198.

[90] Dimopoulos MA, Kastritis E, Rosinol L, Bladé J, Ludwig H. Pathogenesis and Treatment of Renal Failure in Multiple Myeloma. Leukemia 2008;22 1485-1493.

[91] Batuman V. Drersbach AW, Cyran J. Light-Chain Binding Sites on Renal Brush Border Membranes. American Journal of Physiology 1990;258(5) F1259-F1265.

[92] Batuman V, Guan S. Receptor-Mediated Endocytosis of Immunoglobulin Light Chains by Renal Proximal Tubular Cells. American Journal of Physiology 1997;272(4) F521-F530.

[93] Batuman V, Verroust PJ, Navar GL, Kaysen JH, Godo FO, Campbell WC, Simon E, Pontillon F, Lyles M, Bruno J, Hammond TC. Myeloma Light Chains are Ligands for Cubilin (pg280). American Journal of Physiology 1998;275(2) F246-F254.

[94] Santosfetano M, Zanchelli F, Zaccaria A, Poletti G, Fusaroli M. The Ultrastructural Basis of Renal Pathology in Monoclonal Gammopathies. Journal of Nephrology 2005;18(6) 659-675.

[95] Huang ZQ, Sanders PW. Biochemical Interaction between Tamm-Horsfall Glycoprotein and Ig Light Chains in the Pathogenesis of Cast Nephropathy. Laboratory Investigation 1995;73(6) 810-817.

[96] Huang ZQ, Saunders PW. Localization of a Single Binding Site for Immunoglobulin Light Chains on Human Tamm-Horsfall Glycoprotein. Journal of Clinical Investigation 1997;99 (4)732-736.

[97] Ying WZ, Sanders PW. Mapping the Binding Domain of Immunoglobin Light Chains for Tamm-Horsfall Protein. American Journal of Pathology 2001;158(5) 1859-1866.

[98] Sanders PW, Booker BB, Bishop JB, Cheung HC. Mechanisms of Intranephronal Proteinaceous Cast Formation by Low Molecular Weight Proteins. Journal of Clinical Investigation 1990;85(2) 570-576.

[99] Sanders PW, Booker BB. Pathobiology of Cast Nephropathy from Human Bence-Jones Proteins. Journal of Clinical Investigation 1992; 89(2) 630-639.

[100] Solomon A, Weiss DT, Kattine AA. Nephrotoxic Potential of Bence-Jones Proteins. New England Journal of Medicine 1991;324(26) 1845-1851.

[101] Batuman V. Proximal Tubular Injury in Myeloma. Contributions in Nephrology 2007; 153 87-104.

[102] Comenzo RL, Zhang Y, Martinez C, Osman K, Herrera GA. The Tropism of Organ Involvement in Primary Systemic Amyloidosis: Contributions of IgV(L) Germ Line Gene Use and Clonal Plasma Burden. Blood 2001;98(3) 714-720.

[103] Keeling J, Herrera GA. The Mesangium as a Target for Glomerulopathic Light and Heavy Chains: Pathogenic Considerations in Light and Heavy Chain-Mediated Glomerular Damage. Contributions in Nephrology 2007;153 116-134.

[104] Sanders DW, Herrera GA, Galla JH. Human Bence-Jones Protein Toxicity in Rat Proximal Tubular Epithelium in vivo. Kidney International 1987;32(6) 851-861.

[105] Ma CX, Locy MQ, Rompala JF, Dispenzier A, Rajkumar SV, Greipp PR, Fonseca R, Kyle RA, Gertz MA. Acquired Fanconi Syndrome is an Indolent Disorder in the Absence of Overt Multiple Myeloma. Blood 2004;104(1) 40-42.

[106] Savary KC, Price GS, Vaden SL. Hypercalcemia in Cats: A Retrospective Study of 71 Cases (1991-1997). Journal of Veterinary Internal Medicine 2000;14(2) 184-189.

[107] Kogika MM, Lustoza MD, Notomi MK, Wirthl VA, Mirandola RH, Hagiwara MK. Serum Ionized Calcium in Dogs with Chronic Renal Failure and Metabolic Acidosis. Veterinary Clinical Pathology 2006;35(4) 441-445.

[108] Messenger JS, Windham WR, Ward CR. Ionized Hypercalcemia in Dogs: A Retrospective Study of 109 Cases (1998-2003). Journal of Veterinary Internal Medicine 2009;23(3) 514-519.

[109] Woldemeskel M. A Concise Review of Amyloidosis in Animals. Veterinary Medicine International 2012;2012:427296. Epub 2012, Mar 15

[110] Escorsell A, López-Guillermo A, Blade J, Villamor N, Massanes F, Montserrat G, Rozman C. Meningeal Infiltration in Multiple Myeloma. Study of a New Case and Literature Review. Revista Clínica Española 1992;191(9) 479-480.

[111] Schluterman KO, Fassas AB, Van Hemert RL, Hank SI. Multiple Myeloma Invasion of the Central Nervous System. Archives of Neurology 2004;61(9) 1423-1429.

[112] Vermeiren P, Vantilborgh A, Offmer F. Myeloma of the Central Nervous System: Report of a Single Center Case Series. Acta Clinica Belgica 2011;66(3) 205-208.

[113] Marjanovic S, Mijuskovic Z, Stamatovic D, Madjaro L, Ralic T, Trimceu J, Stojanovic J, Radovic V 2nd. Multiple Myeloma Invasion of the Central Nervous System. Vojnosanitetski Pregled. Military Medical and Pharmaceutical Review 2012;69(2) 209-213.

[114] Braund KG, Everett M, Bartels E, DeBysscher E. Neurologic Complications of IgA Multiple Myeloma Associated with Cryoglobulinemia in a Dog. Journal of American Veterinary Medical Association 1979;174(12) 1321-1325.

[115] Van Bree H, Pollet L, Cousement W, Van der Stock J, Mattheeuws D. Cervical Cord Compression as a Neurologic Complication of an IgG Multiple Myeloma in a Dog. Journal of American Animal Hospital Association 1983;19 317-323.

[116] Hammer AS, Couto CG. Complications of Multiple Myeloma. Journal of American Animal Hospital Association 1994;30 9-14.

[117] Malhotra P, Choudhary PP, Lal V, Varma N, Suri V, Varma S. Prevalence of Peripheral Neuropathy in Multiple Myeloma at Initial Diagnosis. Leukemia and Lymphoma 2011;52(11) 2135-2138.

[118] Drappatz J, Batchelor T. Neurologic Complications of Plasma Cell Disorders. Clinical Lymphoma 2004;5(3) 163-171.

[119] Dispenzieri A, Kyle RA. Neurological Aspects of Multiple Myeloma and Related Disorders. Best Practice and Research. Clinical Haematology 2005;18(4) 673-688.

[120] Dernier C, Lozeron P, Adams D, Decaudin D, Isnard-Grivaux F, Lacroix C, Said D. Multifocal Neuropathy due to Plasma Cell Infiltration of Peripheral Nerves in Multiple Myeloma. Neurology 2006;66(6) 917-918.

[121] Bosch EP, Smith BE. Peripheral Neuropathies Associated with Monoclonal Proteins. Medicine Clinics of North America 1993;77(1) 125-139.

[122] Gherardi RK, Authier FJ, Belec L. Pro-Inflammatory Cytokines: A Pathogenic Key of POEMS Syndrome. Review of Neurology (Paris) 1996;152(5) 409-412.

[123] Gherardi RK, Chrétien F, Delfau-Larue MH, Authier FJ, Moulignier A, Roulland-Dussoix D, Bélec L. Neurophaty in Diffuse Infiltrative Lymphocytosis Syndrome: An HIV Neuropathy, not a Lymphoma. Neurology 1998;50(4) 1041-1044.

[124] Ravaglia S, Corso A, Piccolo G, Lozza A, Alfonsi E, Mangiacavalli S, Varettoni M, Zappasodi P, Moglia A, Lazzarino M, Costa A. Immune-Mediated Neuropathies in Myeloma Patients Treated with Bortezomib. Clinical Neurophysiology 2008;119(11) 2507-2512.

[125] Cavaletti G, Gilardini A, Canta A, Rigamonti L, Rodríguez-Menéndez V, Ceresa C, Marmiroli P, Bossi M, Oggioni N, D'Incalci M, De Coster, R. Bortezomib-Induced Peripheral Neurotoxicity: a Neurophysiological and Pathological Study in the Rat. Experimental Neurology 2007;204(1) 317-325.

[126] Mohty B, El-Cheikh J, Yakoub-Agha I, Moreau P, Harousseau JL, Mothy M. Peripheral Neuropathy and New Treatments for Multiple Myeloma Background and Practical Recommendations. Haematologica 2010;95(2) 311-319.

[127] Braund KG. Endogenous Causes of Neuropathies in Dogs and Cats. Veterinary Medicine 1996;91 740-754.

[128] Mariani CL, Shelton SB, Alsup JC. Paraneoplastic Polyneuropathy and Subsequent Recovery Following Tumor Renoval in a Dog. Journal of American Animal Hospital Association 1999;35(4) 302-305.

[129] Cavana P, Sammartano F, Capucchio MT, Catalano D, Valazza A, Farca AM. Peripheral Neuropathy in a Cat with Renal Lymphoma. Journal of Feline Medicine and Surgery 2009;11(10) 869-872.

[130] Mittelman M. The Implications of Anemia in Multiple Myeloma. Clinical Lymphoma 2003;4(1) S23-S29.

[131] Ludwig H, Pohl G, Osterborg A. Anemia in Multiple Myeloma. Clinical Advances in Hematology and Oncology 2004;2(4) 233-241.

[132] Laubach, J. Richardson P, Anderson K. Multiple Myeloma. Annual Review of Medicine 2011;62 249-264.

[133] Madewell BR, Munn RJ, Phillips LP. Endocytosis of Erythrocytes in Vivo and Particulate Substances in Vitro by Feline Neoplastic Mast Cells. Canadian Journal of Veterinary Research 1987;51(4) 517-520.

[134] Darbes J, Majzoub M, Breuer W, Hermanns W. Large Granular Lymphocyte Leukemia/Lymphoma in Six Cats. Veterinary Pathology 1998;35(5) 370-379.

[135] Ezura K, Ezura K, Nomura I, Takahashi T, Shibahara T. Natural Killer-Like T Cell Lymphoma in a Cat. Veterinary Record 2004;154(9) 268-270.

[136] Court EA, Earnest-Koons KA, Barr SC, Gould WI II. Malignant Histiocytosis in a Cat. Journal of American Veterinary Medical Association 1993;203 1300-1302.

[137] Savage DG, Zipin D, Bhagat G, Aloberd B. Hemophagocytic Non-Secretory Multiple Myeloma. Leukemia and Lymphoma 2004;45(5) 1061-1064.

[138] Kanoh T, Fujii H. Phagocytic Myeloma Cells: Report of a Case and Review of the Literature. American Journal of Clinical Pathology 1985;84(1) 121-124.

[139] Kucukkaya RD, Hacihanefioghi A, Yenerei MN, Turgut M, Nalcaci M, Keskin H. CD15-Expressing Phagocytic Plasma Cells in a Patient with Multiple Myeloma. Blood 2001;97(2) 581-582.

[140] San Miguel FJ, Sanchez J, Gonzalez M. Prognostic Factors and Classification of Multiple Myeloma. British Journal of Cancer 1989;59(1) 113-118.

[141] Caro JJ, Salas M, Ward A, Goss G. Anemia as an Independent Prognostic Factor For Survival in Patients with Cancer. Cancer 2001;91(12) 2214-2221.

[142] Fritz E, Ludwig H, Scheithauer W, Sinzinger. Shortened Platelet Half-Life in Multiple Myeloma. Blood 1986;68(2) 514-520.

[143] Falanga A, Rickles FR. Management of Thrombohemorrhagic Syndromes (THS) in Hematologic Malignancies. American Society of Hematology Education Program 2007;2007(1) 165-171.

[144] Chen YH, Marganda MD, Magalhaes C. Hypoalbuminemia in Patients with Multiple Myeloma. Archives of Internal Medicine 1990;150(3) 605-610.

[145] Bataille R, Jourdan H, Zhang XG, Klein B. Serum Levels of Interleukin G, A Potent Myeloma Cell Growth Factor, as a Reflect of Disease Severity in Plasma Cell Dyscrasias. Journal of Clinical Investigation 1989;84(6) 2008-2011.

[146] Lichtenstein A, Tu Y, Fady C, Vescio R, Berenson J. Interleukin-6 Inhibits Apoptosis of Malignant Plasma Cells. Cellular Immunology 1995;162(2) 248-255.

[147] Lim JE, Yoo C, Lee DM, Kim SW, Lee JJ, Suh C. Serum Albumin Level is a Significant Prognostic Factor Reflecting Disease Severity in Symptomatic Multiple Myeloma. Annals of Hematology 2010;89(4) 391-397.

[148] Kyle RA, Greipp RPR. The Laboratory Investigation of Monoclonal Gammopathies. Mayo Clinic Proceedings 1978;53(11) 719-739.

[149] Giraudel JM, Pagés JP, Guelfi JF. Monoclonal Gammopathies in the Dog: A Retrospective Study of 18 cases (1986-1999) and Literature Review. Journal of American Animal Hospital Association 2002;38(2) 135-147.

[150] Harrus W, Waner T, Avidar Y, Bogin E, Peh H, Bark H. Serum Protein Alterations in Canine Ehrlichiosis. Veterinary Parasitology 1996;66(3-4) 241-249.

[151] Taylor SS, Tappin SW, Dodkin SJ, Papasouliotis K, Casamian-Sorrosal D, Tasker S. Serum Protein Electrophoresis in 155 Cats. Journal of Feline Medicine and Surgery 2010;12(8) 643-653.

[152] Tappin SW, Taylor SS, Tasker S, Dodkin SJ, Papasouliotis K, Murphy KF. Serum Protein Electrophoresis in 147 Cats. Veterinary Record 2011;168(17) 456. Epub 2011.

[153] Font A, Closa JM, Mascort J. Monoclonal Gammopathy in a Dog with Visceral Leishmaniasis. Journal of Veterinary Internal Medicine 1994;8(3) 233-235.

[154] Burkhard MJ, Meyer DJ, Rosychuk RA, O'Neil SP, Schultheiss PC. Monoclonal Gammopathy in a Dog with Chronic Pyoderma. Journal of Veterinary Medicine 1995;9(5) 357-360.

[155] De Caprariis D, Sasanelli M, Paradies P, Otranto D, Lia R. Monoclonal Gammopathy Associated with Heartworm Disease of a Dog. Journal of American Animal Hospital Association 2009;45(6) 296-300.

[156] Schwartzman RM. Cutaneous Amyloidosis Associated with a Monoclonal Gammopathy in a Dog. Journal of American Veterinary Medical Association 1984;185(1) 102-104.

[157] Brown G. A Monoclonal Gammopathy-Induced Canine Renal Amyloidosis. Canadian Veterinary Journal 1996;37(2) 105.

[158] Yamada T, Ogura A, Inoue J, Tsujimoto H, Ono K, Goto N, Tomoda I, Fujiwara K, Usui K. A Case of Feline Macroglobulinemia. Japanese Journal of Veterinary Science 1983;45(3) 395-399.

[159] Jaillardon L, Fournell-Fleury C. Waldenström's Macroglobulinemia in a Dog with a Bleeding Diathesis. Veterinary Clinical Pathology 2011;40(3) 351-355.

[160] Hoenig H, O'Brien JA. A Benign Hypergammaglobulinemia Mimicking Plasma Cells Myeloma. Journal of American Animal Hospital Association 1988;24 688-690.

[161] Kyle RA, Raijumar SV. Monoclonal Gammopathies of Undetermined Significance. Hematology and Oncology. Clinics of North America 1999;13 1181-1202.

[162] Kyle RA, Therneau TM, Rajkumar SV, Offord JR, Larson DR, Plavak MF, Melton 3rd J. A Long-Term Study of Prognosis in Monoclonal Gammopathy in Undetermined Significance (comment). New England Journal of Medicine 2002;346 564-669.

[163] Vaerman JP, Fudenberg HH, Vaerman C, Mandy WJ. On the Significance of the Heterogeneity in Molecular Size of Human Serum γA Globulins. Immunochemistry 1965a;2(3) 263-272.

[164] Vaerman JP, Johnson LB, Mandy W, Fudenberg HH. Multiple Myeloma with Two Paraprotein Peaks: An Instructive Case: An Instructive Case. Journal of Laboratory Clinical Medicine 1965b;65 18-25.

[165] Rudders RA, Yakulis V, Heller P. Double Myeloma. American Journal of Medicine 1973;55(2) 215-221.

[166] Kyle RA, Robinson RA, Katzmann JA. The Clinical Aspects of Biclonal Gammopathies. American Journal of Medicine 1981;71(6) 999-1008.

[167] Jacobs RM, Couto CG, Wellman RL. Biclonal Gammopathy in a Dog with Multiple Myeloma and Cutaneous Lymphoma. Veterinary Pathology 1986;23(2) 211-213.

[168] Larsen AE, Carpenter JL. Hepatic Plasmacytoma and Biclonal Gammopathy in a Cat. Journal of American Veterinary Medical Association 1994;205(5) 708-710.

[169] Riches PG, Hobb JR. Mechanisms in Secondary Hypogammaglobulinemia. Journal of Clinical Pathology 1997;13 15-22.

[170] Kyle RA. Sequence of Testing for Monoclonal Gammopathies. Archives of Patholo-gy- Laboratory Medicine 1999;123(2) 114-118.

[171] Wang H, Gao C, Xu L, Yang Z, Zhao W, Kong X. Laboratory Characterizations on 2007 Cases of Monoclonal Gammopathies in East China. Cellular and Molecular Immunology 2008;5(4) 293-298.

[172] O'Connell TX, Horita TJ, Kastavi B. Understanding and Interpreting Serum Protein Electrophoresis. American Family Physician 2005;71(1) 105-112.

[173] Serra MM, Mant MJ, Ruether Ba, Ledbetter JA, Pilarski LM. Selective Loss of CD4+ CD45+ T Cells in Peripheral Blood of Multiple Myeloma Patients. Journal of Clinical Immunology 1988;8 259-265.

[174] Walchner M, Wick M. Elevations of CD8+ CD11b+ Leu-8- T Cells is Associated with the Humoral Immunodeficiency in Myeloma Patients. Clinical and Experimental Immunology 1997;109(2) 310-316.

[175] Kluger N, Sirvente J, Rigau V, Guillot B. Extensive Thrombotic Purpura Revealing Multiple Myeloma Associated Type 1 Cryoglobulinemia. British Journal of Haematology 2011;154(1) Epub 2011.

[176] Payet J, Livartowski H, Kavian N, Chndesris O, Duplin N, Wallet N, Karras A, Salliot C, Suárez F, Avet-Loiseau H, Alyanakian MA, Nawakill CA, Park S, Tamburini J. Roux C, Bouscary D, Sparsa L. Type I Cryoglobulinemia in Multiple Myeloma, a Rare Entity: Analysis of Clinical and Biological Characteristics of Seven Cases and Review of the Literature. Leukemia and Lymphoma 2012;Apr. 19 (Epub ahead of print).

[177] Kallemuchikkal U, Gorevic PD. Evaluation of Cryoglobulins. Archives of Pathology and Laboratory Medicine 1999;123(2) 119-125.

[178] Virella G, Slappendel RJ, Goudswaard J. Multiple Myeloma IgA Cryoglobulinemia and Serum Hyperviscosity in a Dog. International Archives of Allergy and Applied Immunology 1977;55 537-541.

[179] Hurvitz AI, MacEwen EG, Middaug CR. Monoclonal Cryoglobulinemia with Macroglobulinemia in a Dog. Journal of American Veterinary Medical Association 1977;170(5) 511-513.

[180] Traub-Dargatz J, Bertone A, Bennett D, Jones RL, Weingand K, Hall R, Demartini JC, Lavach JD, Roberts SM. Monoclonal Aggregating Immunoglobin Cryoglobulinemia in a Horse with Malignant Lymphoma. Equine Veterinary Journal 1985;17(6) 470-473.

[181] Sabnis SG, Gunson DE, Antonovych TT. Some Unusual Features of Mesangioproliferative Glomerulonephritis in Horses. Veterinary Pathology 1984;21(6) 574-581.

[182] Maede Y, Inaba M, Amano Y, Murase T, Goto I, Itakura C. Cryoglobulinemia in a Horse. Journal of Veterinary Medical Science 1991;53(3) 379-383.

[183] Nagata M, Nanko M, Hashimoto K. Cryglobulinaemia: A Comparison of Canine and Human Cases. Veterinary Dermatology 1998;9 277-281.

[184] Foester J. Cryoglobulins and Cryoglobulinemia. In: Lee GR, Bithell TC, Foersten J (ed). Wintrobe's Clinical Hematology. Philadelphia: Lea and Febiger; 1993. p2284-2293.

[185] Merlini G, Zorzoli I, Anesi C, Perfetti V, Marinone G. Immunochemical Characterization of the Cryoglobulins: Pathophysiologic Implications. Clinical and Experimental Rheumatology 1995;13(13) 571-573.

[186] Oken MM. Multiple Myeloma. Medical Clinics of North America 1984;68 757-787.

[187] Mundy GR, Raisz LG, Cooper RA, Schechter GP, Salmon SE. Evidence for the Secretion of an Osteoclast Stimulating Factor in Myeloma. New England Journal of Medicine 1974;291 1041-1046.

[188] Bataille R, Manolagas SC, Berenson JR. Pathogenesis and Management of Bone Lesions in Multiple Myeloma. Hematology/Oncology Clinics of North America 1997;11(2) 349-361.

[189] Roodman GD. Pathogenesis of Myeloma Bone Disease. Leukemia 2009;23(3) 435-441.

[190] Sezer O. Mieloma Bone Disease: Recent Advances in Biology, Diagnosis and Treatment. Oncologist 2009;14(3) 276-283.

[191] Farrugia AN, Atkins GJ, Bik L, Pan B, Horvath N, Kostakis P, Findlay DM, Bardy P, Zannettino ACW. Receptor Activator of Nuclear Factor-κB Ligand Expression by Human Myeloma Cells Mediates Osteoclast Formation In Vitro and Correlates With Bone Destruction In Vivo. Cancer Research 2003;1(63) 5431-5445.

[192] Care A, Abbas S Ousey J. The Relationship between the Concentration of Ionised Calcium and Parathyroid Hormone-Related Protein (PTHrP I-34) in Milk of Mares. Equine Veterinary Journal 1997;29 186-189.

[193] Wysolmerski J, Stewart A. The Pathophysiology of Malignancy: Diagnosis and Treatment. Compendium on Continuing Education for the Practicing Veterinarian 2003;25 129-136.

[194] Vasilopulos RJ, Mackin A. Humoral Hypercalcemia of Malignancy: Pathophysiology and Clinical Signs. Compendium on Continuing Education for the Practicing Veterinarian 2003;25(2) 122-128.

[195] Van der Kolk JH. Humoral Hypercalcaemia of Malignancy or Pseudohyperparathyroidism in the Horse. Equine Veterinary Education 2007;19(7) 384-386.

[196] Foley P, Shaw D, Runyon C, McConkay S, Ikede B. Serum Parathyroid Hormone-Related Protein Concentration in a Dog with a Thymoma and Persistent Hypercalcemia. Canadian Veterinary Journal 2000;41(11) 867-870.

[197] Anderson GM, Lane I, Fischer J, Lopez A. Hypercalcemia and Parathyroid Hormone-Related Protein in a Dog with Indifferentiated Nasal Carcinoma. Canadian Veterinary Journal 1999;40(5) 341-342.

[198] Martin CK, Tannehill-Gregg SH, Wolfe TD, Rosol TJ. Bone-Invasive Oral Squamous Cell Carcinoma in Cats: Pathology and Expression of Parathyroid Hormone-Related Protein. Veterinary Pathology 2011;48(1) 302-312.

[199] Gajanayake I, Priestnall SL, Benigni L, English K, Summers BA, Garden OA. Paraneoplastic Hypercalcemia in a Dog with Benign Renal Angiomyxoma. Journal of Veterinary Diagnostic Investigation 2010;22(5) 775-780.

[200] Bae BK, Kim CW, Choi US, Choi EW, Jee H, Kim DY, Lee CW. Hypercalcemia and High Parathyroid Hormone-Related Peptide Concentration in a Dog with a Complex Mamary Carcinoma. Veterinary Clinical Pathology 2007;36(4) 376-378.

[201] Bollinger AP, Graham PA, Richard V, Rosol TJ, Nachreiner RF, Refsal KR. Detection of Parathyroid Hormone-Related Protein in Cats with Humoral Hypercalcemia of Malignancy. Veterinary Clinical Pathology 2002;31(1) 3-8.

[202] Kubota A, Kano R, Mizuno T, Tisasue M, Moore PF, Watari T, Tsujimoto H, Hawegawa A. Parathyroid Hormone-Related Protein (PTHrP) Produced by Dog Lymphoma Cells. Journal of Veterinary Medical Science 2002;64(9) 835-837.

[203] Mellanby RJ, Craig R, Evans H, Herrtage ME. Plasma Concentrations of Parathyroid Hormone-Related Protein in Dogs with Potential Disorders of Calcium Metabolim. Veterinary Record 2006;159(25) 833-838.

[204] Pressler BM, Rotstein DS, Law J, Rosol TJ, LeRoy B, Keene BW, Jackson MW. Hypercalcemia and High Parathyroid Hormone-Related Protein Concentration Associated with Malignant Melanoma in a Dog. Journal of American of Veterinary Medical Association 2002;221(2) 263-265.

[205] Bienzle D, Jacobs RM, Lumsden JH. Relationship of Serum Total Calcium to Serum Albumin in Dogs, Cats, Horses and Cattle. Canadian Veterinary Journal 1993;34(6) 360-364.

[206] Duncan PH, Wills MR, Smith BJ, Savory J. Clinical Studies of Protein-Bound Calcium in Various Diseases. Clinical Chemistry 1982;28(4) 672-675.

[207] Center SA, Smith JF. Ocular lesions in a Dog with Serum Hyperviscosity Secondary to an IgA Myeloma. Journal of American Veterinary Medical Association 1982;181(8) 811-813.

[208] Munshi NC, Tricot GJ, Barlogie B. Plasma Cell Neoplasms. In: DeVita VT, Hellman S, Rosenberg SA (eds.). Cancer: Principles and Practice of Oncology. 6th Ed. Philadelphia PA: Lippincott, Williams & Wilkins; 2001. p2465-2499.

[209] Abraham A, Shafi F, Iqbal M, Kollipara R, Rouf E. Syndrome of Inappropriate Antidiuretic Hormone due to Multiple Myeloma. Missoure Medicine 2011;108(5) 377-379.

[210] Sachs J, Bredman B. The Hyponatremia of Multiple Myeloma is True and not Pseudohyponatremia. Medical Hypotheses 2006;67(4) 839-840.

[211] Scollozi R, Boccafogli A, Salmi R, Furlani MR, Guidoboni CA, Vicentini L, Coletti M, Toccheto M. Hypocholesterolemia in Multiple Myeloma. Inverse Relation to the Component M and the Clinical Stage. Minerva Medicine 1983;74(40) 2359-2363.

[212] Yavasoglu I, Tombuloglu M, Kadikoylu G, Donmez A, Cagirgan S, Bolaman Z. Cholesterol Levels in Patients with Multiple Myeloma. Annales of Hematology 2008;87(3) 223-228.

[213] Kimmel SE, Waddell LS, Michel KE. Hypomagnesemia and Hypocalcemia Associated with Protein-Losing Enteropathy in Yorkshire Terriers: Five cases (1992-1998). Journal of American Veterinary Medical Association 2000;217(5) 703-706.

[214] Berent AC, Drobatz KJ, Ziemer L, Johnson VS, Ward CR. Liver Function in Cats with Hyperthyroidism Before and After 131I Therapy. Journal of Veterinary Internal Medicine 2007;21(6) 1217-1223.

[215] Lecoindre P, Chevallier M, Guerret S. Protein-Losing Enteropathy of Non-Neoplastic Origin in the Dog: A Retrospective Study of 34 Cases. Schweizer Archiv für Tierheilkunde 2010;152(3) 141-146.

[216] Perry MC, Kyle RA. The clinical Significance of Bence Jones Proteinuria. Mayo Clinic Proceedings 1975;50(5) 234-238.

[217] Uchida M, Kamata K, Okubo M. Renal Dysfunction in Multiple Myeloma. Internal Medicine 1995;34(5) 364-370.

[218] Bladé J, Fernández-Llama P, Bosch F, Montoliu J, Lens XM, Montoto S, Cases A, Darnell A, Rozman C, Montserrat E. Renal Failure in Multiple Myeloma: Presenting Features and Predictors of Outcome in 94 Patients from a Single Institution. Archives of Internal Medicine 1998;158(17) 1889-1893.

[219] Cengic M, Robovic Z, Rasic S, Goleman S. Relation Between Certain Parameters of Renal Function and Prognosis in Multiple Myeloma. Medicinski Arhiv 2001;55(4) 193-195.

[220] Corso A, Zappasodi P, Lazzarino M. Urinary Proteins and Renal Dysfunction in Patients with Multiple Myeloma. Biomedicine and Pharmacotherapy 2002;56(3) 139-143.

[221] Eleutherakis-Papaiakovou V, Bamias A, Gika D, Simeonidis A, Pouli A, Anagnostopoulos A, Michali E, Economopoulos T, Zervas K, Dimopoulos MA. Renal Failure in Multiple Myeloma: Incidence, Correlations, and Prognostic Significance. Leukemia and Lymphoma 2007;48(2), 337-341.

[222] Morcos SK, El-Nahas AM, Brown P, Haylor J. Effect of Iodinated Water Soluble Contrast Media on Urinary Protein Assays. British Medical Journal 1992;305(4) 29.

[223] Grogan TM. Plasma Cell Myeloma Marrow Diagnosis Including Morphologic and Phenotypic Features. Seminars in Diagnostic Pathology 2003;20(3) 211-215.

[224] Hyun BH, Kwa D, Gabaldon H, Ashton JK. Reactive Plasmacytic Lesions of the Bone Marrow. American Journal of Clinical Pathology 1976;65(6) 921-928.

[225] Borgatti A. Plasma Cell Tumors. In: Weiss DJ, Wardrop KJ (Ed.). Schalm's Veterinary Hematology. Wiley-Blackwell: Iowa, 2010; p511-519.

[226] Ludwig H, Hajek R, Tóthová E, Drach J, Adam Z, Labar B, Egyed M, Spicka I, Gisslinger H, Greil R, Kuhn I, Zojer N, Hinke A. Thalidomide-Dexamethasone Com-

pared with Melphalan-Prednisolone in Elderly Patients with Multiple Myeloma. Blood 2009;113(15) 3435-3442.

[227] Eom HS, Kim YK, Chung JS, Kim K, Kim HJ, Kim HY, Jin JY, Do YR, Oh SJ, Suh C, Seong CM, Kim CS, Lee DS, Lee JH. Bortezomib, Thalidomide, Dexamethasone Induction Therapy Followed by Melphalan, Prednisolone, Thalidomide Consolidation Therapy as a First Line of Treatment for Patients with Multiple Myeloma who Are Non-Transplant Candidates: Results of the Korean Multiple Myeloma Working Party (KMMWP). Annales of Hematology 2010;89(5) 489-497.

[228] Picot J, Cooper K, Bryant J, Clegg AJ. The Clinical Effectiveness and Cost-Effectiveness of Bortezomib and Thalidomide in Combination Regimens with an Alkylating Agent and a Corticosteroid for the First-Line Treatment of Multiple Myeloma: A Systematic Review and Economic Evaluation. Health Technological Assessment 2011;15(41) 1-204.

[229] Begum M, Akther A, Khan KH, Kaiser MS, Rahman MJ, Alam MN. Melphalan plus Prednisolone in the Treatment of Multiple Myeloma. Myemensigh Medical Journal 2012;21(1) 93-97.

[230] Kabir AL, Rahman MJ, Begum M, Dipta TF, Baqui MN, Aziz A, Rahman F, Debnath RC, Habib MA. Response of Vincristine, Melphalan, Cyclophosphamide and Prednisolone in Refractory Multiple Myeloma. Myemensigh Medical Journal 2012;21(1) 114-119.

[231] Lee JI, Burckart GJ. Nuclear Factor Kappa B: Important Transcription Factor and Therapeutic Target. Journal of Clinical Pharmacology 1998;38(11) 981-993.

[232] Ling J, Kumar R. Crosstalk Between NFκB and Glucocorticoid Signaling: A Potential Target of Breast Cancer Therapy. Cancer Letters 2012;322(2) 119-126.

[233] Fan TM, Kitchell BE, Dhaliwall RS. Hematological Toxicity and Therapeutic Efficacy of Lomustine in 20 Tumor-Bearing Cats: Critical Assessment of a Practical Dosing Regimen. Journal of American Animal Hospital Association 2002;38(4) 357-363.

[234] Burton JH, Mitchell L, Thamm DH, Dow SW, Biller BJ. Low-Dose Cyclophosphamide Selectively Decreases Regulatory T Cells and Inhibits Angiogenesis in Dogs with Soft Tissue Sarcoma. Journal of Veterinary Internal Medicine 2011;25(4) 920-926.

[235] Sato M, Yamazaki J, Goto-Koshina Y, Takahaski M, Fujino Y, Ohno K, Tsujimoto H. Evaluation of Cytoreductive Efficacy of Vincristine, Cyclophosphamide, and Doxorubicin in Dogs with Lymphoma by Measuring the Number of Neoplastic Lymphoid Cells with Real-Time Polymerase Chain Reaction. Journal of Veterinary Internal Medicine 2011;25(2) 285-291.

[236] Warry E, Hansen RJ, Gustafson DL, Lana SE. Pharmacokinetics of Cyclophosphamide after Oral and Intravenous Administration to Dogs with Lymphoma. Journal of Veterinary Internal Medicine 2011;25(4) 903-908.

[237] Mitchell L, Thamm DH, Biller BJ. Clinical and Immunomodulatory Effects of Toceranib Combined with Low-Dose Cyclophosphamide in Dogs with Cancer. Journal of Veterinary Internal Medicine 2012;26(2) 355-362.

[238] Wu P, Davies FE, Horton C, Jenner MW, Krishnan B, Alvares CL, Saso R, McCormack R, Dines S, Treleaven JG, Potter MN, Ethell ME, Morgan GJ. The Combination of Cyclophosphamide, Thalidomide and Dexamethasone is an Effective Alternative to Cyclophosphamide-Vincristine-Doxorubicin-Methylprednisolone as Induction Chemotherapy prior to Autologous Transplantation for Multiple Myeloma: a Case Matched Analysis. Leukemia and Lymphoma 2006;47(11) 2335-2338.

[239] Dadacaridou M, Papanicolaou X, Maltesas D, Megalakaki C, Patos P, Panteli K, Repousis P, Mitsouli-Mentzikof C. Dexamethasone, Cyclophosphamide, Etoposide and Cisplatin (DCEP) for Relapsed or Refractory Multiple Myeloma Patients. Official Journal of Balkan Union of Oncology 2007;12(1) 41-44.

[240] Mellqvist UH, Lenhoff S, Johnsen HE, Hjorth M, Holmberg E, Juliusson G, Tangen JM, Westin J. Cyclophosphamide plus Dexamethasone is an Efficient Initial Treatment before High-Dose Melphalan and Autologous Stem Cell Transplantation in Patients with Newly Diagnosed Multiple Myeloma: Results of a Randomized Comparison with Vincristine, Doxorubicin, and Dexamethasone. Cancer 2008;112(1) 129-135.

[241] San Miguel JF, Mateos MV, Ocio E, García-Sanz R. Multiple Myeloma: Treatment Evolution. Hematology 2012;17(1) S3-S6.

[242] Flory AB, Rassnick KM, Erb HN, Garrett LD, Northrup NC, Selting KA, Phillips BS, Locke JE, Chretin JD. Evaluation of Factors Associated with Second Remission in Dogs with Lymphoma Undergoing Retreatment with a Cyclophosphamide, Doxorubicin, Vincristine, and Prednisone Chemotherapy Protocol: 95 Cases (2000-2007). Journal of American Veterinary Medical Association 2011;238(4) 501-506.

[243] Regan RC, Kaplan MS, Bailey DB. Diagnostic Evaluation and Treatment Recommendations for Dogs with Substage-A High-Grade Multicentric Lymphoma: Results of a Survey of Veterinarians. Veterinary Comparative Oncology 2012; Epub ahead of print.

[244] Mandelli F, Avvisati G, Amadori S, Boccadoro M, Gernone A, Lauta VM, Marmont F, Petrucci MT, Tribalto M, Vegna ML, Dammacco F, Pileri A. Maintenance Treatment with Recombinant Interferon Alfa-2b in Patients with Multiple Myeloma Responding to Conventional Induction Chemotherapy. New England Journal of Medicine 1990;322 1430-1434.

[245] Cunningham D, Powles R, Malpas J, Raje N, Milan S, Viner C, Montes A, Hickish T, Nicolson M, Johnson P, Treleaven J, Raymond J, Gore M. Randomized Trial of Maintenance Interferon Following High Dose Chemotherapy in Multiple Myeloma: Long-Term Follow-Up Results. British Journal of Haematology 1998;102(2) 495-502.

[246] Attal M, Harousseau JL, Stoppa AN, Sotto JJ, Fuzibet JG, Rossi JF, Casassu P, Maisonneuve H, Facon T, Ifrah N, Payen C, Bataille R. A Prospective, Randomized Trial of Autologous Bone Marrow Transplantation and Chemotherapy in Multiple Myeloma. New England Journal of Medicine 1996;335 91-97.

[247] Gianni AM, Bregni M, Siena S, Brambilla C, Di Nicola M, Lombardi F, Gandola L, Corrado T, Pileri A, Ravagnani F, Valagussa P, Bonadonna G. High-Dose Chemotherapy and Autologous Bone Marrow Transplantation Compared with MACOP-B in Aggressive B-Cell Lymphoma. New England of Medicine 1997;336 1290-1298.

[248] Fermand JP, Ravaud P, Chevret S, Divine M, Leblond V, Belanger C, Macro M, Pertuiset E, Dreyfus F, Mariette X, Boccacio C, Brouet JC. High-Dose Therapy and Autologous Peripheral Blood Stem Cell Transplantation in Multiple Myeloma: Up-Front or Rescue Treatment?. Results of a Multicenter Sequential Randomized Clinical Trial. Blood 1998;92(9) 3131-3136.

[249] Kröger N, Schwerdtfeger R, Kiehl M, Sayer HG, Renges H, Zabelina T, Fehse B, Tögel F, Wittkowsky G, Kuse R, Zander AR. Autologous Stem Cell Transplantation Followed by a Dose-Reduced Allograft Induces High Complete Remission Rate in Multiple Myeloma. Blood 2002;100(3) 755-760.

[250] Child JA, Morgan GJ, Davies FE, Owen RG, Bell SE, Hawkins K, Brown J, Drayson MT, Selby PJ. High-Dose Chemotherapy with Hematopoietic Stem Cell Rescue for Multiple Myeloma. New England Journal of Medicine 2003;348 1875-1883.

[251] Deeg HJ, Appenlbaum FR, Weiden PL, Hackman RC, Graham TC, Storb RC. Autologous Marrow Transplantation as Consolidation Therapy for Canine Lymphoma: Efficacy and Toxicity of Various Regimens of Total Body Irradiation. American Journal of Veterinary Research 1985;46(9) 2016-2018.

[252] Gasper PW, Rosen DK, Fulton R. Allogeneic Marrow Transplantation in a Cat with Acute Myeloid Leukemia. Journal of American Veterinary Medical Association 1996;208(8) 1280-1284.

[253] Frimberger AE, Moore AS, Rassnick KM, Cotter SM, O'Sullivan JL, Quesenberry PJ. A Combination Chemotherapy Protocol with Dose Intensification and Autologous Bone Marrow Transplant (VELCAP-HDC) for Canine Lymphoma. Journal of Veterinary Internal Medicine 2006;20(2) 355-364.

[254] Berenson JR, Lichtenstein A, Porter L, Dimopoulos MA, Bordoni R, George S, Lipton A, Keller A, Ballester O, Kovacs MJ, Blacklock HA, Bell R, Simeone J, Reitsma DJ, Heffernan M, Seaman J, Knight RD. Efficacy of Pamidronate in Reducing Skeletal Events in Patients with Advances Multiple Myeloma. New England Journal of Medicine 1996;334 488-493.

[255] Berenson JR, Hillner BE, Kyle RA, Anderson K, Lipton A, Yee GC, Biermann JS. American Society of Clinical Oncology-Clinical Practice Guidelines: The Role of Bisphosphonates in Multiple Myeloma. Journal of Clinical Oncology 2002;20(17) 3719-3736.

[256] Berenson JR, Lichtenstein A, Porter L, Dimopoulos MA, Bordoni R, George S, Lipton A, Keller A, Ballester O, Kovacs M, Blacklock H, Bell R, Simeone JF, Reitsma DJ, Heffernan M, Seaman J, Knight RD. Long-Term Pamidronate Treatment of Advances Multiple Myeloma Patients Reduces Skeletal Events. Journal of Clinical Oncology 2008;16(2) 593-602.

[257] Body JJ, Bartl R, Burckhardt P, Delmas PD, Diel IJ, Fleisch H, Kanis JA, Kyle RA, Mundy GR, Paterson AH, Ruben RD. Current Use of Bisphosphonates in Oncology. Journal of Clinical Oncology 1998;16(12) 3890-3899.

[258] Fan TM. Intravenous Aminobisphosphonates for Managing Complications of Malignant Osteolysis in Companion Animals. Topics in Companion Animal Medicine 2009;24(3) 151-156.

[259] Fan TM, Charney SC, De Lorimier LP, Garrett LD, Griffon DJ, Gordon-Evans WJ, Wypij JM. Double-Blind Placebo-Controlled Trial of Adjuvant Pamidronate with Palliative Radiotherapy and Intravenous Doxorubicin for Canine Appendicular Osteosarcoma Bone Pain. Journal of Veterinary Internal Medicine 2009;23(1) 152-160.

[260] Hafeman SD, Varland D, Dow SW. Bisphosphonates Significantly Increase the Activity of Doxorubicin or Vincristine against Canine Malignant Histiocytosis Cells. Veterinary Comparative Oncology 2012;10(1) 44-56.

[261] Ural AU, Avcu F. Bisphosphonates may Potentate Effects of Thalidomide-Dexamethasone Combination in Advances Multiple Myeloma. American Journal of Hematology 2006;81(5) 385-386.

[262] Morgan GJ, Davies FE, Gregory WM, Szubert AJ, Bell SE, Drayson MT, Owen RG, Ashcroft AJ, Jackson GH, Child JA. Effects of Induction and Maintenance plus Long-Term Bisphosphonates on Bone Disease in Patients with Multiple Myeloma: The Medical Research Council Myeloma IX Trial. Blood 2012;119(23) 5374-5383.

[263] Moehler T, Goldschmidt H. Therapy of Relapsed and Refractory Multiple Myeloma. Recent Results in Cancer Research 2011;183 239-171.

[264] Ahn JS, Yang DH, Jung SH, Park HC, Moon JH, Sohn SK, Bae SY, Kim YK, Kim HJ, Lee JJ. A Comparison of Bortezomib, Cyclophosphamide, and Dexamethasone (Vel-CD) Chemotherapy without and with Thalidomide (Vel-CTD) for the Treatment of Relapsed or Refractory Multiple Myeloma. Annales of Hematology 2012;91(7) 1023-1030.

[265] Offidani M, Polloni C, Cavallo F, Liberati MA, Ballanti S, Pulini S, Catarini M, Alesiani F, Corvatta L, Gentili S, Caraffa P, Boccadoro M, Leoni P, Palumbo A. Phase II Study of Melphalan, Thalidomide and Prednisone Combined with Oral Panobinostat in Patients with Relapsed/Refractory Multiple Myeloma. Leukemia and Lymphoma 2012;53(9) 1722-1727.

[266] Hideshima T, Richardson P, Chauhan D, Palombello VJ, Elliot PJ, Adams J, Anderson KC. The Proteasome Inhibitor PS-341 Inhibits Growth, Induces Apoptosis, and Over-

comes Drug Resistance in Human Multiple Myeloma. Cancer Research 2001;61 3071-3077.

[267] Drazner TH. Multiple Myeloma in the Cat. Compendium on Continuing Education for the Veterinary Practitioner 1982;4 206-216.

[268] Hawkins EC, Feldman BF, Blanchard PC. Immunoglobulin A Myeloma in a Cat with Pleural Effusion and Serum Hyperviscosity. Journal of American Veterinary Medical Association 1986;188 876-878.